AF443303

Diabetes in the New Millennium

Diabetes in the New Millennium

Edited by

UMBERTO DI MARIO
University of Rome "La Sapienza", Italy

FRIDA LEONETTI
University of Rome "La Sapienza", Italy

GIUSEPPE PUGLIESE
University of Rome "La Sapienza", Italy

PAOLO SBRACCIA
University of Rome "Tor Vergata", Italy

and

ALBERTO SIGNORE
University of Rome "La Sapienza", Italy

JOHN WILEY & SONS, LTD
Chichester • New York • Weinheim • Brisbane • Singapore • Toronto

Other Wiley Editorial Offices

John Wiley & Sons, Inc., 605 Third Avenue,
New York, NY 10158-0012, USA

WILEY-VCH Verlag GmbH, Pappelallee 3,
D-69469 Weinheim, Germany

Jacaranda Wiley, Ltd., 33 Park Road, Milton,
Queensland 4064, Australia

John Wiley & Sons (Asia) Pte, Ltd., 2 Clementi Loop #02-01,
Jin Xing Distripark, Singapore 129809

John Wiley & Sons (Canada), Ltd., 22 Worcester Road,
Rexdale, Ontario M9W 1L1, Canada

British Library Cataloguing in Publication Data

A catalogue record for this book is available from the British Library

ISBN   0-471-49299-X

Typeset in 10/12pt Times from the authors' disks by Dobbie Typesetting Ltd., Tavistock, Devon.
Printed and bound in Great Britain by Biddles Ltd., Guildford and King's Lynn.
This book is printed on acid-free paper responsibily manufactured from sustainable forestry,
in which at least two trees are planted for each one used for paper production.

Contents

Contributors

AVOGARO, Angelo *Department of Clinical and Experimental Medicine, Cattedra di Malattie del Metabolismo, Via Giustiniani 2, 35128 Padova, Italy*

BACH, Jean-François *Hôpital Necker, Immunologie Clinique, 161 rue de Sevres, 75743 Paris Cedex 15, France*
E-mail: bach@necker.fr

BELFIORE, Antonino *Cattedra di Endocrinologia e Malattie del Matabolismo, Dipartimento di Medicina Sperimentale e Clinica, University of Catanzaro 'Magna Graecia', Policlinico Mater Domini, Catanzaro, Italy*

BERGER, Michael *Department of Metabolic Disease and Nutrition (WHO Collaborating Centre for Diabetes), Heinrich-Heine University, Moorenstrasse 5, D-40225 Düsseldorf, Germany*
E-mail: bergermi@uni-duesseldorf.de

BOLLI, Geremia B. *Dipartimento di Medicina Interna e Scienze Endocrine e Metaboliche, Università di Perugia, Via E. dal Pozzo, 06126 Perugia, Italy*

BOMPIANI, Gian Domenico *Internal Medicine, Institute of Clinica Medica, University of Palermo, Piazza delle Cliniche 2, 90127 Palermo, Italy*

BORRELLO, Esmeralda *Policlinico Umberto I, Clinica Medica II, 00161 Roma, Italy*

BOTTAZZO, Gianfranco *Ospedale Bambin Gesù, P.za Onofreo, 6, 00165 Rome, Italy*

BRENDEL, Mathias *Third Medical Department and Policlinic, University of Giessen, Rodthohl 6, 35385 Giessen, Germany*
E-mail: konrad.federlin@innere.med.uni-giessen.de

BRETZEL, Reinhard G. *Third Medical Department and Policlinic, University of Giessen, Rodthohl 6, 35385 Giessen, Germany*

BRUFANI, Claudia *Division of Endocrinology, Department of Clinical Sciences, La Sapienza University, Viale del Policlinico 155, 00161 Rome, Italy*

BRUNETTI, Paolo *Dipartimento di Medicina Interna e Scienze Endocrine e Metaboliche, Università di Perugia, Via E. dal Pozzo, 06126 Perugia, Italy*
E-mail: brunetti@dimisem.med.unipg.it

CAVALLO, Maria Gisella   *University La Sapienza, 00161 Rome, Italy*

CIPRIANI, Rosalba   *Division of Endicrinology, Department of Clinical Sciences, La Sapienza University, Viale del Policlinico 155, 00161 Rome, Italy*

CITTERIO, Franco   *Servizio di Diabetologia, Policlinico Universitario A. Gemelli, Università Cattolica, Rome, Italy*
E-mail: dhdiabetologia@rm.unicatt.it.md3173@mclink.it

CORDONE, Samantha   *Division of Endicrinology, Department of Clinical Sciences, La Sapienza University, Viale del Policlinico 155, 00161 Rome, Italy*

CREPALDI, Gaetano   *University of Padua, Via Giustiniani 2, I-35128 Padua, Italy*

DAVALLI, Alberto   *Instituto Scientifico and Università, Vita e Salute, Università degli Studi di Milano, San Raffaele, Milan, Italy*

DE FRONZO, Ralph   *Health Science Center at San Antonio, Diabetes Division, 7703 Floyd Curl Dr., 78284-7886 San Antonio, TX USA*
E-mail: Gonzalese1@uthscsa.edu

DEL PRATO, Stefano   *Department of Clinical and Experimental Medicine, Cattedra di Malattie del Metabolismo, Via Giustiniani 2, 35128 Padova, Italy*

DI BIASE, Nicolina   *Policlinico Umberto I, Clinica Medica II, 00161 Roma, Italy*

DIETERLE C.   *Diabetes Center, Department of Internal Medicine, Innenstadt, University of Munich, Ziemssenstrasse 1, D-80336 Munich, Germany*

DI MARIO, Umberto   *Division of Endicrinology, Department of Clinical Sciences, La Sapienza University, Viale del Policlinico 155, 00161 Rome, Italy*
E-mail: umbertod@dem.it

EISENBARTH, George S.   *Barbara Davis Center, UCHCS, Box B140/ Childhood Diabetes, 4200 E 9th Ave, Denver, CO 80224, USA*
E-mail: george.eisenbarth@uchsc.edu

ELLIOT, Sharon J.   *Renal Cell Biology Laboratory, Vascular Biology Institute and Renal Cell Biology Unit, University of Miami School of Medicine, PO Box 016960 (R126), Miami, FL 33101, USA*

FALQUI, Luca   *Instituto Scientifico and Università, Vita e Salute, Università degli Studi di Milano, San Raffaele, Milan, Italy*

FALLUCCA, Francesco   *Policlinico Umberto I, Clinica Medica II, 00161 Roma, Italy*

FEDERICI, Massimo   *Department of Internal Medicine, University of Rome Tor Vergata, Rome, Italy*

FEDERLIN, Konrad   *Third Medical Department and Policlinic, University of Giessen, Rodthohl 6, 35385 Giessen, Germany*
E-mail: konrad.federlin@innere.med.uni-giessen.de

FRITTITTA, Lucia   *University of Catania, Italy*

GABRIELE, Annarita   *Division of Endocrinology, Department of Clinical Sciences, La Sapienza University, Viale del Policlinico 155, 00161 Rome, Italy*

GALLUZZO, Aldo *Endocrinology Section, Institute of Clinica Medica, University of Palermo, Piazza delle Cliniche 2, 90127 Palermo, Italy*
E-mail: agalluz@unipa.it

GERHARDINGER, Chiara *Schepens Eye Research Institute, Harvard Medical School, 20 Staniford Street, Boston, MA 02114, USA*

GHIRLANDA, Giovanni *Servizio di Diabetologia, Policlinico Universitario A. Gemelli, Università Cattolica, Rome, Italy*
E-mail: dhdiabetologia@rm.unicatt.it.md3173@mclink.it

GIORDANO, Carla *Endocrinology Section, Institute of Clinica Medica, University of Palermo, Piazza delle Cliniche 2, 90127 Palermo, Italy*
E-mail: egiordan@unipa.it

GIORGINO, Ricardo *Medicinal Interna, Endocrinologie e Malattie Metaboliche, Dipartimento dell'Emergenza e dei Trapianti di Organi, Università degli Studi, Bari, Italy*
E-mail: r.giorgino@endo.uniba.it

GOLDFINE, Ira D. *University of California at San Francisco, CA 94155, USA*
E-mail: idg@itsa.ucsf.edu

GREINER, Dale L. *University of Massachusetts Medical School, Division of Diabetes, Department of Medicine, Biotech 2, 373 Plantation Street, Suite 218, Worcester, MA 01605, USA*

GRUDEN, G. *Department of Diabetes, Endocrinology and Internal Medicine, Division of Medicine, GKT School of Medicine, 5th Floor, Thomas Guy House, KCL Guy's Hospital Campus, London SE1 9RT, UK*
E-mail: gabriella.gruden@kcl.ac.uk

IDO, Yasuo *Boston University Medical Center Hospital, Diabetes and Metabolism Unit, 88 East Newton Street, Boston, MA 02118-2393, USA*

KARL, Michael *Vascular Biology Institute and Division of Diabetes, Endocrinology and Metabolism, University of Miami School of Medicine, PO Box 016960 (R126), Miami, FL 33101, USA*

KOLB, Hubert *German Diabetes Research Institute, Auf'm Hennekamp 65, 40225 Düsseldorf, Germany*
E-mail: kolb@godot.dfi.uni-duesseldorf.de

KOLB-BACHOFEN, Victoria *Research Group Immunobiology, MED-Heinrich-Heine-University of Düsseldorf, Düsseldorf, Germany*

LANDGRAF, R. *Diabetes Center, Department of Internal Medicine, Innenstadt, University of Munich, Ziemssenstrasse 1, D-80336 Munich, Germany*
E-mail: rlandgra@medinn.med.uni-muenchen.de

LAURO, Renato *Department of Internal Medicine, University of Rome Tor Vergata, Rome, Italy*

LEFÈBVRE, Pierre J. *Division of Diabetes, Nutrition and Metabolic Disorders, Department of Medicine, CHU Sart Tilman (B35), B-4000 Liège 1, Belgium*
E-mail: Pierre.Lefebvre@ulg.ac.be

LESLIE, David *Department of Diabetes and Metabolism, St Bartholomew's Hospital, 3rd Floor, Dominion House, 59 Bartholomew Close, West Smithfield London EC1A 7BE, UK*
E-mail: R.D.Leslie@mds.qmw.ac.uk

LETO, Gaetano *Division of Endicrinology, Department of Clinical Sciences, La Sapienza University, Viale del Policlinico 155, 00161 Rome, Italy*

LORENZI, Mara *Schepens Eye Research Institute, Harvard Medical School, 20 Staniford Street, Boston, MA 02114, USA*
E-mail: lorenzi@vision.eri.harvard.edu

MADDUX, Betty *UCSF Box 1616, San Francisco, CA 94143-1616, USA*
E-mail: bmaddux@itsa.ucsf.edu

MANZATO, Enzo *University of Padua, Via Giustiniani 2, I-35128 Padua, Italy*

MENZINGER, Guido *Endocrinologia, Università di Tor Vergata, Via della Pineta Sacchetti 506, 00168 Rome, Italy*
E-mail: md4593@mclink.it

MOGENSEN, Carl Erik *Department of Diabetes and Endocrinology, Aarhus University Hospitals, DK-800 Aarhus, Denmark*
E-mail: cem@afdm.au.dk

MORDES, John P. *University of Massachusetts Medical School, Division of Diabetes, Department of Medicine, Biotech 2, 373 Plantation Street, Suite 218, Worcester, MA 01605, USA*

MUGGEO, Michele *Ospedale Civile Maggiore, Divisione di Endocrinologia, 37126 Verona, Italy*

MÜHLHAUSER, Ingrid *Unit for Health Sciences and Education, University of Hamburg, Germany*

MÜLLER-FELBER, W. *Diabetes Center, Department of Internal Medicine, Innenstadt, University of Munich, Ziemssenstrasse 1, D-80336 Munich, Germany*

NAPOLI, Angela *Policlinico Umberto I, Clinica Medica II, 00161 Roma, Italy*

NERUP, Jorn *Steno Diabetes Center, Niels Steensens Vej 2, DK-2820 Gentofte, Denmark*
E-mail: Jne@novo.dk

PIEHLMEIER, W. *Diabetes Center, Department of Internal Medicine, Innenstadt, University of Munich, Ziemssenstrasse 1, D-80336 Munich, Germany*

POTIER, Mylene *Renal Cell Biology Laboratory, Vascular Biology Institute and Renal Cell Biology Unit, University of Miami School of Medicine, PO Box 016960 (R126), Miami, FL 33101, USA*

POZZA, Guido *Instituto Scientifico and Università, Vita e Salute, Università degli Studi di Milano, San Raffaele, Milan, Italy*
E-mail: sovs@dibit.hsr.it

POZZILLI, Paolo *Unità per la Prevenzione del Diabete d delle Malattie Metaboliche, Università Campus Biomedico, Via Longoni 83, 00155 Rome, Italy*
E-mail: p.pozzilli@caspur.it

PRICCI, Flavia *Laboratory of Metabolism and Pathological Biochemistry, Istituto Superiore di Sanita, Rome, Italy*

RAJBHANDARI, S. M. *Diabetes Centre, The Central Sheffield University Hospital, Royal Hallamshire Hospital, Glossop Road, Sheffield S10 2JF, UK*
E-mail: MDP95SMR@sheffield.ac.uk

ROMEO, Guilio *Division of Endicrinology, Department of Clinical Sciences, La Sapienza University, Viale del Policlinico 155, 00161 Rome, Italy*

ROSSINI, Aldo A. *Diabetes Division, University of Massachusetts Medical School, 373 Plantation Street, Suite 218, Worcester, MA 01605, USA*
E-mail: aldo.rossini@umassmed.edu

ROTH, Jesse *149-37 Powells Cove Blvd, 11357 Whitestone, NY USA*
E-mail: jesserothmd@hotmail.com

SABBATINI, Angela *Policlinico Umberto I, Clinica Medica II, 00161 Roma, Italy*

SBRACCIA, Paolo *Dipartimento di Medicina Interna, University of Rome, "Tor Vergata", Italy*
E-mail: sbraccia@med.unicoma2.it

SCHEEN, André J. *Division of Diabetes, Nutrition and Metabolic Disorders, Department of Medicine, CHU Sart Tilman (B35), B-4000 Liège 1, Belgium*
E-mail: Andre.Scheen@chu.ulg.ac.be

SCIULLO, Erneste *Policlinico Umberto I, Clinica Medica II, 00161 Roma, Italy*

SECCHI, Antonio *Instituto Scientifico and Università, Vita e Salute, Università degli Studi di Milano, San Raffaele, Milan, Italy*

SERRANO-RIOS, Manuel *Hosp. Univ. De San Carlos, CEA Bermudex 66-5, 28003 Madrid, Spain*
E-mail: uinvest7@hcsc.es

SPALLONE, Vincenza *Endocrinologia, Università di Tor Vergata, Via della Pineta Sacchetti 506, 00168 Rome, Italy*
E-mail: vispa@mclink.it

STRIKER, Gary E. *Vascular Biology Institute and Renal Cell Biology Unit, University of Miami School of Medicine, PO Box 016960 (R126), Miami, FL 33101, USA*
E-mail: gstriker@miami.edu

STRIKER, Liliane J. *Renal Cell Biology Laboratory, Vascular Biology Institute and Renal Cell Biology Unit, University of Miami School of Medicine, PO Box 016960 (R126), Miami, FL 33101, USA*

THOMAS, S. M. *Department of Diabetes, Endocrinology and Internal Medicine, Division of Medicine, GKT School of Medicine, 5th Floor, Thomas Guy House, KCL Guy's Hospital Campus, London SE1 9RT, UK*

TIENGO, Antonio *Department of Clinical and Experimental Medicine, Cattedra di Malattie del Metabolismo, Via Giustiniani 2, 35128 Padova, Italy*
E-mail: atiengo@ux1.unipd.it

TREVISAN, Roberto *Diabetes Section, Ospedali Riuniti di Bergamo, Largo Barozzi 1, Bergamo, Italy*
E-mail: roby.trevisan@tin.it

VIBERTI, Giancarlo *Department of Diabetes, Endocrinology and Internal Medicine, Division of Medicine, GKT School of Medicine, 5th Floor, Thomas Guy House, KCL Guy's Hospital Campus, London SE1 9RT, UK*
E-mail: giancarlo.viberti@kcl.ac.uk

VIGNERI, Riccardo *Cattedra di Endocrinologia, Istituto di Medicina Interna, Malattie Endocrine e del Metabolismo, University of Catania, Ospedale Garibaldi, Piazza S. Maria di Gesù, 95123 Catania, Italy*

VLASSARA, Helen *Mount Sinai School of Medicine, Box 1640 One Gustave L. Levi Pl., 10029-6574 New York, NY USA*
E-mail: HELEN.VLASSARA@smtplink.mssm.edu

WALDHÄUSL, Werner *Division of Endocrinology and Metabolism, Department of Medicine III, Wahringer Gurtel 18-20, A-1090 Vienna, Austria*
E-mail: werner-klaus.waldhaeusl@univie.ac.at

WARD, J. D. *Central Sheffield University Hospital, Royal Hallamshire Hospital, Glossop Road, Sheffield, S10 2JF, UK*

WILLIAMSON, Joseph R. *Boston University Medical Center Hospital, Diabetes and Metabolism Unit, 88 East Newton Street, Boston, MA 02118-2393, USA*

ZIPRIS, Danny *University of Massachusetts Medical School, Division of Diabetes, Department of Medicine, Biotech 2, 373 Plantation Street, Suite 218, Worcester, MA 01605, USA*

Preface

This book goes beyond being an update in the field of basic and clinical research in type 1 and type 2 diabetes and their complications. It aims at providing a clear overview on what has been done so far and, in particular, it is a state-of-the-art account of diabetes research, with emphasis on the scientific goals to achieve in the next century. These topics have been reviewed and discussed in Rome, in the year of the 50th Jubilee of the Catholic Church, by distinguished scientists convened from all over the world, and the outcome of this 'Jubilee Symposium' has been collected in the pages of this book.

The pathogenesis of type 1 diabetes and new advances in type 1 diabetes therapy are described. Three chapters are dedicated to studies in animal models of type 1 diabetes and to the immunological network controlling the progression of the disease. Particular emphasis has been given also to the epidemiology and genetics of type 1 diabetes and to new therapeutic strategies at diabetes onset and in long-standing diabetes, such as tissue and organ transplants, to achieve the important goal of better controlling hyperglycaemia. Other chapters deal with the pathophysiology of type 2 diabetes, with important contributions on glucose and lipid metabolism, insulin action and insulin resistance. The management of patients with type 2 diabetes has been clearly stated in two chapters, also in the light of recent results obtained from large multicentre studies (such as the UKPDS and the DCCT). Further chapters focus on recent achievement in the pathophysiology and therapy of diabetic vascular, ocular, renal and neurological complications, and diabetes complications in pregnancy.

But this book is not just that. Scientists convened in Rome decided to dedicate the book to Professor Domenico Andreani, Emeritus Professor at the University 'La Sapienza' of Rome, who pioneered diabetes research in Italy and spent his career in promoting research and clinical activities in several fields. In his 50 years of work in research he has devoted most of his work to diabetes, he has been President of the European Association for the Study of

Diabetes (EASD), and he has received the prestigious Claude Bernard Award of this society.

As organizers of the 'Jubilee Symposium On Diabetes' we are proud to have managed to gather these leading experts in the field of diabetes and we are therefore grateful to all those who have enthusiastically accepted to prepare an outstanding manuscript for this book.

Umberto Di Mario
Frida Leonetti
Giuseppe Pugliese
Paolo Sbraccia
Alberto Signore

1

Animal Models of Type 1 Diabetes: Concordances, Discordances, Lessons

DANNY ZIPRIS, JOHN P. MORDES,
DALE L. GREINER and ALDO A. ROSSINI
University of Massachusetts Medical School, Division of Diabetes, Department of
Medicine, Biotech 2, 373 Plantation Street, Suite 218, Worcester, MA 01605, USA

Type 1 or 'juvenile' diabetes mellitus results from the selective destruction of pancreatic β cells. Both genetic and environmental factors play a role in the pathogenesis of the disease, and there is little doubt that the final instrument of β cell destruction is the afflicted person's own immune system. Although our understanding of these processes is extensive, it remains incomplete. Continuing efforts to improve our understanding rely on analyses not only of affected children but also of animals with similar diseases. This review focuses on the information gained — the 'lessons learned' — from animal models that have allowed us to formulate a working hypothesis of the pathogenesis of type 1 diabetes.

HUMAN DIABETES MELLITUS

Type 1 or 'juvenile' diabetes is characterized by selective destruction of pancreatic β cells, absolute insulin deficiency and hyperglycemia. It is generally agreed that the final agent of β cell destruction is the patient's own immune system, but viruses, stress, toxins and immune system abnormalities have all been implicated as etiologic factors (1). Scientific information about this

Diabetes in the New Millennium. Edited by U. Di Mario, F. Leonetti, G. Pugliese, P. Sbraccia and A. Signore.
© 2000 John Wiley & Sons, Ltd.

disease has accrued steadily, but our understanding remains inchoate. Type 1 diabetes today is neither preventable nor easily curable.

Our inability to intervene successfully in type 1 diabetes is due, in part, to ethical and technical constraints on our ability to study it effectively. The diseased tissues are inaccessible; the populations at risk are outbred; obtaining approval for novel therapies is difficult. The study of animal models of the disease helps circumvent these constraints. In animal models the disease-related organ systems are accessible. The disorder can intentionally be induced, tissues recovered for analyses, and new therapies readily tested. Not only can animals be bred to manipulate inheritance, but their genome can also be altered.

The scientific database derived from studies of diabetic animals is extensive, and the 'lessons' they offer have led directly to experimental human therapeutics. These have included completed trials of immunosuppressive agents in children with new onset type 1 diabetes and ongoing disease prevention trials based on parenteral tolerance, oral tolerance and immuno-modulation using agents like nicotinamide (2). This is the ideal outcome of animal model research, but it is unlikely that all of the strategies being translated from rodents to humans will succeed. As scientists and clinicians work to develop progressively better strategies, they need also consider as additional 'lessons' the discordances between the animal and human diseases (see Table 1.1).

OVERVIEW: ANIMAL MODELS OF TYPE 1 DIABETES

Animals with spontaneous insulitis and hyperglycemia

The two major animal models of spontaneous onset type 1 diabetes are the non-obese diabetic (NOD) mouse (3–5) and the diabetes-prone BB (BBDP) rat (6,7). The clinical presentation and microscopic islet pathology observed in both rodent diabetes syndromes provide the fundamental underlying concordances that have engendered continuing intense scientific interest. In both rodents, spontaneous islet inflammation (insulitis) is the prelude to selective β cell destruction, insulin deficiency and hyperglycemia, all of which can be prevented by immunosuppression and immunomodulation.

A few important differences between type 1 diabetes in humans and these rodents are obvious. BBDP rats are severely lymphopenic; humans and NOD mice are not. The risk of diabetes in NOD mice is far greater in females; this is not true of humans or BB rats. Ketoacidosis in humans and BBDP rats is more severe and more rapid in onset than in NOD mice. These simple differences in phenotype clearly imply the existence of limits to the 'lessons' that can be learned from these rodent disease states.

Two other animal models in this category are the LETL (Long Evans Tokushima lean) rat and the BBZ/Wor rat, a cross of the BB and Zucker fatty rats. Neither has been analyzed in detail.

Animals with inducible type 1 diabetes-like syndromes

The expression of type 1 diabetes in humans appears often to involve environmental factors (1), and many strategies have been developed similarly to induce diabetes in the context of insulitis in animals. One class of models is based on toxins and infectious agents (8). A widely studied toxin-induced model is the mouse treated with multiple sub-diabetogenic doses of streptozotocin (STZ) (9). Virus-induced models include mice infected with encephalomyocarditis (EMC) or Coxsackie B virus (10) and the diabetes-resistant (BBDR) subline of the BB rat infected with Kilham rat virus (KRV) (6,7). A second class of induced autoimmune diabetes models has been generated by manipulation of the immune system. Examples include diabetes in thymectomized, sublethally irradiated PVG rats (11) and BBDR rats treated with a monoclonal antibody to deplete ART2$^+$ regulatory T cells, plus the immune system activator polyinosinic:polycytidylic acid (poly I:C) (6). Transgenic and knockout technology has provided a third class of induced mouse models (12). Although inherently 'unnatural', these engineered models provide tools for dissecting and studying discrete components of the immune system relevant to type 1 diabetes.

TYPE 1 DIABETES AND ITS ANIMAL MODELS: GENETICS

Human Type 1 Diabetes

Human type 1 diabetes mellitus is familial but non-Mendelian (1). It is associated with permissive HLA haplotypes, particularly with the HLA-DQB1 gene, which encodes the β chain of the HLA-DQ heterodimer. The amino acid at position 57 in the HLA-DQβ chain plays a critical role in diabetes susceptibility in Caucasian populations; an aspartate residue at this position exerts a strong protective effect. Molecular analyses suggest that variation in the efficiency of peptide binding to various HLA-DQ gene products associated with type 1 diabetes bias the immune system towards or away from autoimmunity (13). Another susceptibility locus, IDDM2, is located in the variable number of tandem repeats (VNTR) 5′ to the insulin gene or possibly the insulin gene itself. Results of a genome-wide search for human type 1 diabetes genes have in addition identified 18 loci with at least suggestive linkage to the disease—although more recent analyses dispute the strength of those linkages (14). The clearest 'genetic lesson' from animal models of type 1

Table 1.1. Experimental immunotherapies for autoimmune diabetes

	Human (2)	NOD mouse (5)	BBDP Rat (6,7)	Induced BBDR rat diabetes (6,7)
Diet				
Modified protein intake	TRIGR trial of reduced cow's milk protein to prevent is under way	Hydrolyzed casein and other diets prevent diabetes but cow's milk protein-free diets specifically do not	Hydrolyzed casein and other diets reduce diabetes frequency	No documented protective dietary effect
Vitamins D & E, caloric restriction caramel food coloring, Japanese 'Kampo'	–	Prevent diabetes	Unknown	Unknown
Parenteral Peptide Immunization				
Insulin	Parenteral insulin at diabetes onset may have metabolic benefit. DPT-1 trial of parenteral insulin for prevention under way	Insulin prevents diabetes even at doses that do not produce hypoglycemia. Insulin B chain prevents diabetes	Prevents diabetes at doses that cause hypoglycemia	Prevents diabetes at doses that cause hypoglycemia
Other peptides	Trials of insulin B chain and HSP-65 for prevention under way	HSP, glucagon, GAD, viral peptides prevent diabetes	Unknown	Unknown
Mucosal tolerance induction				
Insulin	DIPP and DPT-1 trials of oral insulin for prevention under way	Oral insulin prevents diabetes	Insulin does not prevent diabetes	Insulin does not prevent diabetes
Other peptides	Nasal proinsulin prevention trial under way	GAD65 prevents diabetes	Unknown	Unknown

Selective immunosuppression with monoclonal antibodies	Various OKT3 mAbs, anti-CD5-ricin immunoconjugate, anti-CD4 mAb, anti-blast CBL1 and an IL-2R-targeted fusion protein have been tested in a few patients	Prevention by antibodies directed against T cells, MHC molecules, cytokines, cytokine receptors, and other molecules	Prevention by antibodies against CD8, ASGM1, CD3	Prevention by anti-CD8
Azathioprine	Minimal benefit	Prevents diabetes	Unknown	Unknown
Linomide	Some metabolic benefit at diabetes onset	Prevents diabetes	Unknown	Unknown
Nicotinamide	Marginal or no effect in new onset disease; ENDIT and DENIS placebo controlled prevention trials are under way	Prevents diabetes	Does not prevent diabetes	Unknown
Cytokine therapy	Oral IFNα trial for prevention under way	IL-1, IL-4, TNFα, IFNα, IFNγ, IL-10 prevent diabetes	Unknown	Unknown
Immunostimulation/adjuvant therapy				
BCG	Ineffective at diabetes onset	Prevents diabetes	Prevents diabetes	Unknown
CFA	–	Prevents diabetes	Prevents diabetes	Unknown
Poly I:C	–	Prevents diabetes	Accelerates onset at high doses; prevents at low doses	Induces diabetes
Miscellaneous				
Androgen	–	Prevents diabetes in females	Does not prevent diabetes	Unknown
NO inhibitors	–	Prevent diabetes	Delays onset	Unknown

Partial listing of immunological interventions tested in humans and rodents with spontaneous and induced autoimmune diabetes. TRIGR, trial to reduce incidence of diabetes in genetically at risk; DPT-1, diabetes prevention trial of type 1 diabetes; DIPP, diabetes prediction and prevention project; HSP, heat shock protein; GAD, glutamic acid decarboxylase; IL-2R, interleukin-2 receptor; ASGM1, anti-asialoGM1; ENDIT, European Nicotinamide Diabetes Intervention Trial; DENIS, Deutsch Nicotinamide Diabetes Intervention Study; IFN, interferon; TNF, tumor necrosis factor; BCG, Bacille Calmette–Guèrin; CFA, complete Freund's adjuvant; poly I:C, polyinosinic:polycytidylic acid; NO, nitric oxide.

diabetes is the relative strength of the major histocompatibility complex (MHC) association in comparison with all other associations.

BB rat

Autoimmune diabetes in both BBDP and BBDR rats involves at least one gene, *iddm2*, associated with the rat MHC (6). Disease expression requires at least one class II $RT1^u$ allele. The enrichment for $DQ\beta$ chain alleles with uncharged amino acids at position 57 observed in diabetic Caucasian humans is not observed in the BB rat. The region around position 57 of the class II β chains of normal LEW and BUF rats is identical to that found in both BBDP and BBDR rats.

In BBDP rats, a second locus, designated *lyp/iddm1*, has been identified. The *lyp/iddm1* gene is responsible for peripheral T cell lymphopenia in these animals (6) and is permissive to the expression of spontaneous hyperglycemia, but it is not required for the underlying predisposition to diabetes (15). Two additional susceptibility loci in BBDP rats of Worcester origin have been mapped in a (WF × BBDP/Wor) × WF backcross, in which diabetes was induced with poly I:C and anti-ART2 monoclonal antibody (mAb) (16). Loci with significant linkage to insulitis and hyperglycemia, respectively, were mapped to chromosomes 4 (*iddm4*) and 13 (*iddm5*). The *iddm4* gene is located in a region containing other major autoimmunity loci in the rat (15). Among these are *cia* and *aia* loci, which are associated with susceptibility to autoimmune arthritis. Another locus, *iddm3*, may be associated with disease resistance (6).

NOD mice

Investigators have analyzed in detail the loci associated with diabetes susceptibility and resistance in NOD mice (17). The analyses reveal at least 18 loci on 11 different chromosomes that associate with diabetes or insulitis. Most diabetes-associated loci identified in the NOD mouse are associated with susceptibility; *idd—7* is the best-defined resistance locus. Loci on chromosome 17 are MHC-associated. Analogous to the human IDDM1 locus, *idd1* in the mouse has been assigned to an MHC class II-associated region. Interestingly, the rare $A\beta^{g7}$ class II β chain allele of the NOD mouse encodes amino acids that render it homologous to the non-asp57 class II DQ alleles associated with human type 1 diabetes susceptibility (17).

Congenic NOD mice

Congenic NOD mouse strains provide another set of models for genetic analysis (17). For instance, the unique $H2^{g7}$ haplotype of the NOD, the strongest susceptibility locus, has been moved to disease-resistant strains. The absence of diabetes in the congenic animals documents the critical role of non-MHC genes in disease expression. In another example, the NOD.B2m^{null} congenic mouse expresses I-A^{g7} NOD class II but does not express MHC class I molecules. It is also resistant to diabetes, clearly defining a previously ambiguous role for MHC class I in diabetes pathogenesis. Congenic NOD mice are being used to fine-map additional *idd* susceptibility loci, and it is hoped that this strategy will eventually lead to their identification.

TYPE 1 DIABETES AND ITS ANIMAL MODELS: ENVIRONMENT

Human type 1 diabetes

Expression of type 1 diabetes in human populations is modified by environmental perturbants (1). Concordance in monozygotic twins, for example, averages only about 50%, depending on the HLA haplotype. The data suggest the action of an environmental agent, but the exact nature of the genetic–environmental interaction is unknown. Epidemiological studies also offer additional evidence for an environmental influence on diabetes expression, indicating that the prevalence of type 1 diabetes is increasing in many populations at a rate that cannot be accounted for by 'genetic drift' (1).

Environmental toxins, stress, dietary components, and childhood vaccination have all been indicted as potential environmental influences on the expression of diabetes, but convincing evidence is lacking. The strongest evidence implicates viral infection as the most probable and important perturbant (1,10). Perhaps the most striking 'environmental lesson' from animal models is how complex and intractable this problem is.

Environmental factors: viruses

Viral infection is temporally associated with many cases of type 1 diabetes but the mechanism by which infection concatenates with predisposition to yield disease is unknown (10). Molecular mimicry and direct β cell cytotoxicity could, in theory, both be important mechanisms, but evidence for the latter is not strong (18). Direct cytotoxicity has been modeled extensively in mice infected with EMC and Coxsackie B viruses (10,19), but strong evidence of direct cytotoxicity as a common factor in human type 1 diabetes is lacking (10).

Compared with mice raised in 'conventional' animal facilities, Caesarian-derived NOD mice reared in a germ-free environment become diabetic more often and at a younger age (4). Infections with vaccinia, lactate dehydrogenase, mouse hepatitis, Sendai, Pichinde or lymphocytic choriomeningitis (LCM) viruses all decrease the incidence of diabetes in NOD mice (20). The data suggest that these viral infections of the NOD mouse may not model the parallel process in humans.

In the BBDP/Wor rat, diabetes occurs in gnotobiotic animals, but viral pathogens modulate the frequency and age at onset of spontaneous disease (6). As in the NOD mouse, LCMV infection decreases the frequency of diabetes in BBDP rats. This virus is hypothesized to function by infecting and downregulating a subset of regulatory peripheral T cells. More interestingly, BBDR/Wor rats housed in virus-free facilities remain free of spontaneous diabetes, but when deliberately infected with Kilham rat virus (KRV) many become diabetic. Naturally occurring infection, transmitted by close contact, induces diabetes in $\sim 1\%$ of animals; direct injection of KRV induces $\sim 30\%$ of animals to become diabetic, and the combination of KRV and depletion of ART2$^+$ regulatory cells induces diabetes in nearly all animals (6). Disease induction does not involve infection of the pancreatic β cells.

These findings in NOD mice and BB rats clearly illustrate the complex interaction of genetics and environment. They also emphasize the need for rigorous definition of colony-of-origin and environmental status when describing and interpreting experimental results.

One last intriguing set of data relevant to viral infection and diabetes derives from transgenic models designed to explore the concept of molecular mimicry. The expression of LCMV glycoprotein on the surface of β cells is by itself incapable of inducing insulitis or diabetes, even if T cells expressing a T cell receptor specific for the glycoprotein are present (21). Actual infection with LCMV in both model systems does, however, induce diabetes, but a cautionary 'lesson' is present. These results in engineered rodents contrast starkly with the *protection* from diabetes associated with naturally occurring LCMV infection in both NOD mice (22) and BB rats (6).

Environmental factors: diet

The importance of diet, particularly cow's milk proteins, in the pathogenesis of human type 1 diabetes is controversial (23). In part, this line of research has been stimulated by reports that food, particularly its protein content, can alter the expression of diabetes in NOD mice and BB rats (Table 1.1). The observations argue that complex natural ingredients absent in semi-purified chow can be diabetogenic. The 'lessons' are not entirely straightforward, however. Feeding NOD mice a variety of dietary supplements or feeding a conventional diet every other day decreases the frequency of diabetes (24), effects not observed in BB rats. In addition, in the NOD mouse model of diabetes, neither milk powder nor BSA exert a diabetogenic effect (25).

In the BB rat, diets including wheat gluten flour and soybean meal yield the maximum frequency of diabetes (6), whereas semi-synthetic and certain processed diets reduce the incidence of diabetes and delay the age at onset. The agency of protection is not the elimination of cow's milk proteins. The mechanisms are unknown. Diets deficient in essential fatty acids also reduce the frequency of diabetes in both **BBDP** and **ART2**-depleted **BBDR** rats (6).

The 'dietary lesson' from the study of animals is confusing. The impact of diet on these syndromes is clear, but the mechanism and hence the relevance to human diabetes remains obscure. Dietary intervention trials in human infants under way in Europe will provide insight into the instructiveness of animals as models of the interaction of diet and autoimmunity (2).

TYPE 1 DIABETES AND ITS ANIMAL MODELS: IMMUNOPATHOGENESIS

The exact pathophysiological process that follows the interaction of genetics and environment interact to induce type 1 diabetes in humans is unclear. In this area, 'lessons' taught by animal studies have been invaluable in advancing our understanding and complementing the available human data.

Stem cells

Pluripotent hematopoietic stem cells give rise to all the lymphohematopoietic lineages implicated in the pathogenesis of type 1 diabetes. At least nine instances of the inadvertent adoptive transfer of type 1 diabetes after allogeneic bone marrow transplantation have been reported, suggesting that the genetic predisposition to the disease may initially be expressed in stem cells (26). Animal data are consistent with this hypothesis, but point to a variety of possible relevant mechanisms.

In the BB rat many laboratories have shown by adoptive transfer into irradiated recipients that the predisposition to diabetes (and also to lymphopenia) resides in bone marrow cells (6,7). Comparable but more detailed analyses have shown that adoptively transferred NOD bone marrow can induce diabetes in *scid* mice (27). These analyses do not, however, specify the mechanism of disease induction.

Thymus

The predisposition of human, NOD mouse, or BB rat bone marrow to generate autoreactive T cells could represent a defect in T cell precursors or a more complex defect involving intrathymic T cell development. In the BB rat the importance of intrathymic events was recognized in early thymectomy studies (6). Subsequently, defects in bone marrow-derived antigen-presenting cells, intrathymic effector cell precursors and intrathymic regulatory cell precursors have all been documented. Reciprocal bone marrow and thymus transplants have been used to document the existence of a thymic microenvironmental defect of bone marrow origin. Thymocytes from BBDR/Wor rats can adoptively transfer diabetes to athymic recipients, but only if development of ART2$^+$ T cells in the recipient is prevented.

These observations demonstrate that abnormal intrathymic cell populations predisposed to autoreactivity and an intrathymic developmental defect could lead to type 1 diabetes in humans, but to date only the animal data can be brought to bear on this issue.

Autoreactive cells

The identity of the β cell cytotoxic autoreactive cell in humans with type 1 diabetes is unknown. Only a few studies have identified possible islet-cell reactive populations, and no cell lines or clones are available. Animal data suggest possible candidate populations.

One proposed autoreactive T cell population in the BBDP rat has a CD8$^+$NKR-P1$^-$ α/βTcR$^+$ ART2$^-$ phenotype (6,7). This population may in part be comprised of long-lived CD8^{low} T cells. Adoptive transfer studies suggest that CD4$^+$ART2$^-$ and CD8$^+$ART2$^-$ cells acting synergistically are required for efficient disease induction. The data suggest that cell types be involved in the initiation of autoreactivity could differ from recruited cytotoxic cell populations involved in the actual implementation and amplification of β cell killing. A requirement for synergy among different cell types could account in part for the difficulties encountered by scientists attempting to identify comparable populations in humans.

One interesting lesson from animal studies is that autoreactive T cells are present in normal rat strains that do not spontaneously develop autoimmunity (11). Cell populations with autoreactive potential may be present in small numbers or in a functionally inactive state, and some degree of risk for development of autoimmune disease may be relatively common.

Splenocytes from adult NOD mice can adoptively transfer diabetes to MHC-compatible, immunodeficient recipients; as in the BB rat, efficient transfer requires both CD4$^+$ and CD8$^+$ T cells (27). Congenic β2-microglobulin knockout NOD mice, which lack MHC class I-restricted CD8$^+$ T cells, fail to become spontaneously diabetic. Additional studies based on these observations suggest that CD8$^+$ cells are involved in the initiation of the autoimmune diathesis and that CD4$^+$ cells may amplify that response (28). Islet specific CD4$^+$ and CD8$^+$ T cell clones have been obtained from affected NOD mice; these can induce diabetes in appropriate recipients (27).

Pancreatic β cells

There has been speculation that an intrinsic β cell abnormality could contribute to the predisposition to autoimmune diabetes. No data support this contention in the case of human type 1 diabetes. In the rat, islets prepared from normal rats and transplanted into BBDP animals can be the target of autoimmune attack, suggesting that these rat β cells are not antigenically unique (6).

Analysis of both islets and the 'β cell environment' has been a major focus of the application of transgene and knockout technology to the study of type 1 diabetes (12). The clearest 'lesson' from studies of transgenic mice may be that the isolated presence of a neoantigen or the hyperexpression of a self antigen on β cells is not enough to cause autoimmune diabetes. Some antigens are completely quiescent, others are associated with non-autoimmune pathology. Mice engineered to hyperexpress MHC class I antigen on β cells become diabetic but do so in the absence of islet inflammation. Mice that express class II molecules on the β cell surface develop islet atrophy without an inflammatory component.

Transgenic NOD and non-NOD mice that express high local concentrations of cytokines in pancreatic islets have been created (12). Non-NOD transgenic mice expressing the pro-inflammatory Th1 cytokines IFNγ or IL-2 develop diabetes, and transgenic NOD mice expressing IL-2 in islets experience accelerated onset of disease. In contrast, non-NOD mice expressing either TNFα or TNFβ develop insulitis without diabetes. Transgenic mice expressing the Th2 cytokine IL-10 on a normal background develop pancreatitis without insulitis or diabetes, but NOD mice transgenic for islet expression of IL-10 experience accelerated disease. If there is a 'lesson' in these analyses of supraphysiological cytokine concentrations in the islets, it may be that no one cytokine can be implicated as the determinant of the balance between autoimmunity and tolerance.

In the standard NOD mouse, antigens associated with the β cell can 'immunize' against the disease (5). These include both oral and parenteral insulin. Diabetes in the BB rat can be prevented by parenteral insulin, but only at doses that cause hypoglycemia, suggesting that 'β cell rest' has led to concealment of the immununological target. Oral insulin does not prevent diabetes in the BB rat and may exacerbate the disorder (6). The 'β cell lessons' from animals treated with prophylactic insulin for tolerization are conflicting. Which 'lesson' will prove to have been instructive for juvenile diabetes prevention will be decided by the outcome of human trials now under way (Table 1.1).

Autoantibodies

In humans, autoantibodies are a hallmark of type 1 diabetes, but few investigators believe that they play a role in pathogenesis (e.g. via antibody-dependent cellular cytotoxicity or ADCC) (29). Rather, these autoantibodies are regarded as possible markers of the inciting autoantigen and as powerful tools for predicting the onset of disease in at-risk populations. The 'autoantibody lessons' from rodents are consistent with the view that their role is indirect.

Not all the autoantibodies important in human type 1 diabetes appear to have counterparts in BB rats (6). Insulin autoantibodies (IAA) have been reported in BB/W/D rats, but their presence could not be confirmed in BB/Wor rats. The human anti-IA-2 antibody is either absent or present only at low titer in BB rats. Anti-glutamic acid decarboxylase (GAD) antibodies are reportedly absent in BB/d and other BB rats, but may be present in BB/OK animals. Autoantibodies against heat shock protein 65 (HSP-65) are absent in BB rats.

Anti-GAD autoantibodies are detectable in the NOD mouse, but levels of both anti-GAD and anti-insulin antibodies appear to be low. As is true of the BB rat, the importance of humoral immune factors, if any, in the pathogenesis of NOD diabetes remains to be determined. In NOD mice, however, data do indicate that B lymphocytes functioning as antigen-presenting cells are critical to the development of diabetes (27). They may act by 'trapping' islet antigens present at low concentration for presentation to autoreactive T cells and by providing important costimulatory signals.

Regulatory cells

The concept of peripheral regulation of autoreactive cells has continued to gain adherents among scientists investigating autoimmune disease states (30). In the BB rat, the expression of diabetes appears to be a function of the relative balance between ART2$^-$ autoreactive cells and ART2$^+$ regulatory cells (6,7). Supportive observations include the fact that lymphocyte transfusions prevent disease in lymphopenic, ART2-deficient BBDP/Wor rats if CD4$^+$ART2$^+$ donor T cells become engrafted. Conversely, diabetes resistant BBDR rats have normal numbers of ART2$^+$ T cells. They do not become diabetic spontaneously, but in vivo depletion of these cells in combination with poly I:C induces diabetes in >90% of treated animals.

In the NOD mouse, there is no definitive marker of regulatory T cells relevant to diabetes expression. There are data that do, however, suggest that such populations must exist. Certain cell populations can adoptively prevent diabetes in NOD mice (30) and recent data suggest that they express a CD4$^+$CD25$^+$ (31) and perhaps a CD62L^{high} phenotype (32). In addition, the induction of IL-4 and TGFβ-secreting 'bystander suppressor cells' has been advanced as the mechanism underlying the prevention of NOD diabetes by parenteral and oral tolerance induction.

In humans with diabetes there are as yet no definitive data that document the phenotype or function of regulatory cells, although in the case of monozygotic twins discordant for the disease, asymmetric peripheral regulation has been suggested as one possibility to account for the discordance. The primate equivalent of the rat ART2 gene is a pseudogene. It is now known, however, that ART2 proteins are ADP-ribosyltransferases (ARTs) (33). ARTs may participate in immune system modulation by several mechanisms, and ribosyltransferase activity (rather than any one specific enzyme) may prove to be important in the peripheral regulation of autoimmunity (33). The animal data continue to provide an impetus to identify comparable regulatory cell populations in humans, and the concept of 'bystander suppression' is one of the theoretical underpinnings of some tolerance-based human diabetes prevention trials (Table 1.1).

TYPE 1 DIABETES AND ITS ANIMAL MODELS: PREVENTION

The 'lessons' from animal models of type 1 diabetes have one paramount purpose: to guide the development of therapies that will prevent and cure the disease that is being modeled. As we have pointed out, however, the lessons are not always consistent or clear. The available data from the NOD mouse demonstrate that type 1 diabetes can be prevented by more than 125 interventions of many different types (5). The data from the BB rat suggest that the type 1 diabetes syndrome in these animals is difficult to prevent or reverse (6). Clearly, many caveats apply to the extrapolation of data sets derived from one species to another. But clinical scientists are obligated to seek a better life for their patients and persons at risk. The 'clinical lessons' from NOD mice and BB rats, and their implementation in human clinical trials are summarized in Table 1.1. Reading across the roles of the table, comparing observations in animals and the corresponding hopeful undertakings in children, afford the clearest indication that some of the 'clinical lessons' taught by animal diabetes could be spurious.

CONCLUSION: THE PATHOGENESIS OF TYPE 1 DIABETES

Scientific understanding of type 1 diabetes in humans is a work in progress. Based on the data available from all the sources we describe above, we have developed a working hypothesis of the pathogenesis of type 1 diabetes. This is summarized in Figure 1.1. The MHC and additional non-MHC loci confer genetic predisposition. Environmental factors then lead to the development of cells that are either in balance (tolerant) or in disequilibrium (leading to diabetes). We view the interrelationship between effector and regulatory cell populations as a critical determinant of disease expression in susceptible individuals. Our working hypothesis is that the expression of diabetes depends on the relative balance between the autoreactive (A) cells and populations of regulatory (R) cells that should normally prevent β cell destruction.

Once the balance has been tipped in favor of autoreactivity, we hypothesize that β cell destruction proceeds as a two-component process. The first, or primary, component initiates β cell damage. The secondary component

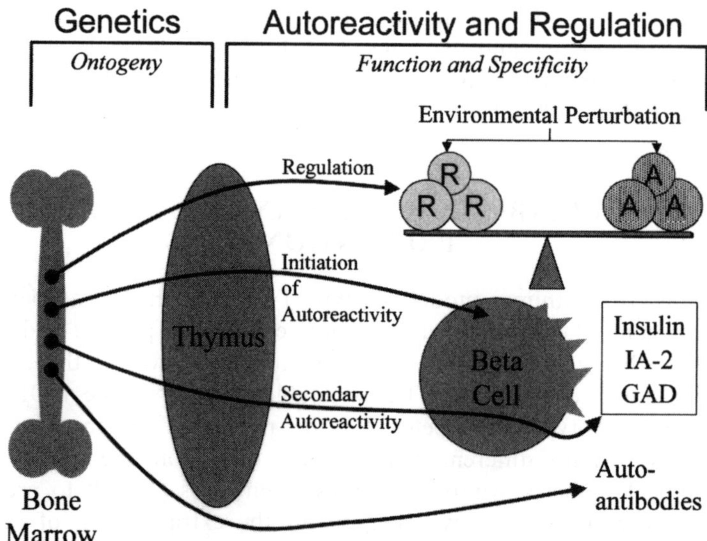

Figure 1.1. Working hypothesis of the pathogenesis of type 1 diabetes mellitus

amplifies the destructive process and results in inter- and intra-molecular determinant spreading of the immune response.

This hypothesis is based in part on human data and in part on data from two decades of study of animal models. There is much more to be learned. A major goal of animal model research in the future will be to identify the 'initiator' cell population, to determine its specificity, to learn how it is activated, and to distinguish it from cell populations that secondarily participate in autoimmune destruction. The hoped for final 'lesson' will teach us how safely to prevent these cells from causing diabetes.

ACKNOWLEDGEMENTS

This work was supported in part by Center Grant DK32520 and Grants DK25306, DK36024 and DK49106 from the National Institutes of Health. The contents of this publication are solely the responsibility of the authors and do not necessarily represent the official views of the National Institutes of Health.

DEDICATION

This review is dedicated to Professor D. Andreani, who has devoted his life to the struggle against diabetes. We are reminded of Newton's letter of 1675 to Robert Hooke in which he stated, 'If I have seen further—than you and Descartes—it is by standing on the shoulders of giants'. It gives us equal pleasure to acknowledge the parallel contribution of Professor Andreani to the vision of his fellow scientists in this area of medical research.

REFERENCES

1. Park Y, Eisenbarth GS: The natural history of autoimmunity in type 1A diabetes mellitus. In *Diabetes Mellitus. A Fundamental and Clinical Text.* LeRoith D, Taylor SI, Olefsky JM, Eds. Philadelphia, PA: Lippincott Williams & Wilkins, 2000, pp. 347–362.
2. Skyler JS, Marks JB: Immune intervention. In *Diabetes Mellitus. A Fundamental and Clinical Text.* LeRoith D, Taylor SI, Olefsky JM, Eds. Philadelphia, PA: Lippincott Williams & Wilkins, 2000, pp. 500–506.
3. Delovitch TL, Singh B: The nonobese diabetic mouse as a model of autoimmune diabetes: immune dysregulation gets the NOD. *Immunity* 7:727–738, 1997.
4. Leiter EH: NOD mice and related strains: origins, husbandry, and biology. In *NOD Mice and Related Strains: Research Applications in Diabetes, AIDS, Cancer and Other Diseases.* Leiter EH, Atkinson MA, Eds. Austin, TX: R.G. Landes, 1998, pp. 1–36.
5. Atkinson M, Leiter EH: The NOD mouse model of insulin dependent diabetes: As good as it gets? *Nature Med* 5:601–604, 1999.
6. Mordes JP, Bortell R, Groen H, Guberski DL, Rossini AA, Greiner DL: Autoimmune diabetes mellitus in the BB rat. In *Frontiers in Animal Diabetes Research. Primer on Animal Models of Diabetes.* Sima AAF, Shafrir E, Eds. Reading, UK: Harwood Academic, 2000 (in press).
7. Crisá L, Mordes JP, Rossini AA: Autoimmune diabetes mellitus in the BB rat. *Diabetes/Metab Rev* 8:9–37, 1992.
8. Karounos DG: Convergence of genetic and environmental factors in the immunopathogenesis of type 1 diabetes mellitus. *J Clin Ligand Assay* 21:262–271, 1998.
9. Herold KC, Vezys V, Koons A, Lenschow D, Thompson C, Bluestone JA: CD28/B7 costimulation regulates autoimmune diabetes induced with multiple low doses of streptozotocin. *J Immunol* 158:984–991, 1997.
10. Yoon JW, Jun H-S: Role of viruses in the pathogenesis of type 1 diabetes mellitus. In *Diabetes Mellitus. A Fundamental and Clinical Text.* LeRoith D, Taylor SI, Olefsky JM, Eds. Philadelphia, PA: Lippincott Williams & Wilkins, 2000, pp. 419–429.
11. Seddon B, Mason D: The third function of the thymus. *Immunol Today* 21:95–99, 2000.
12. Grewal IS, Flavell RA: New insights into insulin dependent diabetes mellitus from studies with transgenic mouse models. *Lab Invest* 76:3–10, 1997.
13. Nepom GT, Kwok WW: Molecular basis for HLA-DQ associations with IDDM. *Diabetes* 47:1177–1184, 1998.
14. Concannon P, Gogolin-Ewens K, Hinds DA, Wapelhorst B, Morrison VA, Stirling B, Mitra M, Farmer J, Williams SR, Cox NJ, Bell GI, Risch N, Spielman RS: A second-generation screen of the human genome for susceptibility to insulin-dependent diabetes mellitus. *Nature Genet* 19:292–296, 1998.
15. Martin A-M, Maxson MN, Leif J, Mordes JP, Greiner DL, Blankenhorn EP: Diabetes-prone and diabetes-resistant BB rats share a common major diabetes susceptibility locus, *iddm4*: additional evidence for a 'universal autoimmunity locus' on rat chromosome 4. *Diabetes* 48:2138–2144, 1999.
16. Martin A-M, Blankenhorn EP, Maxson MN, Zhao M, Leif J, Mordes JP, Greiner DL: Non-major histocompatibility complex-linked diabetes susceptibility loci on

chromosomes 4 and 13 in a backcross of the DP BB/Wor rat to the WF rat. *Diabetes* 48:50–58, 1999.

17. Leiter E: Genetics and immunogenetics of NOD mice and related strains. In *NOD Mice and Related Strains: Research Applications in Diabetes, AIDS, Cancer, and Other Diseases.* Leiter E, Atkinson M, Eds. Austin, TX: R.G. Landes, 1998, pp. 37–69.

18. Atkinson MA: Molecular mimicry and the pathogenesis of insulin-dependent diabetes mellitus: still just an attractive hypothesis. *Ann Med* 29:393–399, 1997.

19. Horwitz MS, Bradley LM, Harbertson J, Krahl T, Lee J, Sarvetnick N: Diabetes induced by Coxsackie virus: initiation by bystander damage and not molecular mimicry. *Nature Med* 4:781–785, 1998.

20. Karasik A, Hattori M: Use of animal models in the study of diabetes. In *Joslin's Diabetes Mellitus.* Kahn CR, Weir GC, Eds. Malvern, PA: Lea & Febiger, 1994, pp. 317–350.

21. Oldstone MBA, Von Herrath M, Evans CF, Horwitz MS: Virus-induced autoimmune disease: Transgenic approach to mimic insulin-dependent diabetes mellitus and multiple sclerosis. *Curr Top Microbiol Immunol* 206:67–83, 1996.

22. Oldstone MBA: Viruses as therapeutic agents. I. Treatment of nonobese insulin-dependent diabetes mice with virus prevents insulin-dependent diabetes mellitus while maintaining general immune competence. *J Exp Med* 171:2077–2089, 1990.

23. Schrezenmeir J, Jagla A: Milk and diabetes. *J Am Coll Nutr* 19:176S–190S, 2000.

24. Yoon J-W, Elliott RB: Discussion. Environmental factors: viruses and diet. In *Frontiers in Diabetes Research. Lessons from Animal Diabetes III.* Shafrir E, Ed. London: Smith-Gordon, 1991, pp. 198–203.

25. Kolb H: On the aetiopathogenesis of type 1 diabetes: key roles for innate immunity and dietary antigens? *Exp Clin Endocrinol Diabetes* 107:S13–S16, 1999.

26. Sorli CH, Greiner DL, Mordes JP, Rossini AA: Stem cell transplantation for treatment of autoimmune diseases. *Graft* 1:71–81, 1998.

27. Serreze DV: The identity and ontogenic origins of autoreactive T lymphocytes in NOD mice. In *NOD Mice and Related Strains: Research Applications in Diabetes, AIDS, Cancer and Other Diseases.* Leiter E, Atkinson M, Eds. Austin, TX: R.G. Landes, 1998, pp. 71–100.

28. Graser RT, DiLorenzo TP, Wang FM, Christianson GJ, Chapman HD, Roopenian DC, Nathenson SG, Serreze DV: Identification of a CD8 T cell that can independently mediate autoimmune diabetes development in the complete absence of CD4 T cell helper functions. *J Immunol* 164:3913–3918, 2000.

29. Greenbaum CJ, Palmer JP: Autoantibodies and the disease process of type 1 diabetes mellitus. In *Diabetes Mellitus. A Fundamental and Clinical Text.* LeRoith D, Taylor SI, Olefsky JM, Eds. Philadelphia, PA: Lippincott Williams & Wilkins, 2000, pp. 374–382.

30. Rashba EJ, Reich E-P, Janeway CA, Sherwin RS: Type 1 diabetes mellitus: an imbalance between effector and regulatory T cells? *Acta Diabetol* 30:61–69, 1993.

31. Salomon B, Lenschow DJ, Rhee L, Ashourian N, Singh B, Sharpe A, Bluestone JA: B7/CD28 costimulation is essential for the homeostasis of the $CD4^+CD25^+$ immunoregulatory T cells that control autoimmune diabetes. *Immunity* 12:431–440, 2000.

32. Lepault F, Gagnerault MC: Characterization of peripheral regulatory $CD4^+$ T cells that prevent diabetes onset in nonobese diabetic mice. *J Immunol* 164:240–247, 2000.

33. Bortell R, Kanaitsuka T, Stevens LA, Moss J, Mordes JP, Rossini AA, Greiner DL: The RT6 (Art2) family of ADP-ribosyltransferases in rat and mouse. *Mol Cell Biochem* 193:61–68, 1999.

2

The Natural History of Insulitis in Autoimmune Diabetes

HUBERT KOLB[1] and VICTORIA KOLB-BACHOFEN[2]

[1]German Diabetes Research Institute and [2]Research Group Immunobiology, MED-Heinrich-Heine-University of Düsseldorf, Düsseldorf, Germany

Detailed molecular studies on the natural course of insulitis presently are only available from two animal models which spontaneously develop type 1-like autoimmune diabetes, the BB rat and the NOD mouse. Initially, focal infiltration of exocrine tissue and of the islet periphery, mostly by macrophages and/or dendritic cells, is observed. This may lead to β cell stress, antigen release and sensitization of autoimmune T cells in draining pancreatic lymph nodes. The subsequent peri-insular infiltration by lymphocytes involves Th2 type T cells as the major component. The progression from benign peri-insular infiltration to destructive intra-insulitis is driven by cells of the innate immune system, by releasing Th1 inducing cytokines, such as IL-12, IL-18 and TNFα. As a consequence, autoaggressive Th1 type T cells dominate during destructive intra-insular infiltration. The analysis of NOD-related but diabetes-resistant mouse strains revealed three checkpoints of insulitis progression, the induction of IL-12/IL-18 expression, the activation of Th1 cells by these cytokines and the concomitant presence or absence of an antagonistic Th2 type immune response in pancreatic lesions.

One major obstacle to research on the pathogenesis of type 1 diabetes at the molecular level is the limited availability of the target tissue. Recently, methods of endoscopy and sample procurement have reached a high standard, so that a new assessment of risks vs. benefits of pancreatic biopsies, if performed in specialized centres, seems warranted. To date, most of our knowledge on the

Diabetes in the New Millennium. Edited by U. Di Mario, F. Leonetti, G. Pugliese, P. Sbraccia and A. Signore.
© 2000 John Wiley & Sons, Ltd.

natural history of insulitis comes from the study of two animal models with spontaneous autoimmune diabetes, the BB rat and the NOD mouse (1,2).

Despite differences in genetics, kinetics and sex dependence of disease development, basic characteristics of islet inflammation are quite similar in BB rats and NOD mice. It therefore appears justified to assume that properties of insulitis in animals are largely shared with characteristics of islet inflammation in human type 1 diabetes, which is supported by the close similarity of disease-associated human and rodent major histocompatibility complex (MHC) class II genes and by the fact that the autoimmune response focuses on identical targets of the β cell in man and rodents, such as the insulin B chain and 65 kDa glutamate decarboxylase.

ORIGIN OF ISLET INFILTRATION

In an early study we had analysed the natural course of insulitis in the BB rat by detailed immunohistochemistry of more than 700 islets (3). Islet infiltration was observed to be asynchronous, i.e. non-infiltrated islets were found in the neighbourhood of islets with early or late infiltration stages. Evaluation of larger pancreatic areas, however, revealed that variations did not occur between individual islets but rather between larger areas of the organ, which either inflamed, as evident from enhanced MHC class I expression in most islets, or appeared largely normal. These areas had recognizable boundaries and represented regions superimposing with one limb of the vasculature (Hanenberg, Kolb-Bachofen and Kolb, unpublished). In nearly 100% of cases first signs of islet inflammation were seen at the periductular pole of the islet, or somewhat dispersed in the islet periphery. Hallmarks of early islet inflammation were the locally enhanced MHC class I antigen expression as well as few infiltrating mononuclear cells, mostly macrophages (3). Studies by other groups have confirmed the early abundance of macrophages and/or of dendritic cells in the infiltrate (4–6).

When considering both findings, i.e. the patchy distribution of islet inflammation and the preponderance of macrophages, islet inflammation appears to be tightly controlled by the vasculature. Inflammatory changes affect islets linked through the same local vascular system and infiltration starts at postcapillary venules located in the islet periphery.

A recent study suggests that the primary activation of autoreactive immune cells occurs outside the islet, i.e. in draining parapancreatic lymph nodes (7). Upon adoptive transfer of diabetogenic T cells to healthy recipients, proliferating cells were initially observed only in pancreatic lymph nodes, well before the onset of insulitis (7). Usually, activation of T cells in draining lymph nodes requires an inflammatory situation in the respective organ and enhanced release of local antigens which then are presented by dendritic cells in the draining lymph nodes. We have therefore proposed that an immune response of the innate immune system to β cells precedes activation of adaptive immunity (8). This early attraction of single macrophages by unknown receptor–ligand interactions has been termed by us have 'single cell insulitis' (9).

Very recently, Drexhage's group (10) have reported on macrophage infiltration of islets and the concomitant formation of mega-islets also in NOD mice with non-functional adaptive immunity, NOD *scid* mice, which lends further support to the concept that the initial stages of islet aggression are T cell-independent. Interestingly, target autoantigens recognized early in the disease process must also be expressed in some exocrine areas distant to islets. This conclusion comes from our study of pancreatic biopsies at an early age of diabetes prone **BB** rats. The earliest morphological change, being highly predictive of later diabetes development was the interstitial infiltration of the exocrine tissue by immunocytes, mostly activated macrophages, with concomitant damage of the surrounding exocrine tissue (11).

One candidate antigen expressed in endocrine cells but also in exocrine tissue is heat shock protein (hsp) 60 (12). In the NOD mouse as well as in diabetic patients, autoreactive T cells recognizing hsp60 are found. Moreover, T cell lines reactive to hsp60 are able to transfer the disease or to inhibit autoimmune diabetes (13–15). Finally, hsp60 appears also to be directly recognized by macrophages via invariant receptors expressed on these cells (16).

BENIGN VS. DESTRUCTIVE INSULITIS

In both animal models, only 50–80% of animals progress to overt diabetes, although all animals develop insulitis. In fact, the number of infiltrating mononuclear cells may be similar in non-diabetic and diabetic NOD mice (17). This led to the concept of two types of islet inflammatory reactions, i.e. benign insulitis vs. destructive insulitis. In islet transplantation studies, benign insulitis was associated with peri-insular infiltration, leaving the β cell rich core of islets largely unaffected. In contrast, destructive insulitis was characterized by the presence of mononuclear cells throughout the grafted islet with β cell destruction as a prominent event (18).

Importantly, immunohistochemistry revealed preferential expression of the Th2 cytokine IL-4 in peri-insular, benign infiltrates, whereas intra-insulitis was associated with a high number of IFNγ-positive immunocytes (18). A subsequent analysis of the course of insulits in NOD or BB pancreas revealed that early peri-insulitis has a dominant component of Th2-type immune reactivity while progression towards intra-islet infiltration and diabetes was characterized by a shift towards the expression of Th1 type cytokines, such as IFNγ (19–24).

It should be noted that not all studies concur that insulitis progresses from a Th2 dominant to a Th1 dominant state. However, immunohistochemical studies must be considered as giving the most reliable information and all of these reports agree on peri-insulitis preceding intra-insulitis in both the NOD mouse and the BB rat. Peri-insulitis was always reported as associated with Th2 type cytokine expression, while staining for IFN γ was prominent in intra-insulitis (18,19,25,26). Results discrepant from this concept were based on the analysis of isolated islets or of leukocytes retrieved from isolated islets, an approach suffering from several problems. The number of islets which can be retrieved from inflamed NOD mouse pancreas is usually 25–50% lower than from pancreas devoid of insulitis, which suggests a preferential loss of damaged islets during the isolation procedure. Moreover, collagenase treatment and subsequent centrifugation steps will enrich for leukocytes within islets as compared with peri-insular or periductular infiltrates. In addition, it is long known that the number of mRNA copies of IFNγ in a Th1 cell by far exceeds the amount of IL-4 copies in a Th2 cell. Taken together, these experimental shortcomings may explain why mRNA analysis of islets shows a predominance of the Th1 cytokine IFNγ also early in the disease (27,28), i.e. at a time, when peri-insulitis and Th2-type cytokines are the dominant features of immuno-histochemical studies.

CONTROL OF PROGRESSION FROM PERI- TO INTRA-INSULITIS

Since the progression of islet infiltration is an asynchronous event, factors controlling the transition from benign to destructive cannot be readily identified. Two different approaches have been used to elucidate the mechanisms involved; both approaches applied methods to synchronize the disease process in pancreatic islets.

One method of insulitis synchronization and acceleration is the application of a single dose of cyclophosphamide. This intervention causes diabetes development in the majority of NOD mice within a few weeks (29). If given at an early age, when peri-insulitis is the dominant stage of islet infiltration, progression towards intra-insulitis is observed within 7–10 days (19). This setting allows to determine which immune reactivities precede the occurrence of intra-islet infiltration.

The first changes we could observe occurred within 24 h after cyclo-phosphamide treatment and are associated with cells of the innate immune system. These changes include downregulation of Th2-associated markers in macrophages such as arginase (H. Rothe, A. Hausmann, H. Kolb, submitted) and, conversely, upregulation of Th1-associated mediators produced by macrophages, such as IL-12 and IL-18 (30,31). Both cytokines are known as key products of antigen presenting cells for the induction of Th1 cell reactivities (32,33). Indeed, targeting IL-12 or IL-18 dependent immunity by various approaches have provided evidence for a decisive role of these cytokines in controlling destructive insulitis (6).

Synchronization of insulitis progression by cyclophosphamide was also used for analysing molecular changes in a simplified mouse model with transgenic expression of the T cell receptor of the highly diabetogenic clone BDC2.5 (34). Again, the cytokines IL-12 and IL-18 as well as TNFα were found pivotal for the transition to β cell destructive insulitis.

Another approach to synchronize islet infiltration is to perform islet grafts. The progression to destructive insulitis was unaffected if grafted islets were deficient in expressing Fas, IFNγ receptor or inducible NO synthase, whereas the lack of the 55 kDa TNFα receptor 1 prevented intra-insulitis and graft destruction but not peri-insulitis (35).

Taken together, three mediators of natural immunity, i.e. IL-12, IL-18 and ligands of TNFα receptor 1, appear critically involved in controlling the switch from benign to destructive insulitis.

A scheme integrating the data discussed above is shown in Figure 2.1. The initial attraction of macrophages/dendritic cells to islets may cause antigen release and activation of autoimmune T cells in draining lymph nodes. Later, the transition from benign to destructive insulitis appears to require antigen presentation within affected islets.

CHECKPOINTS OF INSULITIS PROGRESSION IN PANCREATIC LESIONS

When considering the many events between the initiation of β cell autoimmunity and the manifestation of overt diabetes, it is not surprising that a host of different types of intervention can effectively delay or prevent the disease process at many different levels (36). In order to learn more about physiological defences against aggressive insulitits development, we analysed mouse strains which do not progress to overt diabetes despite some genetic predisposition for β cell autoimmunity and the development of mild or even severe insulitis. Mouse strains expressing different diabetes risk genes of NOD mice were analysed. For the reasons described above, cytokine gene expression was analysed in total pancreas rather than in isolated islets and islet inflammation was synchronized and accelerated by cyclophosphamide treatment.

A comparative analysis of four NOD-related mouse strains revealed three checkpoints of insulitis progression (H. Rothe, Y. Ito, H. Kolb, submitted for publication). The first checkpoint was identified as the lack to express IL-12 and IL-18 in response to cyclophosphamide, as observed in NON and

Focal infiltration of exocrine tissue
(mostly activated macrophages)
and
Focal peri-insular infiltration
(mostly activated macrophages/dendritic cells)

↓

Sensitization of autoimmune cells in
pancreatic lymph nodes

↓

Extended peri-insular infiltration
T cells (major component),
dominant expression of Th2 type cytokines

↓

Enhanced expression of IL-12, IL-18, TNFα

↓

Destructive intra-insulitis,
dominance of Th1 type cytokines

Figure 2.1. Proposed concept of the natural course of insulitis in animal models of type 1 diabetes

NOD.NON-H^{2nb1} mice. In these strains some peri-insulitis was found, but little progression to intra-insulitis. In contrast, the two strains carrying the MHC region of NOD, i.e. NOR and NON.NOD-H^{2g7}, did progress to substantial intra-insulitis concomitant with IL-12 and IL-18 gene expression in response to cyclophosphamide treatment. However, in NON.NODH^{2g7} mice the production of IL-12 and IL-18 failed to activate the Th1 immune response, as evidenced by a complete lack of IFNγ gene expression. In contrast, within pancreas of NOR mice IL-12 and IL-18 expression did induce a Th1 response comparable to that of NOD mice. However, there was a concomitant and sustained expression of the Th2 type cytokine IL-4, which is known to antagonize Th1 reactions and therefore dampened destructive insulitis in NOR mice sufficiently to prevent the development of overt diabetes.

In summary, three checkpoints of insulitis progression were identified (Figure 2.2). The first checkpoint controls the activation of innate immune cells and their production of IL-12 and IL-18. The second checkpoint determines the ability of Th1 lymphocytes to respond to IL-12 and IL-18. The third checkpoint controls the presence or absence of a potent and sustained Th2

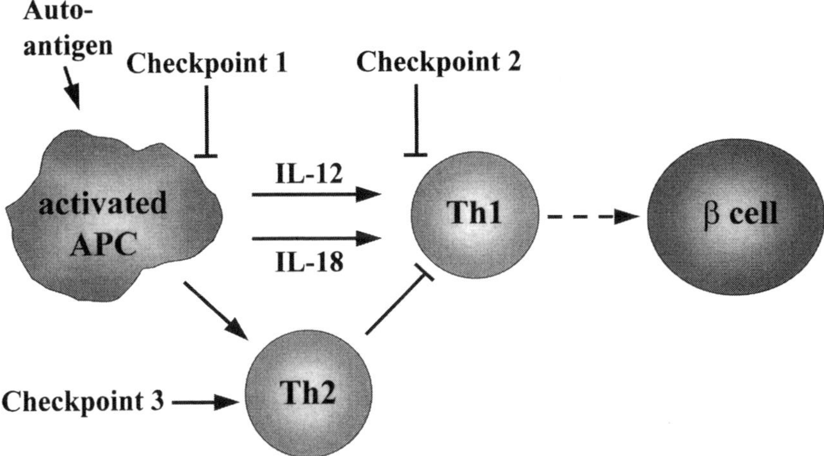

Figure 2.2. Checkpoints of insulitis progression in pancreatic lesions. Mouse strains genetically related to NOD, but not progressing to overt diabetes, either do not express IL-12 and IL-18 in pancreatic lesions (checkpoint 1) or they fail to respond to these cytokines with activation of Th1 immunity (checkpoint 2). A third level of control is the induction an antagonistic Th2-type response (checkpoint 3)

response limiting the pathogenic activity of autoaggressive immune cells in intra-insulitits.

ACKNOWLEDGEMENTS

We thank R. Schreiner for help with preparation of the manuscript. This work was supported by the Deutsche Forschungsgemeinschaft, the Bundesminister für Gesundheit and the Minister für Wissenschaft und Forschung des Landes Nordrhein-Westfalen.

REFERENCES

1. Crisa L, Mordes JP, Rossini AA: Autoimmune diabetes mellitus in the BB rat. *Diabet Metab Rev* 8:4–37, 1992.
2. Delovitch TL, Singh B: The nonobese diabetic mouse as a model of autoimmune diabetes: immune dysregulation gets the NOD. *Immunity* 7:727–738, 1998.
3. Hanenberg H, Kolb-Bachofen V, Kantwerk-Funke G, Kolb H: Macrophage infiltration precedes and is a prerequisite for lymphocytic insulitis in pancreatic islets of prediabetic BB rats. *Diabetologia* 32:126–134, 1989.
4. Lee K-U, Amano K, Yoon J-W: Evidence for initial involvement of macrophage in development of insulitis in NOD mice. *Diabetes* 37:989–991, 1988.

5. Voorby HAM, Jeucken PHM, Kabel PJ, De-Haan M, Drexhage HA: Dendritic cells and scavenger macrophages in the pancreatic islets of prediabetic BB rats. *Diabetes* 38:1623–1629, 1989.

6. Rothe H, Kolb H: The APC 1 concept of type I diabetes. *Autoimmunity* 27:179–184, 1998.

7. Hoglund, P., J. Mintern, C. Waltzinger, W. Heath, C. Benoist, and D. Mathis: Initiation of autoimmune diabetes by developmentally regulated presentation of islet cell antigens in the pancreatic lymph nodes. *J Exp Med* 189:331–339, 1999.

8. Kolb-Bachofen V, Kolb H: A role for macrophages in the pathogenesis of type 1 diabetes. *Autoimmunity* 3:145–155, 1989.

9. Kolb-Bachofen V, Kolb H: New concept of insulitis and B-islet cell destruction. *Diabetes* 32:22A, 1983.

10. Rosmalen JG, Homo-Delarche F, Durant S, Kap M, Leenen PJ, Drexhage HA: Islet abnormalities associated with an early influx of dendritic cells and macrophages in NOD and NODscid mice. *Lab Invest* 80:769–777, 2000.

11. Kolb-Bachofen V, Schraermeyer U, Hoppe T, Hanenberg H, Kolb H: Diabetes manifestation in BB rats is preceded by pan-pancreatic presence of activated inflammatory macrophages. *Pancreas* 5:578–584, 1992.

12. Brudzynski K: Insulitis-caused redistribution of heat-shock protein hsp60 inside β-cells correlates with induction of hsp60 autoantibodies. *Diabetes* 42:908–913, 1993.

13. Elias D, Cohen IR: Treatment of autoimmune diabetes and insulitis in NOD mice with heat shock protein 60 peptide p277. *Diabetes* 44:1132–1138, 1995.

14. Cohen IR: The Th1/Th2 dichotomy, hsp60 autoimmunity, and type 1 diabetes. *Clin Immunol* 84:103–106, 1997.

15. Feili-Hariri M, Frantz MO, Morel PA: Prevention of diabetes in the NOD mouse by a Th1 clone specific for a hsp60 peptide. *J Autoimmun* 14:133–142, 2000.

16. Chen W, Syldath U, Bellmann K, Kolb H: Human 60-kDa heat shock protein: a danger signal to the innate immune system. *J Immunol* 162:3212–3219, 1999.

17. Sadelain MWJ, Qiun H, Lauzon J, Singh B: Prevention of type 1 diabetes in NOD mice by adjuvant immunotherapy. *Diabetes* 39:583–589, 1990.

18. Shedadeh NN, LaRosa F, Lafferty KJ: Altered cytokine activity in adjuvant inhibition of autoimmune diabetes. *J Autoimmun* 6:291–300, 1993.

19. Rothe H, Faust A, Schade U *et al*: Cyclophosphamide treatment of female non-obese diabetic mice causes enhanced expression of inducible nitric oxide synthase and interferon-gamma, but not of interleukin-4. *Diabetologia* 37:1154–1158, 1994.

20. Shimada A, Charlton B, Taylor-Edward C, Fathman CG: Beta-cell destruction may be a late consequence of the autoimmune process in non-obese diabetic mice. *Diabetes* 45:1063–1067, 1996.

21. Rabinovitch A, Sorensen O, Suarez-Pinzon WL, Power RF, Rajotte RV, Bleackley RC: Analysis of cytokine mRNA expression in syngeneic islet grafts of NOD mice: interleukin 2 and interferon gamma mRNA expression correlate with graft rejection and interleukin 10 with graft survival. *Diabetologia* 37:833–837, 1994.

22. Kolb H, Wörz-Pagenstert U, Kleemann R, Rothe H, Rowsell P, Scott FW: Cytokine gene expression in the BB rat pancreas: natural course and impact of bacterial vaccines. *Diabetologia* 39:1448–1454, 1996.

23. Zipris D, Greiner DL, Malkani S, Whalen B, Mordes JP, Rossini AA: Cytokine gene expression in islets and thyroids of BB rats. IFN-gamma and IL-12p40 mRNA increase with age in both diabetic and insulin-treated nondiabetic BB rats. *J Immunol* 156:1315–1321, 1996.

24.	Rabinovitch A, Suarez-Pinzon W, El-Sheikh A, Sorensen O, Power RF: Cytokine gene expression in pancreatic islet-infiltrating leukocytes of BB rats: expression of Th1 cytokines correlates with beta-cell destructive insulitis and IDDM. *Diabetes* 45:749–754, 1996.

25.	Faust A, Rothe H, Schade U, Lampeter EF, Kolb H: Primary nonfunction of islet grafts in autoimmune diabetic NOD mice is prevented by treatment with IL-4 and IL-10. *Transplantation* 62:648–652, 1996.

26.	Hancock WW, Polanski M, Zhang J, Blogg N, Weiner HL: Suppression of insulitis in non-obese diabetic (NOD) mice by oral insulin administration is associated with selective expression of interleukin-4 and -10, transforming growth factor, a prostaglandin-E. *Am J Pathol* 147:1193–1199, 1995.

27.	Rabinovitch A, Suarez-Pinzon WL, Sorensen O, Bleackley RC, Power RF: IFN-gamma gene expression in pancreatic islet-infiltrating mononuclear cells correlates with autoimmune diabetes in nonobese diabetic mice. *J Immunol* 154:4874–4882, 1995.

28.	Fox CJ, Danska JS: IL-4 expression at the onset of islet inflammation predicts nondestructive insulitis in nonobese diabetic mice. *J Immunol* 158:2414–2424, 1997.

29.	Yasunami R, Bach JF: Anti-suppressor effect of cyclophosphamide on the development of spontaneous diabetes in NOD mice. *Eur J Immunol* 18:481–484, 1998.

30.	Rothe H, Burkart V, Faust A, Kolb H: Interleukin-12 gene expression is associated with rapid development of diabetes mellitus in non-obese diabetic mice. *Diabetologia* 39:119–122, 1996.

31.	Rothe H, Jenkins NA, Copeland NG, Kolb H: Active stage of autoimmune diabetes is associated with the expression of a novel cytokine, IGIF, which is located near *Idd2. J Clin Invest* 99:469–474, 1997.

32.	Manetti R, Parronchi P, Giudizi MG *et al*: Natural killer cell stimulatory factor (interleukin-12) induces T helper type 1 (Th1)-specific immune responses and inhibits the development of IL-4-producing Th cells. *J Exp Med* 177:1199, 1993.

33.	Okamura H, Tsutsui H, Komatsu T *et al*: Cloning of a new cytokine that induces IFN-gamma production by T cells. *Nature* 78:88, 1994.

34.	Andre-Schmutz I, Hindelang C, Benoist C, Mathis D: Cellular and molecular changes accompanying the progression from insulitis to diabetes. *Eur J Immunol* 29:245–255, 1999.

35.	Pakala SV, Chivetta M, Kelly CB, Katz JD: In autoimmune diabetes the transition from benign to pernicious requires an islet cell response to tumor necrosis factor α. *J Exp Med* 189:1053–1062, 1999.

36.	Atkinson MA, Leiter EH: The NOD mouse model of type 1 diabetes: as good as it gets? *Nature Med* 5:601–604, 1999.

3

New Genetic Markers

GEORGE S. EISENBARTH

Childhood Diabetes, Barbara Davis Center, UCHCS, Denver, CO, USA

Type 1A (immune-mediated) diabetes mellitus of both man and animal models has become one of the most intensively studied autoimmune disorders. Despite this intensity of study a number of fundamental questions remain unanswered and a molecular understanding of the disease process for any given patient or animal model is incomplete. Despite our incomplete understanding we now have much improved tools for the prediction of the disease, and in animal models diabetes can be prevented with a number of interventions. Trials are under way or planned for the prevention of type 1A diabetes in man. In part these trials depend upon improved understanding of the natural history of type 1 diabetes, which is based to a large extent upon genetic studies coupled with prospective evaluation of individuals at risk for type 1 diabetes. In this review we will emphasize recent studies of both children developing type 1 diabetes and the NOD mouse model of the disease. For both we believe autoimmunity directed at insulin is a key component of the autoimmune process and that genes both within the major histo-compatibility complex and non-class II genes determine diabetes susceptibility as well as susceptibility to a series of associated autoimmune disorders. This review will discuss: (a) the 'natural history' of the disease, including disease prediction for both the NOD mouse and man; (b) type 1 diabetes and genetically associated autoimmune disorders; (c) lessons provided by the study of twins; (d) three non-MHC genetic regions contributing to diabetes susceptibility (the insulin gene, the AIRE mutation on chromosome 21, and the IDDM17 locus on chromosome 10q25.1); and (e) immunologic 'vaccination' for prevention of diabetes in genetically susceptible hosts.

THE 'NATURAL HISTORY' OF THE DISEASE INCLUDING DISEASE PREDICTION FOR BOTH THE NOD MOUSE AND MAN

There are three major hypotheses concerning the islet β cell destruction that precedes the development of type 1A diabetes (1). All three hypotheses recognize that autoimmunity precedes the development of diabetes usually by years in man and by weeks to months in animals models. We favor the hypothesis that following the activation of destructive autoimmunity β cell destruction follows a chronic (almost linear) course, such that disease onset given specific markers of progressive autoimmunity is highly predictable (2). The second hypothesis, favored by Lafferty and coworkers, is that though there is a long prodromal phase, β cell destruction acutely occurs at the onset of diabetes (3). Finally, Palmer and coworkers have championed a more relapsing and remitting course of disease (4). For any given individual a different course may occur, but studies of β cell mass of the NOD mouse (5), and loss of first phase insulin secretion (intravenous glucose tolerance testing) prior to diabetes onset (6) and loss of C-peptide secretion after diabetes onset we believe are strong but not definitive observations consistent with chronic β cell destruction. Loss of insulin secretion and loss of C-peptide secretion usually proceeds over years. The former occurs prior to diabetes and the latter after overt hyperglycemia.

In man the best marker of the process leading to diabetes is the presence of autoantibodies reacting with multiple islet autoantigens and multiple epitopes of these autoantigens (combinatorial autoantibody prediction) (7,8). At present excellent autoantibody assays are now available for three major islet autoantigens, insulin, glutamic acid decarboxylase and ICA512 (IA-2). Autoantibodies to a related molecule IA-2β (also termed phogrin) are usually a subset of ICA512 autoantibodies. The majority of individuals expressing only a single autoantibody do not progress to diabetes. Those expressing two or more autoantibodies have a risk of diabetes exceeding 60% over the next decade. The time to onset of type 1A diabetes amongst individuals with autoantibodies correlates with expression of insulin autoantibodies and loss of first phase insulin secretion (9). Despite NOD mice being inbred and raised in the same environment, phenotypic variation in the age of first expression of insulin autoantibodies correlates with progression to diabetes (10) (Figure 3.1). With fluid phase radioassays we have rarely detected autoantibodies to islet autoantigens other than insulin.

TYPE 1 DIABETES AND GENETICALLY ASSOCIATED AUTOIMMUNE DISORDERS

Type 1A diabetes is strongly associated with a series of autoimmune disorders, including the two polyendocrine autoimmune syndromes, type 1 and type 2. It

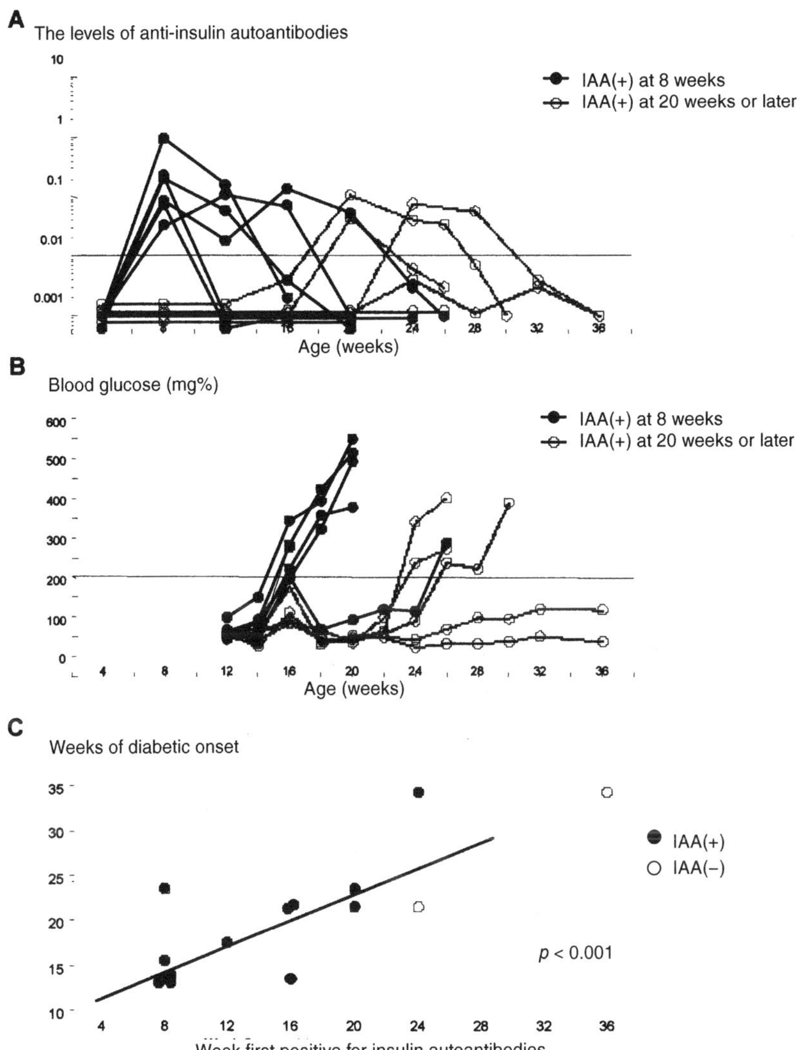

Figure 3.1. Early development of insulin autoantibodies of NOD mice correlates with earlier development of diabetes. From (10), with permission of the National Academy of Sciences, USA

is likely that genes both within and outside of the MHC account for this association. Celiac disease and Addison's disease are both associated with HLA DR3 and DR4 haplotypes, which are also associated with diabetes. The association of these disorders with each other is greater than can be explained by HLA haplotypes. In particular, one in three patients with type 1 diabetes who are DR3/DQ2 homozygous express transglutaminase autoantibodies (11). One half of these individuals have high levels of transglutaminase autoantibodies and celiac disease on biopsy. This very strong association of diabetes with celiac disease suggests that a subset of type 1A diabetes may result from similar immunologic abnormalities, potentially abnormalities of maintaining tolerance upon introduction of dietary peptides. Addison's disease is a much rarer disorder. Our studies of Addison's disease indicates that the disorder is associated with both DR3/DQ2 and DR4/DQ8 haplotypes (12). In addition, and somewhat different from type 1A diabetes, the majority of patients with DR4 and Addison's disease have DRB1*0404 and not DRB1*0401 or DRB1*0402. In addition Sanjeevi and coworkers have found that the MIC-A gene is associated with Addison's disease; the MIC-A 5.1 allele, which lacks the transmembrane domain of the molecule appears to be a major disease determinant (13). We estimate that approximately one in 25 patients with type 1 diabetes with the DQ8/DQ2 haplotype express 21-hydroxylase autoantibodies and one in three of these individuals have, or will develop on follow-up, Addison's disease. This compares to a population risk of approximately 1 in 20 000.

LESSONS PROVIDED BY THE STUDY OF TWINS (TYPE 1A DIABETES HETEROGENEITY)

A major question relating to the genetics of type 1 diabetes is the mode of inheritance. In particular, a leading hypothesis is that, similar to the NOD mouse model, diabetes is of polygenic etiology. Polygenic inheritance indicates that multiple genes, each with a small effect, sum to exceed a 'threshold' which is associated with disease. We hypothesize that type 1A diabetes is not polygenic but rather heterogeneous and oligogenic, with different families potentially having different genetic syndromes leading to diabetes. Of importance is that in most families only two or several major genes, including genes of the major histocompatibility complex, may provide susceptibility. This hypothesis for genetic heterogeneity comes from:

1. Studies of sibling pairs with diabetes which have failed to identify 'major' genes outside of HLA class II genes contributing to diabetes risk (14).
2. Difficulty of replicating loci associated with type 1 diabetes in studies of sibling pairs (15).
3. Existence of several animal models of type 1 diabetes with oligogenic inheritance (e.g. BB rat and Long–Evans rat) (16,17).
4. Existence of 'monogenic' and oligogenic disease inheritance in man (see below).
5. Heterogeneity evidenced by groups of twins (see below).

Studies of monozygotic twins provided the first evidence that, given the presence of islet autoantibodies, loss of first phase insulin secretion on intravenous glucose tolerance testing was progressive and aided in the prediction of the time of onset of diabetes (18). Identical twins can develop type 1A diabetes up to 40 years after their index twin, with approximately one in two initially discordant twins developing diabetes with long-term follow-up (19). Expression of anti-islet autoantibodies is similar to development of diabetes, with dizygotic twins expressing autoantibodies at a frequency similar to siblings, in contrast to monozygotic twins, who have a much greater risk for both diabetes and expression of autoantibodies.

The wide variation amongst patients developing type 1A diabetes is also seen amongst index cases of patients with type 1 diabetes. If an index twin develops diabetes at an older age, as a group concordance rate is much less compared to twins, where the index developed diabetes as a young child. This suggests that groups of identical twins are heterogeneous in terms of their age of developing diabetes, which is related to the eventual concordance, consistent with genetic heterogeneity.

THREE NON-MHC GENETIC REGIONS CONTRIBUTING TO DIABETES SUSCEPTIBILITY (A. INSULIN GENE; B. THE AIRE MUTATION ON CHROMOSOME 21; AND C. THE IDDM17 LOCUS ON CHROMOSOME 10Q25.1)

Three non-MHC loci contributing to type 1A diabetes we have been particularly concerned with are the insulin gene (20), the AIRE gene (autoimmune regulator gene associated with the autoimmune polyendocrine syndrome type 1) (21,22) and a locus termed IDDM17 on chromosome 10q25.1 (23).

A variable nucleotide tandem repeat was associated with type 1 diabetes more than decade ago (20). The longest set of repeats decreases the risk of type 1A diabetes (24). Insulin message, as well as insulin by immunohistochemistry, is expressed both in the thymus and in the spleen. Of note is that the longer repeat is also associated with greater insulin messenger RNA expressed in the thymus (25,26). With the studies of Hanahan and coworkers demonstrating that greater message expression in the thymus of genes driven off the insulin promoter can protect from insulitis (peripheral antigen expressing cells) (27), an attractive hypothesis is that insulin expression in lymphoid organs provides protection.

The autoimmune polyendocrine syndrome type 1 (APS-I) is a remarkable disorder with Addison's disease, hypoparathyroidism and mucocutaneous candidiasis. Approximately 18% of patients with this syndrome develop type 1 diabetes. In this syndrome, HLA alleles do influence risk of Addison's disease

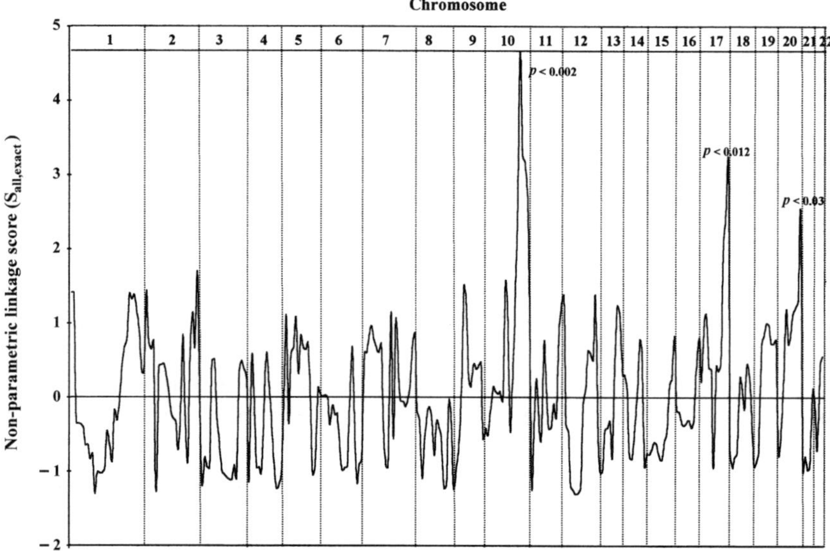

Figure 3.2 Multiple linkage analysis in a Bedouin Arab family. A locus on chromosome 10 associated with diabetes risk. Republished from (23), with permission of *Journal of Clinical Investigation*

(28), or type 1 diabetes (of five rare patients we have observed with DQB1*0602 and type 1 diabetes, one patient has APS-I). The APS-I results from an autosomal recessive mutation of a gene on chromosome 21, termed the 'autoimmune regulator' (AIRE) (21,22). The gene appears to function as a transcription factor and is expressed within infrequent cells (probably macrophage or dendritic) within the thymus (29). How an abnormality of a single gene in relatively few cells of the thymus contributes to so many autoimmune disorders is currently unknown.

With the hypothesis that type 1A diabetes is a genetically heterogeneous disorder, we have begun to study large families where it might be possible to perform linkage analysis within a single family. Pnina Vardi in Israel identified a single family that now has 21 members with type 1A diabetes. In addition, a subset of family members have celiac disease and Graves' disease. Diabetes is associated with DR3 and DR4 haplotypes, similar to studies in other populations. In addition, a locus on chromosome 10 is strongly associated with disease (23) (Figure 3.2).

A detailed map of the region of interest (termed IDDM17) has been compiled and the sequence of a 120 000 bp bacterial artificial chromosome (BAC) obtained. Within this BAC we have identified more than 50 single nucleotide polymorphisms (snps). Three contiguous snps are identical in all diabetic haplotypes and the risk of type 1A diabetes amongst family members homozygous for *iddm17* and with DR3 is 40% vs. 0% for those lacking DR3 or not homozygous at *iddm17*. There are no known genes within the region of interest and a series of expressed sequence tags are being evaluated as a potential 'diabetogene'.

IMMUNOLOGIC 'VACCINATION' FOR PREVENTION OF DIABETES IN GENETICALLY SUSCEPTIBLE HOSTS

The DAISY (Diabetes Autoimmunity Study of the Young) study, headed by Marian Rewers (30), is evaluating infants followed from birth for the expression of anti-islet autoimmunity. Consistent with a number of studies, DR3/DQ2;DR4/DQ8 children with a first-degree relative with type 1 diabetes are at extremely high risk of developing anti-islet autoimmunity (31,32). Approximately 40% of such DR3/DR4 siblings develop anti-islet auto-antibodies prior to age 3. No other group has such a high risk of developing autoimmunity. For most children (but not all), insulin autoantibodies are the first antibody detected. We have recently modified the protein A antibody radioassay of Williams and coworkers (33) to a 96-well filtration plate format (10). With this format it is possible rapidly to analyze the expression of insulin autoantibodies. Both young children and NOD mice developing diabetes express high levels of insulin autoantibodies. Of five children persistently expressing insulin autoantibodies prior to 1 year of age, four are already diabetic, while in contrast only one other child followed from birth has developed diabetes (of approximately 900). For NOD mice, the mice which expressed insulin autoantibodies early developed diabetes earlier. The prominence of insulin autoantibodies in NOD mice is consistent with the studies of Wegmann and coworkers of T cells which recognize insulin (34,35). Approximately half of the lymphocytes infiltrating islets reacted with insulin (34), and the great majority of these CD4 insulin-reactive T cells react with the B:9–23 peptide of insulin (36). The majority of T cells reacting with the B:9–23 peptide have a restricted T cell repertoire with dominant use of the α chain AV13.3 (37). Despite the α-chain restriction, the V-J junction is variable and the β-chain is variable. Two epitopes are present within the B:9-23 sequence (38) (Figure 3.3).

The T cells which recognize this α-chain are able to transfer diabetes and 'immunization' with the B:9-23 peptide or altered peptide ligands of B:9-23 prevent the development of diabetes in NOD mice (39). In addition to CD4 T cells, Wong and coworkers have reported that their CD8 diabetogenic clone reacts with the insulin peptide B:15-23 (40,41).

A number of molecules when administered to NOD mice are able to prevent the development of diabetes, including adjuvants (42), heat shock proteins (43,44) and islet autoantigens, insulin and glutamic acid decarboxylase. Insulin

 Diabetes in the New Millennium

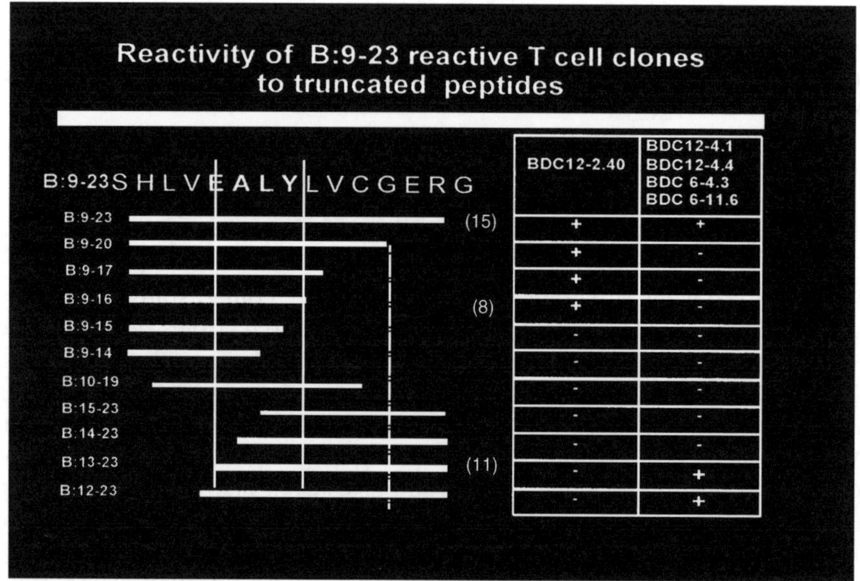

Figure 3.3. T cell clones from NOD mice recognize two different epitopes within the B:9-23 insulin sequence. Republished from (38), with permission of Academic Press

and peptides of insulin have been administered orally, subcutaneously and intra-nasally with diabetes prevention. For example, the whole B-chain, but not the A-chain of insulin when administered subcutaneously in incomplete Freund's adjuvant, prevents the bulk of diabetes (45). In a similar manner, the B:9-23 peptide is effective for diabetes prevention (39). It is thought that such immunization prevents diabetes by expanding clones of T cells able to target islets because of their reactivity with insulin. These clones produce cytokines that prevent rather than accelerate the development of diabetes (46,47).

Given the development of a series of antigenic 'vaccines' for the prevention of diabetes in NOD mice, related studies are beginning in man. The first such studies utilize insulin itself, with either oral or parenteral administration. A small pilot trial from the Joslin and Barbara Davis Diabetes Centers evaluating parenteral insulin administration provided pilot data that such therapy might delay the development of diabetes of autoantibody-positive first-degree relatives (48). The large DPT-1 (Diabetes Prevention Trial-1) is under way, with more than 70 000 first degree relatives of patients with type 1 diabetes screened for autoantibody expression. Relatives found to autoantibody positive are staged with glucose tolerance testing (intravenous and oral), HLA typing (to rule out the presence of DQB1*0602) and determination of insulin autoantibodies. Based upon high or moderate risk of diabetes, these relatives are then randomized to either parenteral or oral insulin therapy, respectively.

From studies in animals it is likely that the preventive effects of insulin do not depend upon utilization of biologically active insulin with its risk of hypoglycemia. Thus a number of peptides of autoantigens are entering phase I clinical trials for disease prevention. These include altered peptide ligands of insulin B:9-23 (Neurocrine), Heat shock protein 60 peptide (Peptor) (44), and glutamic acid decarboxylase (Diamyd) (49,50). Initial trials target individuals with new onset type 1 diabetes or high-risk relatives already expressing anti-islet autoantibodies. With observations that anti-islet autoantibodies develop early in life and children rapidly develop a series of anti-islet autoantibodies, it is likely that disease prevention will be more efficacious if therapy is begun prior to the development of these autoantibodies (10). Initial trials would need to study individuals with very high genetic risk. As reviewed above, the only group currently identifiable with such a genetic risk are first-degree relatives expressing DQ8/DQ2. Hopefully as non-MHC genes contributing to diabetes risk are identified and effective therapies developed, individuals from the general population (non-relatives) will be identifiable who might benefit from preventive therapy. This is obviously a long-term goal, with information needed in terms of the safety, efficacy and ability to monitor immunologic therapies.

ACKNOWLEDGEMENTS

Supported by Grants DK32083, DK32493 and DK55969 from the National Institutes of Health, and grants from the American Diabetes Association, the Juvenile Diabetes Foundation and the Children's Diabetes Foundation, and Grant M01 RR00069 from the General Clinical Research Program, National Centers for Research Resources.

REFERENCES

1. Robles DT, Eisenbarth GS: Immunology of diabetes and related autoimmune diseases clinical immunology. Rich R, Fleisher T, Kotzin B, Shearer W, Shroeder H 2000. (GENERIC) Ref Type: unpublished work.
2. Eisenbarth GS: Type 1 diabetes mellitus. A chronic autoimmune disease. *N Engl J Med* 314:1360–1368, 1986.
3. Dilts SM, Lafferty KJ: Autoimmune diabetes: the involvement of benign and malignant autoimmunity. *J Autoimmun* 12:229–232, 1999.
4. Greenbaum CJ, Sears KL, Kahn SE, Palmer JP: Relationship of B-cell function and autoantibodies to progression and nonprogression of subclinical type 1 diabetes. *Diabetes* 48:170–175, 1999.

5. Sreenan S, Pick AJ, Levisetti M, Baldwin AC, Pugh W, Polonsky KS: Increased β-cell proliferation and reduced mass before diabetes onset in the nonobese diabetic mouse. *Diabetes* 48:989–996, 1999.

6. Bleich D, Jackson RA, Soeldner JS, Eisenbarth GS: Analysis of metabolic progression to type I diabetes in ICA[+] relatives of patients with type I diabetes. *Diabetes Care* 13:111–118, 1990.

7. Verge CF, Gianani R, Kawasaki E *et al*: Prediction of type I diabetes in first-degree relatives using a combination of insulin, GAD, and ICA512bdc/IA-2 autoantibodies. *Diabetes* 45:926–933, 1996.

8. Bingley PJ, Christie MR, Bonifacio E *et al*: Combined analysis of autoantibodies improves prediction of IDDM in islet cell antibody-positive relatives. *Diabetes* 43:1304–1310, 1994.

9. Eisenbarth GS, Gianani R, Yu L *et al*: Dual parameter model for prediction of type 1 diabetes mellitus. *Proc Assoc Am Physicians* 110:126–135, 1998.

10. Yu L, Robles DT, Abiru N *et al*: Early expression of anti-insulin autoantibodies of man and the NOD mouse: evidence for early determination of subsequent diabetes. *Proc Natl Acad Sci USA* 97:1701–1706, 2000.

11. Bao F, Yu L, Babu S *et al*: One third of HLA DQ2 homozygous patients with type 1 diabetes express celiac disease associated transglutaminase autoantibodies. *J Autoimmun* 13:143–148, 1999.

12. Yu L, Brewer KW, Gates S *et al*: DRB1*04 and DQ alleles: expression of 21-hydroxylase autoantibodies and risk of progression to Addison's disease. *J Clin Endocrinol Metab* 84:328–335, 1999.

13. Gambelunghe G, Falorni A, Ghaderi M *et al*: Microsatellite polymorphism of the MHC class I chain-related (MIC-A and MIC-B) genes marks the risk for autoimmune Addison's disease. *J Clin Endocrinol Metab* 84:3701–3707, 1999.

14. Mein CA, Esposito L, Dunn MG *et al*: A search for type 1 diabetes susceptibility genes in families from the United Kingdom. *Nature Genet* 19:297–300,1998.

15. Concannon P, Gogolin-Ewens KJ, Hinds DA *et al*: A second-generation screen of the human genome for susceptibility to insulin-dependent diabetes mellitus. *Nature Genet* 19:292–296, 1998.

16. Martin AM, Maxson MN, Leif J, Mordes JP, Greiner DL, Blankenhorn EP: Diabetes-prone and diabetes-resistant BB rats share a common major diabetes susceptibility locus, iddm4: additional evidence for a universal autoimmunity locus on rat chromosome 4. *Diabetes* 48:2138–2144, 1999.

17. Yokoi N, Kanazawa M, Kitada K *et al*: A non-MHC locus essential for autoimmune type I diabetes in the Komeda diabetes-prone rat. *J Clin Invest* 100:2015–2021, 1997.

18. Srikanta S, Ganda OP, Eisenbarth GS, Soeldner JS: Islet cell antibodies and beta cell function in monozygotic triplets and twins initially discordant for type I diabetes mellitus. *N Engl J Med* 308:322–325, 1983.

19. Redondo MJ, Rewers M, Yu L *et al*: Genetic determination of islet cell autoimmunity in monozygotic twin, dizygotic twin, and non-twin siblings of patients with type 1 diabetes: prospective twin study. *Br Med J* 318:698–702, 1999.

20. Bell GI, Horita S, Karam JH: A polymorphic locus near the human insulin gene is associated with insulin-dependent diabetes mellitus. *Diabetes* 33:176–183, 1984.

21. Aaltonen J, Björses P, Perheentupa J *et al*: An autoimmune disease, APECED, caused by mutations in a novel gene featuring two PHD-type zinc-finger domains. *Nature Genet* 17:399–403, 1997.

22. Bjorses P, Aaltonen J, Horelli-Kuitunen N, Yaspo ML, Peltonen L: Gene defect behind APECED: a new clue to autoimmunity. *Hum Mol Genet* 7:1547–1553, 1998.
23. Verge CF, Vardi P, Babu S *et al*: Evidence for oligogenic inheritance of type 1A diabetes in a large Bedouin Arab family. *J Clin Invest* 102:1569–1575, 1998.
24. Bennett ST, Wilson AJ, Cucca F *et al*: *IDDM2-VNTR*-encoded susceptibility to type 1 diabetes: dominant protection and parental transmission of alleles of the insulin gene-linked minisatellite locus. *J Autoimmun* 9:415–421, 1996.
25. Pugliese A, Zeller M, Fernandez A *et al*: The insulin gene is transcribed in the human thymus and transcription levels correlate with allelic variation at the INS VNTR-IDDM2 susceptibility locus for type I diabetes. *Nature Genet* 15:293–297, 1997.
26. Vafiadis P, Bennett ST, Todd JA *et al*: Insulin expression in human thymus is modulated by INS VNTR alleles at the IDDM2 locus. *Nature Genet* 15:289–292, 1997.
27. Hanahan D: Peripheral-antigen-expressing cells in thymic medulla: factors in self-tolerance and autoimmunity. *Curr Opin Immunol* 10:656–662, 1998.
28. Neufeld M, Maclaren NK, Blizzard RM: Two types of autoimmune Addison's disease associated with different polyglandular autoimmune (PGA) syndromes. *Medicine (Baltimore)* 60:355–362, 1981.
29. Heino M, Peterson P, Kudoh J *et al*: Autoimmune regulator is expressed in the cells regulating immune tolerance in thymus medulla. *Biochem Biophys Res Commun* 257:821–825, 1999.
30. Rewers M, Bugawan TL, Norris JM *et al*: Newborn screening for HLA markers associated with IDDM: diabetes autoimmunity study in the young (DAISY). *Diabetologia* 39:807–812, 1996.
31. Eisenbarth GS, Elsey C, Yu L, Rewers M: Infantile anti-islet autoimmunity: DAISY study. *Diabetes* 47:A210 (Abstr), 1998.
32. Schenker M, Hummel M, Ferber K *et al*: Early expression and high prevalence of islet autoantibodies for DR3/4 heterozygous and DR4/4 homozygous offspring of parents with type I diabetes: the German BABYDIAB study. *Diabetologia* 42:671–677, 1999.
33. Williams AJK, Bingley PJ, Bonifacio E, Palmer JP, Gale EAM: A novel micro-assay for insulin autoantibodies. *J Autoimmun* 10:473–478, 1997.
34. Wegmann DR, Norbury-Glaser M, Daniel D: Insulin-specific T cells are a predominant component of islet infiltrates in pre-diabetic NOD mice. *Eur J Immunol* 24:1853–1857, 1994.
35. Wegmann DR, Gill RG, Norbury-Glaser M, Schloot N, Daniel D: Analysis of the spontaneous T cell response to insulin in NOD mice. *J Autoimmun* 7:833–843, 1994.
36. Daniel D, Gill RG, Schloot N, Wegmann D: Epitope specificity, cytokine production profile and diabetogenic activity of insulin-specific T cell clones isolated from NOD mice. *Eur J Immunol* 25:1056–1062, 1995.
37. Simone E, Daniel D, Schloot N *et al*: T cell receptor restriction of diabetogenic autoimmune NOD T cells. *Proc Natl Acad Sci USA* 94:2518–2521, 1997.
38. Abiru N, Wegmann D, Kawasaki E, Gottlieb P, Simone E, Eisenbarth GS: Dual overlapping peptides recognized by insulin peptide B:9–23 reactive T cell receptor AV13S3 T cell clones of the NOD mouse. *J Autoimmun* 2000. (in press).
39. Daniel D, Wegmann DR: Protection of nonobese diabetic mice from diabetes by intranasal or subcutaneous administration of insulin peptide B-(9-23). *Proc Natl Acad Sci USA* 93:956–960, 1996.

40. Wong FS, Janeway CAJ: The role of CD4 vs. CD8 T cells in IDDM. *J Autoimmun* 13:290–295, 1999.

41. Wong FS, Visintin I, Wen L, Flavell RA, Janeway CA: CD8 T cell clones from young nonobese diabetic (NOD) islets can transfer rapid onset of diabetes in NOD mice in the absence of CD4 cells. *J Exp Med* 183:67–76, 1996.

42. Qin HY, Singh B: BCG vaccination prevents insulin-dependent diabetes mellitus (IDDM) in NOD mice after disease acceleration with cyclophosphamide. *J Autoimmun* 10:271–278, 1997.

43. Elias D, Cohen IR: Treatment of autoimmune diabetes and insulitis in NOD mice with heat shock protein 60 peptide p277. *Diabetes* 44:1132–1138, 1995.

44. Elias D, Meilin A, Ablamunits V *et al*: Hsp60 peptide therapy of NOD mouse diabetes induces a Th2 cytokine burst and downregulates autoimmunity to various β-cell antigens. *Diabetes* 46:758–764, 1997.

45. Muir A, Peck A, Clare-Salzler M *et al*: Insulin immunization of nonobese diabetic mice induces a protective insulitis characterized by diminished intra-islet interferon-gamma transcription. *J Clin Invest* 95:628–634, 1995.

46. Zekzer D, Wong FS, Wen L *et al*: Inhibition of diabetes by an insulin-reactive CD4 T-cell clone in the nonobese diabetic mouse. *Diabetes* 46:1124–1132, 1997.

47. Tian J, Chau C, Kaufman DL: Insulin selectively primes Th2 responses and induces regulatory tolerance to insulin in pre-diabetic mice. *Diabetologia* 41:237–240, 1998.

48. Keller RJ, Eisenbarth GS, Jackson RA: Insulin prophylaxis in individuals at high risk of type I diabetes. *Lancet* 341:927–928, 1993.

49. Tisch R, Wang B, Serreze DV: Induction of glutamic acid decarboxylase 65-specific Th2 cells and suppression of autoimmune diabetes at late stages of disease is epitope dependent. *J Immunol* 163:1178–1187, 1999.

50. Tian J, Lehmann PV, Kaufman DL: Determinant spreading of T helper cell 2 (Th2) responses to pancreatic islet autoantigens. *J Exp Med* 186:2039–2043, 1997.

4

Restoring Self-tolerance in Diabetics

JEAN-FRANÇOIS BACH

INSERM U 25, Hôpital Necker, Paris, France

Insulin-dependent diabetes mellitus (IDDM) is an autoimmune disease secondary to the loss of tolerance to β cell autoantigens, which results in an aggressive T cell-mediated islet specific autoimmune response (1). The limitations of insulin therapy, with the common onset of degenerative complications due to imperfect metabolic control, have prompted the idea of treating diabetics, or better prediabetics, with methods aiming at the control of such autoimmune response.

It has thus been shown that cyclosporin A, a T cell selective agent, is able to induce long-term remission of recently diagnosed IDDM (2). This approach was, however, confronted with several hurdles: (a) the drug effect stops when the treatment is terminated; (b) the drug shows direct toxicity, namely nephrotoxicity; and (c) the drug may be at the origin of manifestations of overimmunosuppression (tumours, infections). Hopefully, treatments administered to diabetics were not given at a sufficient dosage for a sufficient period of time to induce such hazards, but the risk clearly exists if the treatment was pursued in conditions required for a long-term effect. The best approach to circumvent these difficulties is to restore tolerance to β cell autoantigens. The goal of this paper is to review the various approaches that can be taken in this direction.

Diabetes in the New Millennium. Edited by U. Di Mario, F. Leonetti, G. Pugliese, P. Sbraccia and A. Signore.
© 2000 John Wiley & Sons, Ltd.

TOLERANCE TO β CELL AUTOANTIGENS

Non-diabetic healthy individuals are operationally tolerant to their β cells. This does not imply that they do not harbour β cell-reactive T cells, but if such T cells are present they do not induce any clinically meaningful β cell lesions.

The mechanisms of self-tolerance have been a matter of intensive debate over recent decades. Three main orders of mechanisms have been demonstrated in experimental models and are likely to operate in humans.

Deletion of autoreactive T cells does take place in the thymus (defect in negative selection). Negative selection plays a major role in the constitution of the T cell repertoire. However, that this selection essentially applies to T cells expressing T cell receptors with high affinity for the corresponding peptides, which explains how low-affinity T cells escape the thymus. Low-affinity organ-specific autoreactive T cells that seed to the periphery are perfectly able to mount an aggressive autoimmune response if adequately stimulated. In other words, deletion is probably not an exclusive mechanism explaining the protection from autoimmunity of normal subjects. More precisely, thymic deletion could represent a mechanism limiting the number of autoimmune diseases (that could be more common or more severe in its absence), but there is much experimental evidence to indicate that the autoreactive T cells that are responsible for autoimmune diseases are present (although in reduced number) in normal subjects. This point is illustrated by the ease with which one may derive T cell lines reactive to myelin basic protein (3) or glutamic acid decarboxylase from normal subjects (4).

Anergy is another important, although less well-defined, mechanism. Anergy may be considered as a state of T cell paralysis, rendering it unable to proliferate in the presence of the specific peptide. Anergy is classically reversed by IL-2 addition but this feature does not appear as central as it used to be. In fact, the definition of anergy has recently been widened, creating some confusion with the regulatory T cells that will be discussed in the next paragraph. Anergy is considered here as an intrinsic antigen-specific paralysis and is probably an important mechanism in the maintenance of self-tolerance. Its intimate mechanisms remain obscure and its relevance to physiological conditions uncertain. Most convincing data were obtained in transgenic mice, where either or both the autoantigen and/or the autoreactive TCR are overexpressed to an unphysiological extent, which prompts cautious interpretation (5).

Immunoregulation, also named dominant or active tolerance, is another very attractive mechanism. The concept of T cell-mediated suppression (the former term for regulatory T cells) was quasi-abandoned in the 1980s, when most of the data and concepts dealing with these T cell subsets were duly questioned. However, evidence has accumulated over the last decade to suggest that physiological autoimmunity is placed under the tight control of $CD4^+$ regulatory T cells. Such T cells are not yet fully characterized, but it appears that their selective depletion (not affecting effector autoreactive T cells) leads readily to a state of pathologic autoimmunity, as demonstrated after thymectomy performed at an early* age of reconstitution of immuno-incompetent rodents with T cells depleted in regulatory T cells defined by one of their markers, CD45RA, CD25 or CD62L (6,7). Direct evidence for such regulatory T cells can be obtained by showing the capacity of regulatory T cell-enriched populations to protect from autoimmune disease.

The nature of these regulatory T cells is still ill-defined and possibly not unique. Several phenotypes have been described, including both cytokine producing cells (Th2 cell producing IL-4, IL-10 and IL-13, Th3 cells producing TGF b) and Tr1 cells (producing IL-10) but also non-cytokine-producing cells.

Loss of self-tolerance in diabetes could be due to a defect in one of the mechanisms described above: defect in negative selection, breakdown of anergy or loss of regulatory T cell control.

Alternatively, one can hypothesize that the main event is the overriding of the control mechanism by a major autoantigen-driven effector immune response secondary to operationally increased immunogenicity of the antigenic peptides (8).

THE AUTOANTIGEN APPROACH

Rationale

It has been shown possible in animal models to protect from diabetes by inducing tolerance to β cell autoantigens (9–11). The tolerance appears to be of the active type, rather than being secondary to deletion or anergy. In fact, using either insulin, GAD or hsp60, a clear Th2 polarization was demonstrated (12,13), suggesting that the tolerant state was the result of immune deviation. Thus, in the case of GAD, IL-4 knock-out mice that are defective in their capacity to mount Th2 responses are resistant to tolerance induction (14).

Advantages

The strategy is very attractive, since one may expect very limited toxicity of the autoantigen preparation. There is no risk of overimmunosuppression, since in most straightforward protocols the autoantigen is used alone, in the absence of concomitant immunosuppressive treatment. It is not expensive, particularly when synthetic peptides are used in place of the whole recombinant molecules.

Pitfalls

These differ in prediabetic and recently diagnosed subjects. In the first case (prediabetes), the main risk is that of acceleration of diabetes onset due to undesirable idiosyncratic sensitization, rather than tolerance. In the second case (recently diagnosed diabetes), the question is that of possibly insufficient efficacy at an advanced stage of the disease, or perhaps the long time needed for tolerance to take place.

Ongoing trials

Several clinical trials have been launched using various autoantigens and clinical settings. *Insulin* has been used using the nasal route in prediabetics at a small scale. Parenteral or oral insulin have been used in a large-scale preventive protocol (DPT1). Results of these trials are not yet available. Oral insulin has also been used in recently diagnosed diabetics with little or no effect.

GAD. Phase I trials are being performed with the whole recombinant molecule in Sweden.

Hsp60. The p277 peptide of hsp 60 is being used in Phase I/II trials in recently diagnosed diabetics with promising data. No acceleration of diabetes progression was seen.

CD3 ANTIBODY

Rationale

Anti-CD3 monoclonal antibodies were first used as conventional immuno-suppressive agents. It was initially shown in human renal transplantation that OKT3 was a potent immunosuppressant both capable of preventing and curing rejection episodes. Two sets of data indicated that anti-CD3 antibodies could do more than providing a non-antigen-specific suppression of immune responses. First, several anti-T cell antibodies, including CD3 antibodies as well as CD4 or CD40L antibodies, were shown to induce long-term tolerance to allografts in mice and non-human primates. Second, we showed in the NOD mouse that administration of low doses of CD3 antibody for only 5 consecutive days induced a long-term (quasi-definitive) remission of established diabetes, inasmuch as the antibody was given soon after the diagnosis of the disease (15). Interestingly, in both settings (transplantation and diabetes) tolerance was associated with induction or boosting of regulatory circuits involving CD4 T cells (16). In other words, the antibodies acted not only by blocking their target but also, perhaps more importantly, by providing positive signalling to regulatory T cells. The nature of the regulatory T cells in question is still the matter of debate and investigation.

Several data suggest that they are antigen-specific and one may assume that their activation results from the combined effect of the antigen present *in situ* and of the antibody.

Ongoing trials

Two clinical trials have been started to evaluate the effect of CD3 antibodies in recently diagnosed diabetics. In both trials, the antibody is administered for a short period of time (less than a month). The antibody has been humanized by genetic engineering to ensure: (a) that it is not mitogenic and thus does not lead to the massive cytokine release observed after the first injection of OKT3 (with severe clinical symptoms) (17); and (b) that is not immunogenic. The end points are endogenous insulin production (C peptide) and, to a lesser degree, insulin requirement (U/kg).

Main advantages

The CD3 approach is very attractive because its effects are immediate through the clearing of insulitis that follows the initiation of the treatment even if the major mode of action (associated with stimulation of regulatory T cells) develops more slowly. The treatment works at its best in already established disease, even at a relatively advanced stage. The treatment is of short duration, which reduces the risk of overimmunosuppression and the cost.

Pitfalls

The antibody administered induces an initial state of immunosuppression (with limited risks, however, because of the absence of long-term immunosuppression and the short duration of treatment). The risk of a cytokine release syndrome is minimal, due to the antibody molecule modification, but cannot be formally excluded.

Other approaches

No approach other than those described above have been shown to induce long-term protection when the autoimmune process is started. The only exceptions deal with some manoeuvres shown to work in mice injected with diabetogenic T cells from fully diabetic mice, or in diabetic mice receiving a syngeneic islet graft. This is notably the case of IL-4 gene therapy using a retroviral vector recombinant for the IL-4 gene and spleen cells from diabetic mice as missiles to guide them towards the islets (Yamamoto AM, Chatenoud L, submitted). Interestingly, we could show using this approach that the cells providing IL-4 intra-islet delivery were the regulatory T cells mentioned above ($CD4^+$ $CD62L^+$).

Other methods affording long-term protection, and hence prevention of the loss of self-tolerance to islet antigens, are listed in Table 4.1. It should be made clear that none of these methods is readily applicable in human diabetes for the time being. We will have to wait until the identification of subjects at risk of diabetes but without any ongoing autoimmune response (even islet autoantibodies) becomes sufficiently reliable. Even then, we will have to limit ourselves to totally innocuous treatments.

Table 4.1. Long-term prevention of diabetes after treatment of young NOD mice

	NOD mouse	Man
Chemical immunosuppression		
Cyclosporin A	+	+ (R)
Azathioprine	+	+ (R)
FK 506	+	
Rapamycin	+	
Deoxyspergualine	+	
Monoclonal antibodies	+	
Anti-CD3	+	+ (O)
Anti-CD4	+	
Anti-CD8	+	
Anti-CD40L	+	
Anti-IFNγ	+	
Anti-MHC class II	+	
Anti-lymphocyte serum	+	
Antigens	+	
Insulin		
Native molecule s.c.	+	+ (O/R)
oral	+	+ (O/R)
intranasal	+	+ R
B chain (i.m. + adjuvant)	+	
Peptide (intranasal)	+	
APL	+	
Glutamic acid decarboxylase		
Native molecule	+	+ (O)
Peptide	+	
Heat shock protein 60 (p277)	+	+ (O)
Miscellaneous		
Nicotinamide	+	+ (O)
Vaccine therapy		
CFA/BCG	+	+ (O)
Q fever vaccine	+	
Streptococcal extract	+	
CTLA4-Ig	+	

O, open; R, randomized.

Table 4.2. Tolerance clinical trials in human diabetics and prediabetics

Insulin		
Subcutaneous insulin	Prediabetics	DPT1
Oral insulin	Prediabetics	DPT1
	Recently diagnosed diabetics	France
		Florida, USA
		Italy
Nasal insulin	Prediabetics	Australia
GAD		
Recombinant molecule intradermal injection	Volunteers (Phase I)	Sweden
Hsp 60 p277		
Parenteral injection + adjuvant	Diabetics	Israel
CD3 antibodies		
Short-term treatment	Diabetics	USA
		Belgium

REFERENCES

1. Bach JF: Insulin-dependent diabetes mellitus as an autoimmune disease. *Endocrine Rev* 15:516–542, 1994

2. Feutren G, Papoz L, Assan R *et al*: Cyclosporin increases the rate and length of remissions in insulin-dependent diabetes of recent onset. Results of a multicentre double-blind trial. *Lancet* 2:119–124, 1986.

3. Shanmugam A, Copie-Bergman C, Caillat S, Bach JF, Tournier-Lasserve E: *In vivo* clonal expansion of T lymphocytes specific for an immunodominant N-terminal myelin basic protein epitope in healthy individuals. *J Neuroimmunol* 59:165–172, 1995.

4. Lohmann T, Leslie RDG, Londei M: T cell clones to epitopes of glutamic acid decarboxylase 65 raised from normal subjects and patients with insulin-dependent diabetes. *J Autoimmun* 9:385–389, 1996.

5. Bercovici N, Delon J, Cambouris C, Escriou N, Debre P, Liblaus RS: Chronic intravenous injections of antigen induce and maintain tolerance in T cell receptor-transgenic mice. *Eur J Immunol* 29:345–354, 1999.

6. Shevach EM: Regulatory T cells in autoimmmunity. *Ann Rev Immunol* 18:423–449, 2000.

7. Bach JF: Immune dysregulation in organ-specific autoimmune diseases: the case of type I diabetes. *Immunologist* 6:158–160, 1998.

8. Bach JF, Koutouzov S, Vanendert PM: Are there unique autoantigens triggering autoimmune diseases? *Immunol Rev* 164:139–155, 1998.

9. Kaufman DL, Clare-Salzler M, Tian J *et al*: Spontaneous loss of T-cell tolerance to glutamic acid decarboxylase in murine insulin-dependent diabetes. *Nature* 366: 69–72, 1993.

10. Tisch R, Yang XD, Singer SM, Liblau RS, Fugger L, McDevitt HO: Immune response to glutamic acid decarboxylase correlates with insulitis in non-obese diabetic mice. *Nature* 366:72–75, 1993.

11. Elias D, Cohen IR: Peptide therapy for diabetes in NOD mice. *Lancet* 343:704–706, 1994.

12. Tian J, Olcott A, Hanssen L, Zekzer D, Kaufman DL: Antigen-based immunotherapy for autoimmune disease: from animal models to humans? *Immunol Today* 20:190–195, 1999.
13. Elias D, Meilina A, Ablamunits V *et al*: Hsp60 peptide therapy of NOD mouse diabetes induces a Th2 cytokine burst and downregulates autoimmunity to various beta-cell antigens. *Diabetes* 46:758–764, 1997.
14. Tisch R, Wang B, Serreze DV: Induction of glutamic acid decarboxylase 65-specific Th2 cells and suppression of autoimmune diabetes at late stages of disease is epitope dependent. *J Immunol* 163:1178–1187, 1999.
15. Chatenoud L, Thervet E, Primo J, Bach JF: Anti-CD3 antibody induces long-term remission of overt autoimmunity in nonobese diabetic mice. *Proc Natl Acad Sci USA* 91:123–127, 1994.
16. Chatenoud L, Primo J, Bach JF: CD3 antibody-induced dominant self tolerance in overtly diabetic NOD mice. *J Immunol* 158:2947–2954, 1997.
17. Chatenoud L, Ferran C, Legendre C *et al*: *In vivo* cell activation following OKT3 administration. Systemic cytokine release and modulation by corticosteroids. *Transplantation* 49:697–702, 1990.

5

Tolerance Induction for Prevention of Type 1 Diabetes

PAOLO POZZILLI and MARIA GISELLA CAVALLO

Unità per la Prevenzione del Diabete e delle Malattie Metaboliche,
Università Campus Biomedico and Dipartimento di Medicina Interna,
Università di Tor Vergata, Rome, Italy

Prevention of type 1 diabetes is a topic of great interest today. Two large multinational trials in genetically and immunologically susceptible subjects to the disease using nicotinamide (ENDIT) and insulin (DPT1) will be concluded in 2003 and 2004.

New trials are planned with the aim of inducing tolerance to specific and non-specific diabetes antigens, such as insulin peptide(s), GAD or GAD peptides and a peptide of heat shock protein 60, following promising results in preventing the disease obtained in the non-obese diabetic mouse model. In this chapter we first review the concept of tolerance induction with particular reference to type 1 diabetes. We then discuss the most promising approaches based on this type of strategy which, in our opinion, are likely to be tested in large preventive trials of human type 1 diabetes because of a solid rationale and the preventive results shown in experimental models.

INDUCTION OF TOLERANCE: STATE OF THE ART

Type 1 diabetes mellitus is characterized by a T cell-mediated autoimmune destruction of pancreatic islet cells, which is believed to develop as a result of a failure of the physiologic mechanisms of self-tolerance to β cell-associated antigens. Although the nature of the initiating antigen in type 1 diabetes is still uncertain, studies in animal models of type 1 diabetes have suggested that at the beginning of the disease process, GAD and insulin are among the earliest β cell antigens targeted by T cells. Only with the progression of the disease does T cell recognition spread to additional β cell molecules, leading to amplification of the β cell destructive process and to development of overt disease (1). Lymphocytes play a major role in the destructive process of β cells in type 1 diabetes. Mature CD4$^+$ T lymphocytes are divided into two major functionally distinct subsets according to their cytokine production pattern in response to antigen stimulation: T helper 1 cells (Th1), which produce predominantly IFNγ, and T helper 2 cells (Th2), secreting IL4 and IL10 (2).

Autoreactive T cells involved in the process leading to type 1 diabetes have been identified as Th1 lymphocytes, which induce rapid progression to diabetes, as opposed to Th2 cells, which seem to mediate protection from the disease (3–4). Thus, an imbalance between these two lymphocyte populations has been proposed to be responsible for at least the stage of progression to type 1 diabetes. The balance between Th1 and Th2 cells during an immune response seems to be regulated by the expression of costimulatory molecules, which also appear to have important implications in the T cell recognition of self-molecules (5).

Recently, great interest has been paid to the possibility of preventing or halting the disease progression through the induction of immune tolerance to β cell-associated self-antigens. Both parenteral and oral administration of autoantigens have been shown to induce regulatory responses which are capable of counteracting pathogenic responses and prevent disease manifestation. Due to the antigen specificity of the immune process underlying type 1 diabetes, this type of strategy, by aiming at inactivating selectively the T cells involved in this process, has the advantage of preserving the function of the immune system in general, as opposed to other immune suppressing strategies. However, since in human type 1 diabetes the initiating autoantigen is unknown, the only feasible approach to achieve a state of immune tolerance is through the generation of immune regulatory cells in subjects who already have an ongoing autoimmune process. With this approach, antigen-induced regulatory responses can downregulate effector T cells in the target organ via a mechanism known as 'bystander suppression' (6), mediated locally by the release of Th2 and Th3 cytokines (7). Thus, after antigen-based immunotherapy, Th2 responses have been shown to spread from the administered autoantigen to different autoantigens expressed in the target tissue (e.g. β cells). The efficacy of antigen administration varies according to a number of variables, including antigen dose, route of administration, frequency of administration and type of antigen. An additional aspect which seems to be crucial for the success of antigen-induced tolerance is the stage of the disease process. It has been shown that the ability to induce regulatory responses declines with the progression of the disease, and this is important to consider for human trials, where the treatment can only be started at relatively late stages of type 1 diabetes progression. Induction of immune tolerance to β cell-associated self-antigens has been attempted in animal models using a variety of antigens or antigen-derived peptides, using different routes and modalities of administration. Trials have been also implemented in humans following the evidence that in animals, this type of strategy could, in many cases, obtain protection from the disease (8).

Tolerance induction through insulin administration

Insulin is considered one of the relevant antigens in inducing the disease process, since T cell clones specific to the β chain are able to adoptively transfer the disease in NOD-*scid* mice (9). In addition, this antigen, when administered orally or parenterally to NOD mice, can protect these animals from developing diabetes (10,11). In this model, protection appears to be mediated by the induction of peripheral tolerance with the stimulation of specific immune regulatory Th2 cells. When NOD mice were gavage-fed 0.5 mg (13–14 units) doses of porcine NPH insulin on alternate days for 2 weeks, and later received 1.0 mg on a bi-weekly basis, the onset of diabetes was delayed by 6–12 weeks in females, while it was not altered in males. Microscopic examination revealed that insulitis was also reduced. It remains unclear whether CD4$^+$ or CD8$^+$ cells are needed for the protective effect on diabetes onset, although in another study CD4$^+$ cells after oral insulin suppressed adoptive transfer of diabetes (12). More recently, an insulin-reactive CD4 T cell clone has been isolated in the NOD mouse, which appears to act locally in the islets by releasing TGF β or other cytokines capable of inhibiting proliferation of toxic lymphocytes. Another study has suggested that treatment with the insulin-containing peptide B9-B23 can protect the NOD mouse more effectively from developing diabetes (13). As far as the mechanism of action is concerned, it has been suggested that insulitis can be prevented through a bystander suppression mechanism that is dependent on the local release of immune regulatory cytokines. Ongoing investigations using insulin or other preventive antigens are therefore addressing cytokine production and cell surface marker expression of islet-infiltrating lymphocytes, β chain epitope mapping and adjuvant effects. In view of the putative bystander actions in response to oral insulin treatment, the effect of immunization with other islet antigens, either alone or in combination, should be tested. It still remains to be established whether reduction of insulitis is necessary for protection from diabetes, as very often, prevention of hyperglycaemia is obtained in animal models also in the presence of insulitis. Also, in humans, the administration of parenteral insulin before the onset of hyperglycemia in high-risk individuals has been shown to slow down or prevent disease onset (14). A large clinical trial, the DPT 1 trial, is currently under way in the USA as an open trial involving individuals at risk for type 1 diabetes.

The DPT-1 trial is designed to evaluate whether antigen-based immune intervention with insulin, which has been shown to be effective in animals, can delay the onset of type 1 diabetes. The DPT-1 was designed to screen approximately 60 000 relatives at a rate of 15 000 yearly for 4 years, yielding 540 per year for staging at an ICA-positive frequency of 3.6%. The sensitivity of the trial was to test the rescue of one-third of those treated with insulin in the parenteral trial, and one-half of those who were given oral insulin. Recombinant human insulin is given parenterally (twice daily subcutaneously as Ultralente at 0.25 IU/kg/day and yearly by infusion as regular insulin for 4 days), or orally as encapsulated regular insulin at 7.5 mg/day. Parenteral insulin is given to high-risk relatives (risk > 50% by 5 years) in a non-placebo-based randomized trial; this arm started in 1994, whereas the oral arm began in September 1996. In this US multicenter trial, 10 centres, 144 affiliates and 210 satellites are involved (15). Recently, a multicenter double-blind trial with oral insulin in patients with recent onset type 1 diabetes has been completed, and showed that administration of oral insulin, at a dose of 5 mg/day for 1 year, starting at the time of disease diagnosis, had no effect on residual β cell function, as assessed by C-peptide secretion (16).

TOLERANCE INDUCTION THROUGH GAD ANTIGEN ADMINISTRATION

The 65 kDa isoform of GAD65 has been shown to be an important autoantigen in type 1 diabetes, therefore there is a potential for GAD-based therapy to treat and/or prevent type 1 diabetes. This possibility is reinforced by the findings of both proliferative and cytotoxic T cell responses to GAD65 in prediabetics and in patients with recent onset disease (17,18). GAD65-reactive T cells have been shown to be involved in early destruction of β cells (1) and the injection of GAD65 or GAD peptides via a variety of routes induces tolerance to GAD65, thus delaying or preventing insulin dependence (19–21). More recently, β cell-specific suppression of GAD expression in two lines of antisense GAD transgeneic NOD mice was shown to prevent these mice from developing the disease (22). Furthermore, it is of interest, in case GAD is used for prevention, that immunization with GAD65 did not induce lymphocytic infiltration in the islets in different non-diabetes-prone mouse strains (23). In our own experience, a single subcutaneous injection to NOD male mice of GAD65 did not increase the disease rate (24).

At present, there are two GAD-based immunotherapeutic strategies, i.e. passive tolerance aimed to inactivate or preventing the priming of autoreactive T cells, and active tolerance aimed at inducing a protective immune response (25). In the NOD mouse model, both passive and active tolerance induction via the administration of GAD65 have protected against diabetes insurgence (26).

Active tolerance was associated with immune deviation of T cell responses to GAD65 from diabetogenic Th1 to protective Th2 responses (27). In the BB rat model, GAD65 therapy reduced the number of IFNγ producing thymocytes (12), suggesting that such therapy has the potential to immunomodulate. One key question is the dose and timing of GAD administration to induce tolerance in humans. A phase 1 study has been carried out in healthy volunteers involving the subcutaneous injections of four ascending doses of recombinant GAD65, up to a maximum of 0.5 mg/subject. No adverse effects were reported and, most important, antibodies to GAD65, insulin or IA-2 were not detected following the administration of GAD65. Phase II trials may start soon in patients with recent onset type 1 diabetes and patients with late autoimmune diabetes of the adult (LADA) using recombinant GAD65 formulated with alum as adjuvant.

TOLERANCE INDUCTION WITH DiaPep277 PEPTIDE

The strategy underlying the DiaPep277 approach in preventing type 1 diabetes is that of antigen-specific suppression. Two animal models of autoimmune diabetes were used to show that hsp60-specific autoimmunity precedes the onset of clinical hyperglycemia in the NOD mouse and the low-dose streptozotocin (STZ) model (28,29). The T cells that recognize hsp60 were derived from pre-diabetic NOD spleens and were capable of adoptively transferring insulitis and hyperglycemia to young prediabetic NOD mice, thus demonstrating that the autoimmune response to hsp60 is not just an epiphenomenon, but plays a role in the pathogenesis of diabetes. The diabetogenic T cells recognize the hsp60 peptide epitope corresponding to positions 437–460, called 'p277'. This peptide contains two cystein residues that are highly sensitive to oxidation. To stabilize the peptide, these cysteins were replaced by valines, and the modified peptide was called DiaPep277. This peptide is fully cross-reactive with the original p277, and has the same biological activity. Based on the high spontaneous reactivity to this peptide at the preclinical stage of diabetes, the feasibility of deviating the autoimmune responses by direct administration of the peptide was studied. The DiaPep277 peptide proved to be a potent inducer of protection from the development of diabetes in the mouse models. NOD mice were treated shortly before the onset of hyperglycemia or, at the time of onset, with a single dose of DiaPep277 in adjuvant. The DiaPep277-treated NOD mice were protected from diabetes, 70% remaining normoglycemic if treated before onset, while all the control mice developed diabetes (30). The successful treatment was accompanied by significant reduction in the level of destructive insulitis (31). NOD mice that were untreated, or treated with a control peptide, progressed to intra-islet insulitis that accompanied the onset of diabetes. On the other hand, the pancreas of DiaPep277-treated mice manifested islets that were either clear of infiltrating lymphocytes, or the infiltrate was restricted to the periphery of the islet, as observed at early pre-clinical stages of the disease. The reduced inflammatory response in the islets was accompanied by a dramatic change in the immune responses that are typical of the NOD mouse. The spontaneous autoimmune responses to self-antigens such as hsp60, GAD65 and insulin were suppressed in the DiaPep77-treated mice. The effect was detected on both the cellular responses (T cell proliferative responses) and autoantibody production. Moreover, in analysing the cytokine responses before and after the treatment, a Th1 to Th2 shift was observed in the DiaPep277-specific T cells. Although this shift was observed in the DiaPep277-stimulated response, it can explain the suppression of the Th1 response to GAD65 and insulin by bystander suppression. DiaPep277 treatment was also effective in suppression of the inflammatory Th1 response in the pancreatic lesions. Thus, DiaPep277, a self-epitope in autoimmune diabetes, could be effectively used to shut down destructive insulitis, deviate the pro-inflammatory Th1 responses to a non-pathogenic Th2 mode and, probably through suppressive Th2 cytokines, downregulate the autoimmune responses to a panel of self-antigens that are related to diabetes. Phase 1 trials with DiaPep277 have been carried out safely in normal volunteers and pilot trials have begun in recent-onset young type 1 diabetes patients to see whether β cell mass can be preserved. Of particular interest is the group of patients with LADA as target for therapy with DiaPep277. This is a relatively newly defined subpopulation of type 2 diabetes. Patients that show autoimmune features similar to type 1 diabetes and become insulin-dependent within a few years after diagnosis. As this group of patients is 8–15% of all type 2 diabetes, it equals in numbers the type I patients. These patients are a highly attractive target population, since they are already diagnosed as diabetics, hence the screening involved in setting up a clinical trial is relatively simple, and the clinical endpoint (prevention of insulin dependency) is straightforward.

CONCLUSIONS

In conclusion, the field of tolerance induction for treatment and prevention of type 1 diabetes is a novel and fascinating one. However, we are at a very preliminary stage and much caution is advised. One particular concern is that therapy with specific antigens or peptide may boost the immune response, thereby promoting rather than arresting the immune process as shown in other autoimmune conditions (32). Therefore we need a careful assessment of the dose to be administered and cautious monitoring of treated patients enrolled in pilot trials.

ACKNOWLEDGEMENTS

The work described in this review performed by the authors is supported by Grants from the Juvenile Diabetes Foundation International, the Ministry of University and Technological Research (Italy) and Centro Internazionale Studi Diabete.

REFERENCES

1. Tisch R *et al*: Immune response to glutamic acid decarboxylase correlates with insulitis in non-obese diabetic mice. *Nature* 366:72–75, 1993.
2. Mossman TR, Coffman RL: Th1 and Th2 cells: different patterns of lymphokine secretion lead to different functional properties. *Annu Rev Immunol* 7:145–173, 1989.
3. Rabinovitch A *et al*: Cytokine gene expression in pancreatic islet-infiltrating leukocytes of BB rats: expression of Th1 cytokines correlates with beta-cell destructive insulitis and IDDM. *Diabetes* 45:749–754, 1996.
4. Tisch R, McDevitt H: Insulin-dependent diabetes mellitus. *Cell* 85:291–297, 1996.
5. Perez VL *et al*: Induction of peripheral T cell tolerance in vivo requires CTLA-4 engagement. *Immunity* 6:411–417, 1997.
6. Miller AM, Lider O, Weiner HL: Antigen-driven bystander suppression after oral administration of antigens. *J Exp Med* 174:791–798, 1991.
7. Weiner HL: Oral tolerance immune mechanisms and treatment of autoimmune disease. *Immunol Today* 18:335–343, 1997.
8. Pozzilli P: Prevention of insulin-dependent diabetes mellitus 1998. *Diabet Metab Rev* 14:69–84, 1998.
9. Daniel D, Gill RG, Schloot N, Wegmann D. Epitope specificity cytokine production profile and diabetogenic activity of insulin-specific T cell clones isolated from NOD mice. *Eur J Immunol* 25:1056–1062, 1995.
10. Zhang I, Davidson L, Eisenbarth G, Weiner HL: Suppression of diabetes in non-obese diabetic mice by oral administration of porcine insulin. *Proc Natl Acad Sci USA* 88:10 252–10 256,1991.
11. Muir A, Ramiya V: New strategies in oral immunotherapy for diabetes prevention. *Diabet Metab Rev* 12:1–14, 1996.
12. Bergerot I, Fabien N, Maguer V, Thivolet C: Oral administration of human insulin to NOD mice generates CD4 + ve cells that suppress adoptive transfer of diabetes. *J Autoimmunity* 7:655–663, 1994.
13. Daniel D, Wegmann DR: Protection of non-obese diabetic mice from diabetes by intranasal or subcutaneous administration of insulin peptide.B9-23. *Proc Natl Acad Sci USA* 93:628–634, 1995.
14. Keller RJ, Eisenbarth GS, Jackson RA: Insulin prophylaxis in individuals at high risk of type 1 diabetes. *Lancet* 341:927–928, 1993.
15. Eisenbarth GS *et al*: Prediction and prevention of type 1 diabetes. *Transplant Proc* 26:361–362, 1994.
16. Pozzilli P, Pitocco D, Visalli N *et al*: No effect of oral insulin on residual B cell function in recent onset type 1 diabetes (the IMDIAB VII). *Diabetologia* (in press).
17. Atkinson MA *et al*: Response of peripheral-blood mononuclear cells to glutamate decarboxylase in insulin-dependent diabetes. *Lancet* 399:458–459, 1992.
18. Atkinson MA *et al*: Cellular immunity to a determinant common to glutamate decarboxylase and Coxsackie virus in insulin-dependent diabetes. *J Clin Invest* 94:2125–2129, 1994.

19. Kaufman DL *et al*: Spontaneous loss of T-cell tolerance to glutamic acid decarboxylase in murine insulin dependent diabetes. *Nature* 366:69–72, 1993.
20. Petersen JS *et al*: Neonatal tolerisation with glutamic acid decarboxylase but not with bovine serum albumin delays the onset of diabetes in NOD mice. *Diabetes* 44:1478–1484, 1994.
21. Tisch R *et al*: Administering glutamic acid decarboxylase to NOD mice prevents diabetes. *J Autoimmun* 7:845–850, 1994.
22. Yoon J-W: Control of autoimmune diabetes in NOD mice by GAD expression or suppression in cells. *Science* 284:1183–1187, 1999.
23. Plesner A *et al*: Immunisation of diabetes-prone or non-diabetes-prone mice with GAD65 does not induce diabetes or islet pathology. *J Autoimmun* 11:335–341, 1998.
24. Beales PE, Liddi R, Rosignoli G, Pozzilli P: Intradermal GAD skin test in NOD mouse *Autoimmunity* (in press).
25. Tian J *et al*: Nasal administration of glutamate decarboxylase(GAD65)peptides induces Th2 responses and prevents murine insulin dependent diabetes. *J Exp Med* 183:17–24, 1996.
26. Tisch R *et al*: Induction of GAD65-specific regulatory T-cells inhibits ongoing autoimmune diabetes in non-obese diabetic mice. *Diabetes* 47:894–899, 1998.
27. Bieg S *et al*: The lymphopenia (lyp) gene controls the intrathymic cytokine ratio in congenic BioBreeding rats. *Diabetes* 40:786–792, 1997.
28. Elias D, Reshef T, Birk OS, Van der Zee R, Walker MD, Cohen IR: Vaccination against autoimmune mouse diabetes with a T-cell epitope of the human 65-kDa heat shock protein. *Proc Natl Acad Sci USA* 88:3088–3091, 1991.
29. Elias D, Cohen IR: The hsp60 peptide p277 arrests the autoimmune diabetes induced by the toxin streptozotocin. *Diabetes* 45:1168–1172, 1996.
30. Elias D *et al*: Hsp60 peptide therapy of NOD mouse diabetes induces a Th2 cytokine burst and downregulates autoimmunity to various beta cell antigens. *Diabetes* 46:758–764, 1997.
31. Elias D, Cohen IR: Treatment of autoimmune diabetes and insulitis in NOD mice with heat shock protein 60 peptide p277. *Diabetes* 44:1132–1138, 1995.
32. Blanas E, Heath WR: Oral administration of antigen can lead to the onset of autoimmune disease. *Int Rev Immunol* 18:217–228, 1999.

6

Clinical Trials in Pre-diabetes: an Overview

CARLA GIORDANO, GIAN DOMENICO BOMPIANI
and ALDO GALLUZZO
Institute of Clinica Medica, Faculty of Medicine, University of Palermo, Italy

Type 1 diabetes is an autoimmune disease in which pancreatic insulin-producing β cells are attacked and destroyed by the body's own immune system (1–3). This erroneous attack could be prevented or stopped by re-educating the immune system and diverging it away from the β cells. Studies initiated in the 1980s demonstrated that short-term remission from the disease could be induced with immunosuppressive therapy (4). Although immunosuppressive drugs can help prolonging clinical remissions after diabetes onset, their adverse effects prevent their long-term use, especially in children. It is essential that intervention in otherwise healthy prediabetic children be free of significant risks and toxicity. Today's prevention strategies aim at diverting the immune response from autoimmunity to self-tolerance in a diabetes-specific manner without using immunosuppressive agents that could compromise the patients' health.

In recent years, progress in molecular biology, gene technology and immunology have contributed extensively to our knowledge of the interaction between the genetic background, environmental factors, and the evolution of the autoimmune mechanisms leading to overt type 1 diabetes. The pathogenesis of type 1 diabetes involves genetic predisposition to the disease. Non-genetic (environmental) factors act as triggers in genetically susceptible individuals and activate immune mechanisms, specifically targeting pancreatic islet β cells (5). The immune response results in a progressive destruction of pancreatic islet β cells and consequent development of type 1 diabetes mellitus. The evolution of this process appears to be slow, often spanning several years, with a long

Diabetes in the New Millennium. Edited by U. Di Mario, F. Leonetti, G. Pugliese, P. Sbraccia and A. Signore.
© 2000 John Wiley & Sons, Ltd.

prediabetic period preceding the onset of overt diabetes, thereby providing a window of opportunity of intervention in those subjects bearing HLA susceptibility markers who are found to have increased diabetes risk using autoantibody testing.

Today, effective prevention strategies aim to:

1. Confer protection to individuals at increased-risk for type 1 diabetes (e.g. GAD autoantibody-positive relatives of diabetic probands).
2. Preserve residual β cell mass in recent-onset type 1 diabetic patients.
3. Prevent or delay type 1 diabetes from developing in those diagnosed with the type 2 form of the disease.
4. Prevent or delay recurrence of the autoimmune disease in type 1 diabetes patients receiving pancreas or islet cell transplantation.

Several strategic approaches have been used and many are currently under investigation. Two large networks — DPT-1 (Diabetes Prevention Trial — Type 1) and ENDIT (European Nicotinamide Diabetes Intervention Trial) — have been established to test interventions that might prevent or delay the development of clinical type 1 diabetes in relatives of individuals with the disease.

In this review, we will focus on different possibilities to confer protection to individuals at high risk for type 1 diabetes. Firstly, we will present data showing what is theoretically possible to preserve islet β cell function in high-risk subjects and evidence suggesting activation of protective and/or repair mechanisms within the β cells in response to the immune attack. Additional strategies for preventing autoimmune diabetes, based on the concept of prevention of the initial injury to β cells, will be summarized.

POTENTIAL PROPHYLACTIC AGENTS

Parenteral insulin

Parenteral insulin therapy has been shown to protect against type 1 diabetes in both the NOD mouse and the BB rat (6–7). In both models, insulin treatment alters and/or decreases the insulitis. The protection provided by insulin is disease-specific because in BB rats the development of thyroiditis is not affected. It remains to be established whether the positive effects are due to the fact that insulin administration contributes to maintain normal blood glucose levels, induces β cell rest, or directly intervenes on the immunological mechanisms of the disease. The Diabetes Control and Complications Trial (DCCT) has unequivocally demonstrated that residual insulin secretion, as dosed by C-peptide levels, continues to play a role in maintaining a better control for a long period of time (8). This observation, together with the knowledge that aggressive insulin treatment of new onset type 1 diabetes in humans increases the frequency and duration of insulin-free remission, strongly suggests that those islets that survive the ongoing destructive autoimmune process may function effectively (9). The β cell destruction of type 1 diabetes may, in part, depend on a balance between β cell injury and β cell defence and repair and/or regeneration. This theory was further supported by results emerging from a pilot study of the prophylactic value of 5 day courses of intravenous insulin given to ICA-positive children at risk for type 1 diabetes every 9 months, combined with a daily low-dose sub-cutaneous insulin therapy; five treated children and none of the untreated control patients maintained their metabolic status after a 3 year period (10). One possible explanation for the prophylactic effect of parenteral insulin is a reduction in β cell secretory activity. The mechanisms underlying the prolongation of islet function with intensive therapy or parenteral insulin may include a reduction in glucotoxicity and/or β cell rest conferring relative slowing of the autoimmune process that destroy β cells. Insulin-induced hypoglycaemia may reduce biosynthesis of insulin, GLUT2 and other putative autoantigens. This sort of masking effect may regulate T cells, particularly favouring the Th2/IL4-mediated response pathway. These data have been demonstrated in both NOD mouse and BB rat. In particular, in the NOD mouse there are many *in vitro* observations indicating the possibility of β cell repair rather than regeneration (4). β Cell repair has also been demonstrated after *in vivo* β cell damage. NOD mice develop, from 5 weeks of age, a progressive mononuclear infiltration in and around the pancreatic islets. Usually this infiltrate evolves into a destructive insulitis in those mice progressing to diabetes. When islets with insulitis were isolated from NOD mice at different ages, the islets showed an abnormal insulin release and defective glucose metabolism that progressively worsened with age. These alterations were completely restored after 1 week of culture, during which infiltrating T cells were depleted. These data suggest that in prediabetic NOD mice, a population of suppressed and/or partially damaged β cells exists (11). If the immune assault is arrested, islets, either by repair mechanisms and/or regeneration, could regain normal function. At present, it is more likely that lower glucose levels in prediabetic subjects resulted in less β cell stimulation (β cell rest) and that this resulted in relative β cell protection as compared with patients of the conventionally treated group (12).

Administration of the β chain of insulin or a metabolically inactive variant of insulin also confers protection (13). Splenocytes from NOD mice immunized with insulin or the β chain of insulin immunization appear to activate regulatory T cells and to reduce IFNγ content in NOD mouse islets. It must also be noted that type 1 diabetes was delayed with somatostatin, an agent that suppresses endogenous insulin production (14). These results suggest that both immunological and metabolic factors may contribute to the beneficial effect of prophylactic insulin therapy in the NOD mouse.

Although DCCT showed that the protective effects on residual β cell function are unlikely to be mediated by an immunological effect of insulin, it appears that lower glucose levels in the intensively treated subjects resulted in a lower β cell stimulation, which is capable of protecting residual β cell function more effectively than conventional treatment. Several experimental data confirm that decreased β cell activity appears to confer protection against β cell destruction. Furthermore, consistent with this hypothesis there is the observation that parenteral insulin may induce a T-helper 1 (Th1) to T-helper 2 (Th2) shift. It is accepted that the Th1 subset of T cells and their cytokine products, IL-2, IFNγ and TNF are the principal protagonists involved in the insulitis process, while Th2 subsets and their cytokine products, IL-4 and IL-10, are downregulated. The insulitis process is initiated by type 1 cytokines but its progression involves also other immune pathways. In fact, type 1 cytokines activate cytotoxic T cells that specifically interact with β cells, thus contributing to their destruction. The shift induced by parenteral insulin is demonstrated by the IAA measurement after subcutaneous insulin, which causes a predominant Th2 response with IgG1, IgG3 and IgG4, whereas insulin autoantibodies associated with type 1 diabetes are predominantly IgG3, indicating a Th1 response (15).

A final hypothesis is based on insulin's capacity to block apoptosis, which is today considered the most probable mechanism involved in β cell death (16).

Oral insulin

Oral administration of relevant autoantigens has been reported to delay or suppress onset of disease in a number of experimental autoimmune disorders, including autoimmune type 1 diabetes. Oral insulin is reported to reduce the severity of lymphocytic infiltration in the pancreatic islets of NOD mice (17). The mechanism by which oral insulin induces tolerance has not been understood. There is no evidence that oral insulin can prevent type 1 diabetes in humans. However, for this approach to be effective, repeated feeding of large amounts of autoantigens is required, limiting the usefulness of this therapy for human use. One new strategy may be the use of small amounts of insulin conjugated to a mucosal carrier protein, i.e. insulin–MCP (cholera toxin B-subunit) (18). Studies in NOD mice have shown that insulin–MCP can delay and prevent spontaneous disease in adult animals and in transgenic mice with virally (LCMV)-induced diabetes. The amount of insulin–MCP required for therapeutic activity in these models was several hundred-fold less than that of insulin alone.

In the DPT-1 trial, the first subject was assigned to the oral study on September 1996, and therefore enrolment projections differ. Since DPT-1 is a masked study, no outcome data will be available until the study is completed (19).

DRUGS INFLUENCING THE IMMUNE SYSTEM

Cyclosporin

Cyclosporin A has been used in subjects at high risk for type 1 diabetes. β Cell responses to the intravenous glucose tolerance test, hyperglycaemic clamp and intravenous glucagon were evaluated before and after a 6 month course of cyclosporin in seven subjects at high risk for type 1 diabetes. The results obtained studying initial insulin secretory responses were markedly positive when compared with healthy control subjects. However, success was only observed during the first months of therapy since, after 6 months of cyclosporin, β cell responses remained markedly abnormal. All the patients became diabetic after 5–36 months. These negative results were confirmed in a French study (4).

Improved treatment for type 1 diabetes did not emerge from the trials of cyclosporin and azathioprine. The major risks included drug-specific effects (irreversible nephrotoxicity for cyclosporin and bone marrow suppression and hepatoxicity for azathioprine) and general effects of chronic immunosuppression (severe infection and neoplasia). The clinical benefit seen in the randomized trials could not justify these potential risks.

Antibodies against CD40L or CD80

CD40–CD40L interactions are responsible for the production of antibodies to T cell-dependent antigens. Furthermore CD40–CD40L signalling stimulates the formation of germinal centres and causes immunoglobulin isotype switching. Through the induction of costimulatory molecules on β cells, CD40–CD40L mediates the expression of adhesion molecules such as B7.1, B7.2 and ICAM. The costimulatory molecules are also induced on the surface of macrophages, activated endothelial cells, dendritic cells and keratinocytes. CD40–CD40L blockade has been shown to ameliorate nephritis in SNF1 lupus mice, to prevent the onset of heavy metal glomerulonephritis, to prevent and treat EAE in mice, etc. (20). The effect of CD40–CD40L blockade has also been shown to promote the acceptance of islet cell allografts in mice and non-human primates, and similar results have been obtained for kidney allografts in monkeys and skin and cardiac allografts in mice. A *Phase I trial* is currently under way to study the effect of a single i.v. dose of a humanized anti-CD40L monoclonal antibody in patients with systemic lupus erythematosus. In type 1 diabetes this monoclonal antibody has been used in islet transplants in primates and the preliminary results are of high interest.

In ongoing immune responses, both *in vitro* and *in vivo* studies indicate that the monoclonal antibody anti-CD80 is effective in blocking T cell activation, IL-2 secretion and antigen-specific antibody production in the presence of

CD86. Toxicology study showed no mortality, clinical adverse effects or abnormalities in serum chemistry or haematology. No change in CD4, CD8 or CD20 cells has been described. However, the results of preliminary experiments are initial results, and a long time will pass before a clinical trial in type 1 diabetes could be planned (18).

ANTIGEN-BASED THERAPY

Insulin B9-B23 peptide

A dominant epitope of the insulin autoantigen resides in the B chain (B9-B23) and has been shown to be recognized by both CD4 and CD8 T cells in NOD mice. Based on this information, a series of soluble altered peptide ligands designed to block or change the activation response of the type 1 diabetes autoimmune T cells have been recently proposed in type 1 diabetes. A novel peptide called NBI-6024 showed ability in binding to the antigen-binding site on the autoimmune T cell blocking activation, but also demonstrated to produce a strong protective Th2 type immunogenic effect. *In vivo* studies in the NOD mouse have also shown a significant reduction in the development of diabetes and histopathological damage in the β cells (18).

GAD65

The clinical presence of autoantibodies to GAD65 is a sensitive and early predictor of type 1 diabetes. In addition, both proliferative and cytotoxic T cell responses to GAD65 have been detected in prediabetic and new onset diabetic patients. These clinical observations are supported by a large number of studies in NOD mice. GAD65-reactive T cells have been shown to be critically involved in early destruction of pancreatic β cells, and the injections of GAD65 or GAD peptides via a variety of routes induce tolerance to GAD65, delaying or preventing insulin dependence. More recently, β cell specific suppression of GAD expression in two lines of antisense GAD transgenic NOD mice was shown to prevent these mice from spontaneously developing the disease. It has also been shown that immunization with GAD65 did not induce islet cell pathology in three non-diabetes-prone mouse strains (21).

Currently, there are two autoantigen-based immunotherapeutic strategies; 'passive' tolerance, aiming at inactivating or preventing priming of autoreactive T cells, and 'active' tolerance, involving induction of protective immune responses. In the NOD mouse model, both passive and active tolerance induction via administration of GAD65 have protected against diabetes development. Active tolerance was associated with immune deviation of T cell responses to GAD65 from diabetogenic Th1 to protective Th2 responses.

There is an ongoing clinical Phase I trial involving subcutaneous injection of four ascending dose levels up to a maximum of 0.5 mg/person in healthy Caucasian male volunteers. The aims of this trial are to study adverse clinical effects, whether the dose is well tolerated, and the behaviour of autoantibodies to GAD65, insulin or IA-2 (4,18).

Peptide 277

The design of such a therapeutically approach is based on understanding how the immune system attacks the β cells. The immune system has two functional arms: innate immunity and adaptive immunity. The innate immunity is the first line of defence against invading pathogens, and consists of macrophages and dendritic cells. These cells secrete pro-inflammatory cytokines and express surface molecules, both necessary for the recruitment and activation of the adaptive immunity that consists of T and B lymphocytes. One potent activator of the innate immune system is hsp60, since it can induce the secretion of pro-inflammatory cytokines such as IL12 and TNFα, and upregulate the expression of adhesion molecules. Hsp60 is considered as a major activating signal for the immune system and is considered to be playing a role in the pathogenesis of different autoimmune diseases. The epitope spanning residues 437–460 of the human hsp60 was found to be linked to type 1 diabetes, in experimental models as well as in patients. Very recently the natural sequence has been used to develop a peptide-based compound as a vaccine for type 1 diabetes. The peptide mode of action is based on the paradigm that the pathogenetic autoimmune T cells that mediate type 1 diabetes are of the Th1 phenotype. This peptide, when tested in animal models, suppresses Th1 responses. Based on these experimental data, one company has produced this peptide in large scale and has carried out pre-clinical toxicology in Phase I and Phase II studies in newly diagnosed type 1 diabetic patients. The immunological monitoring showed that the p277 peptide-treated patients had increased Th2 responses and conserved or even improved their β cell function.

The active ingredient is a 24 amino acid peptide, having the sequence position 437–460 of the human hsp60, in which cysteine residues are replaced by valine. For ethical reasons, the *Phase I* study was conducted in long-term diabetes patients instead of healthy volunteers. Currently, a double-blind placebo-controlled, multiple-dose study was initiated in Belgium in type 1 diabetic patients. Two exploratory *Phase II* studies were initiated in Israel. The preliminary results showed a difference between p277- and placebo-treated groups, both in adults and children, in maintenance of β cell function. The clinical plan for p277 focuses on a fast-track vaccine approach. In conclusion, at present two populations are the principal targets: (a) newly diagnosed type 1 diabetes patients, established; in these patients, p277 vaccination is expected to modulate the destructive pro-inflammatory autoimmune attack on the remaining reserve of β cells, allowing their survival and continued function; (b) late autoimmune diabetes of the adult (LADA), a relatively newly defined subpopulation of type 2 diabetic patients that show autoimmune characteristics similar to type 1 diabetes, and become insulin-dependent within few years after diagnosis (18).

NICOTINAMIDE

Nicotinamide, the amide of nicotinic acid, is a component of NAD^- and $NADP^+$ and is an essential dietary constituent, the recommended daily requirement being approximately 5–20 mg in adults.

It has been shown in animal studies that nicotinamide protects β cells against a variety of noxious stimuli, including streptozotocin, IL-1, TNFα, and IFNγ. It is a free radical scavenger, a potent inhibitor of PARP (4,22). Intravenous administration of nicotinamide before administration of a diabetogenic dose of alloxan prevents diabetes in 60% of rats and nicotinamide prevents diabetes and reduces the severity of insulitis in young NOD mice. Nicotinamide acts increasing intracellular NAD^+ content either by serving as a precursor for its synthesis or by reducing poly- or mono-ADP ribosylation, or both. Nicotimatide stimulates β cell regeneration in 90% of pancreasectomized rats, possibly acting through regenerating genes (23,24). Nicotinamide exerts its protective effect in the NOD mouse by mediating the expression and enzymatic activity of cytokine-induced nitric oxide synthase, therefore resulting in the suppression of nitric oxide formation in the β cells, and thereby resulting in less DNA damage and mithocondrial enzyme inactivation. A therapeutic effect of nicotinamide in preserving residual β cell function when given at diagnosis of type 1 diabetes in addition to insulin has been proven. A 20-nation international clinical trial, the European Nicotinamide Diabetes Intervention Trial (ENDIT), is ongoing. The preliminary results suggest that the onset of type 1 diabetes can be delayed by nicotinamide, particularly if it is begun early enough; 552 patients were enrolled, 111 progressed to diabetes and 123 withdrew from study. Recruitment closed on May 1998 and final results of the trial are expected by 2003.

CONCLUDING REMARKS

DPT-1, ENDIT and the Cow's Milk Avoidance Trial represent the progress characterizing 2000 diabetology. The intervention strategies are numerous and aim at preventing or delaying progression to clinical type 1 diabetes. Blockade of the final common pathway leading to the damage of β cells is considered realistic, but today caution when transferring findings from animal models to the human situation is still strongly to be recommended. type 1 diabetes is a preventable disease and it is now the time to be conscientious diabetologists.

REFERENCES

1. Lernmark A, Falorni A. Immune phenomena and events in the islets in insulin-dependent diabetes diabetes mellitus. In *Textbook of Diabetes*. Pickup J, Williams G, Eds. Oxford, UK: Blackwell Science, 1997, pp. 15.1–15.29.
2. Bain SC, Mijovic CH, Barnett AH: Genetic factors in the pathogenesis of insulin-dependent diabetes mellitus. In *Textbook of Diabetes*. Pickup J, Williams G, Eds. Oxford, UK: Blackwell Science, 1997, pp. 13.1–13.13.
3. Yoon J. Environmental factors in the pathogenesis of insulin-dependent diabetes mellitus. In *Textbook of Diabetes*. Pickup J, Williams G, Eds. Oxford, UK: Blackwell Science Ltd, 1997, pp. 14.1–14.14.
4. Naik RG, Palmer JP: Preservation of β-cell function in type 1 diabetes. *Diabet Rev* 7(3):154–182, 1999.
5. Benoist C, Mathis D: Cellular and molecular changes accompanying the progression from insulitis to diabetes. *Eur J Immunol* 29:245–255, 1999.
6. Gotfredsen CF, Buschard K, Frandsen EK: Reduction of diabetes incidence of BB Wistar rats by early prophylactic insulin treatment of diabetes-prone animals. *Diabetologia* 28:933–935, 1985.
7. Muir A, Peck A, Clare-Saizler M, Song YH, Cornelius J, Luchetta R, Krischer J, Maclaren N: Insulin immunization of nonobese diabetic mice induces a protective insulitis characterized by diminished intra-islet interferon-γ transcription. *J Clin Invest* 95:628–634, 1995.
8. The Diabetes Control and Complications Trial Research Group. The effect of intensive treatment of diabetes on the development and progression of long-term complications in insulin-dependent diabetes mellitus. *N Engl J Med* 329:977–986, 1993.
9. Mirouze J, Selam JL, Pham TC, Mendoza E, Orsetti A: Sustained insulin-induced remission of juvenile diabetes by means of external pancreas. *Diabetologia* 144:223–227, 1978.
10. Keller RJ, Eisenbarth GS, Jackson RA: Insulin prophylaxis in individuals at high risk of type 1 diabetes. *Lancet* 341:927–928, 1993.
11. Mauricio D, Mandrup-Poulsen T: Apoptosis and the pathogenesis of IDDM: a question of life and death. *Diabetes* 47:1537–1543, 1998.
12. Hao W, Linsong L, Mehta V, Lernmark A, Palmer JP: The functional state of the beta cell affects expression of both forms of glutamic acid decarboxylase. *Pancreas* 9:558–562, 1994.
13. Karounos DG, Bryson JS, Cohen DA: Metabolically inactive insulin analog prevents type 1 diabetes in prediabetic NOD mice. *J Clin. Invest* 6:1344–1348, 1997.
14. Bowman MA, Campbell L, Darrow BL, Ellis TM, Suresh A, Atkinson MA: Immunological and metabolic effects of prophylactic insulin therapy in NOD-scid/scid adoptive transfer model of IDDM. *Diabetes* 45:205–208, 1996.
15. Kumar D: Insulin antibodies: reduction in various antiinsulin IgG subclasses with human insulin therapy. *Horm Metabol Res* 25:360–364, 1993.

16. Giordano C, Galluzzo A: Fas-mediated apoptosis in human type 1 diabetes: its possible role in the destruction of pancreatic β-cells. *Diabet Nutr Metab* 10:233–241, 1997.
17. Zhang JA, Davidson L, Eisenbarth GS, Weiner HL: Suppression of diabetes in NOD mice by oral admistration of porcine insulin. *Proc Natl Acad Sci USA* 88: 10 252–10 256, 1991.
18. Workshop on Future Directions in Prevention of Type 1 Diabetes. January 9–10, 2000. Inter-Continental Hotel, Miami, FL, USA.
19. American Diabetes Association: *Update on DPT-1*, Alexandria, VA: American Diabetes Association, 1998.
20. Rossini AA, Greiner DL, Mordes JP: Induction of immunologic tolerance for transplantation. *Physiol Rev* 79:99–141, 1999.
21. Hancock WW, Polanski M, Zhang J, Blogg N, Weiner HL: Suppression of insulitis in non-obese diabetic (NOD) mice by oral insulin administration is associated with selective expression of interleukin-4, and-10, transforming growth factor-beta and prostaglandin-E. *Am J Pathol* 147:1193–1199, 1995.
22. Elliot RB, Chase HP: Prevention or delay of type 1 (insulin-dependent) diabetes mellitus in children using nicotinamide. *Diabetologia* 34:362–365, 1991.
23. Sandler S, Andersson A: Long-term effects of exposure of pancreatic islets to nicotinamide *in vitro* and DNA synthesis, metabolism and β-cell function. *Diabetologia* 29:199–202, 1986.
24. Sandler S, Hellerstrom C, Eizirik DL: Effects of nicotinamide supplementation on human pancreatic islet function tissue culture. *J Clin Endocrinol Metab* 77:1574–1576, 1998.

7

Intensive Insulin Therapy in Type 1 Diabetes

PAOLO BRUNETTI and GEREMIA B. BOLLI
Department of Internal Medicine, University of Perugia, Italy

In 1993, two independent intervention trials conclusively showed that long-term maintenance of near-normoglycaemia, as indicated by the percentage of glycosylated haemoglobin A_{1c} (HbA_{1c}) by intensive insulin therapy, strongly protects against onset and/or progression of long-term microangiopathic complications (1,2). Thus, patients with type 1 diabetes mellitus (T1 DM), especially young patients with recent onset or short duration of the disease, should be treated intensively.

Some barriers still prevent the majority of T1 DM patients from being on intensive treatment. The reasons are multiple. Perhaps the most common are economical and cultural. The local organization of diabetes care also plays a role. Intensive therapy is undoubtedly expensive, especially the cost of blood glucose self-monitoring. However, besides money, a modern culture of treatment of T1 DM by diabetologists and an appropriate structure of diabetes clinics are required. Only deeply motivated diabetologists can motivate T1 DM patients to initiate intensive therapy and carry its burden over the years with belief in preventing catastrophies of single or multiple organ failures. In order to reach this goal, with a few exceptions, general practitioners or family physicians, generally without long-term experience of insulin replacement, should not take care of management of T1 DM. Rather, they should refer their T1 DM patients to experienced diabetologists for appropriate care.

In this review, the modern strategies of insulin replacement in relation to the goal of intensive therapy will be discussed.

Diabetes in the New Millennium. Edited by U. Di Mario, F. Leonetti, G. Pugliese, P. Sbraccia and A. Signore.
© 2000 John Wiley & Sons, Ltd.

RATIONALE OF INSULIN REPLACEMENT IN T1 DM

Physiology teaches that two key approaches are needed to reproduce glucose homeostasis in insulin-deficient T1 DM. First, post-prandial blood glucose control requires a sharp spike of plasma insulin immediately following meal ingestion. Second, the inter-prandial or post-absorptive state requires a flat, peakless plasma insulin concentration until the next meal. Most of the problems of insulin replacement in T1 DM derive from the fact that the subcutaneous (s.c.) route of injection or infusion still has to be used to replace insulin. From the s.c. site of injection, insulin is absorbed into the systemic, not the portal, circulation. More important, the s.c. route retards absorption of insulin, and causes variability of absorption from one injection to another. The latter problem is only partly dependent on the anatomical site of injection, because there is quite a large variability of absorption within the same anatomical area of injection. As it will be discussed later, insulin analogues have been designed to overcome, at least in part, the problem of s.c. absorption.

REPLACEMENT OF INSULIN NEEDS AT MEAL-TIME

S.c. absorption of human regular insulin

Until a few years ago, only human regular insulin was available for postprandial control in T1 DM. Human insulin has a high tendency for self-association to form hexamers, the predominant form present in the insulin vials that patients use. Because insulin is absorbed in monomeric form from the s.c. site of injection by the capillaries into the bloodstream, and because the dissociation rate of human insulin hexamers into monomers in the s.c. tissue is a slow process, absorption of human insulin is also slow. Therefore, administration of regular, short-acting insulin to T1 DM patients does not result in a peak at a time at which there is glucose absorption from the intestine. Because of insulin deficiency, primarily at the portal level, blood glucose increases excessively 1–2 hours after meal ingestion, especially if no time interval is allowed between s.c. injection and meal ingestion (3). When a 30 minute interval is allowed between insulin injection and meal ingestion, the better plasma insulin bioavailability improves post-prandial blood glucose (3). In fact, this is the rationale for suggesting at least a 30 minute interval between s.c. insulin injection and meal ingestion to T1 DM patients, but in practice the rule is only sometimes followed. Four to 5 hours after the s.c. insulin injection, the continuing absorption from the injection site of human or purified pork insulin results in inappropriate hyperinsulinaemia, which increases the risk for hypoglycaemia because by that time meal absorption is nearly complete (3).

Short-acting insulin analogues

In order to overcome the problems of non-physiological pharmacokinetics of human regular insulin, short-acting insulin analogues have been synthesized. The first short-acting insulin analogue was LysB28, ProB-29-human insulin (Eli Lilly & Co). Insulin aspart (NovoNordisk) is an additional short-acting insulin analogue created by replacing proline at position B28 by aspartic acid. The background, structure and physicochemical characteristics, receptor binding, toxicology, pharmacokinetics and dynamics of these two insulin analogues have recently been reviewed (4). Although the primary structure of insulin lispro and insulin aspart differ, from a practical point of view these two molecules result in superimposable pharmacokinetics and dynamics after s.c. injection (4).

Short-acting insulin analogues improve the 1 and 2 hour post-prandial blood glucose as compared to regular human insulin because they peak earlier in the plasma (4). However, short-acting insulin analogues have a shorter duration of action as compared to regular human insulin (5). This results in a more rapid loss of glycaemic control 3–4 hours after s.c. injection of the short-acting analogue, as compared to human regular insulin (Figure 7.1). An exception is patients with new or recent onset T1 DM, in whom the residual endogenous β cell secretion prevents the insulin deficiency later after administration of lispro at mealtime (6).

To solve the problem, a dose of NPH should be added to the lispro dose at mealtime (one-third of the lispro dose) to prevent loss of blood glucose control late after meals. Under these conditions, the combination of lower post-prandial blood glucose and no deterioration of blood glucose in the fasting state, results in long-term improvement of blood glucose (Figure 7.1) (5). Long-term studies have been performed to test the hypothesis that lispro + NPH mixtures at each meal could possibly improve long-term blood glucose control better than regular insulin at each meal, while maintaining the bedtime NPH injection. Several studies with either mixtures of lispro and NPH at each meal or continuous s.c. insulin infusion (CSII) of lispro by a minipump [reviewed in (4)] have indicated that lispro decreases HbA_{1c} by $\sim$0.3–0.5 percentage points more than human regular insulin. This percentage reduction in HbA_{1c} may appear modest, but one should consider that in those studies, human regular insulin was always injected 30 minutes prior to each meal. In reality T1 DM patients often used to take regular insulin at mealtime which deteriorates HbA_{1c} (7). In addition, the improvement in HbA_{1c} in those studies [reviewed in (4)] was observed in patients who started with good values of HbA_{1c} ($< 7.0\%$) at baseline. Thus, it is likely that the improvement in HbA_{1c} in real life of T1 DM patients with long-term use of lispro at mealtime would be greater than 0.3–0.5%.

One important advantage with use of short-acting insulin analogues at meals is the more flexible life-style, because patients can not only inject immediately before the meal and eat, but also better adapt the dose to the carbohydrate intake.

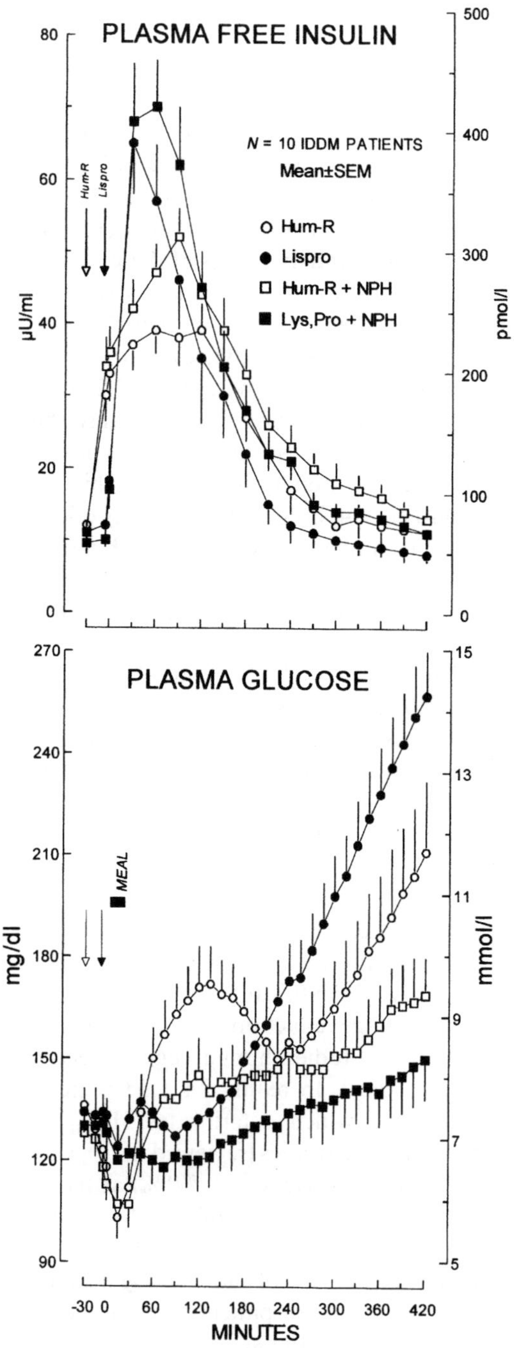
PLASMA FREE INSULIN
80
60
40
20
0
µU/ml
500
400
300
200
100
0
pmol/l
Hum-R
Lispro
N = 10 IDDM PATIENTS
Mean±SEM
Hum-R
Lispro
Hum-R + NPH
Lys,Pro + NPH
PLASMA GLUCOSE
270
240
210
180
150
120
90
mg/dl
15
13
11
9
7
5
mmol/l
MEAL
Hum-R
Lispro
-30 0 60 120 180 240 300 360 420
MINUTES

To maintain an optimal pre-prandial and fasting blood glucose control with mealtime lispro, only few units of NPH at breakfast, lunch and dinner are sufficient (4). In initial studies, the amount of NPH injected at each meal was proportional to the number of hours to the next insulin injection (4). Therefore, the NPH dose at lunch is greater than at breakfast (4). The proportion of the short-acting insulin analogue in the combination with NPH should always be predominant as compared to NPH. However, at breakfast the need for NPH is less than at lunchtime, because the time interval between breakfast and lunch is shorter than that between lunch and dinner, and because in the morning hours there is still a carryover effect of bedtime NPH from the previous night. Also, the need of NPH at dinner is small because the next bedtime NPH injection is administered within 3–4 hours. We have learned from patients that they prefer double injections with pens at each meal, rather than mixing lispro and NPH in a syringe to save one shot. This multiple daily insulin injection regimen is feasible with motivated patients, made motivated by motivated diabetologists. The future availability of pre-mixed formulations of lispro/NPL mixtures (NPL is the protamine-retarded formulation of lispro, with a pharmaco-dynamic profile essentially identical to NPH) will simplify the regimen of lispro + NPH administration at each meal. The most promising mixtures are the 'high-mix' 75/25 (75% lispro/25% NPL) which could be used at breakfast and dinner, and the 'mid-mix' 50/50 (50% lispro/50% NPL) which should be suitable at lunch. This is the basis of the proposal in the present chapter for using 'high-mix' and 'mid-mix' in combination with bedtime NPH as a model of intensive insulin therapy.

The beneficial effects of a few units of NPH added to mealtime short-acting insulin analogue are the result of appropriate plasma insulin concentrations between meals (8). A notable advantage of the multiple small doses of NPH is the low risk for interprandial hypoglycaemia as compared to once or twice daily NPH administration, because with the former approach the units delivered at each administration are fewer, the s.c. insulin depot is lower, and consequently absorption less variable (9). In fact, in a 1 year study, NPH

Figure 7.1. The s.c. injection of the short-acting insulin analogue lispro (full circles) in T1 DM patients results in more rapid appearance of insulin in the plasma, with a greater peak and faster disappearance as compared to human regular insulin (open circles) (upper panel). As a result, the 1 and 2 hour post-prandial blood glucose concentration is lower with lispro (lower panel). However, after 3 hours, hyperglycaemia is greater with lispro as compared to human regular insulin, because of lower plasma insulin concentration. The addition of 0.07 U/kg NPH insulin to mealtime lispro (closed squares) prevents the late post-prandial deterioration of blood glucose observed with lispro. Although an improvement is observed with human regular insulin plus NPH (open squares) as well, the combination lispro + NPH results in better overall post-prandial blood glucose control, as compared to human regular insulin + NPH. From (5), with permission

combined with lispro at each meal has not only decreased the percentage of HbA_{1c} more than human regular insulin at mealtime, but has also decreased the frequency of mild hypoglycaemia by $\sim$35% and improved awareness of, and counterregulation to, hypoglycaemia (10). The observation that a rational regimen of insulin delivery in T1 DM that improves long-term blood glucose control *decreases, not increases* the risk of hypoglycaemia (10) indicates that when the insulin regimen is 'tailored' to the needs of individual patients, HbA_{1c} decreases and the risk for hypoglycaemia decreases as well. This is in contrast with the finding of the DCCT study, in which a decrease in HbA_{1c} was associated with an increase in the frequency of severe hypoglycaemia (2).

REPLACEMENT OF INSULIN NEEDS IN THE POST-ABSORPTIVE STATE (BASAL INSULIN)

Physiology of insulin secretion in the post-absorptive state

In humans who have two or three meals a day, half or even two-thirds of the 24 hour period is 'post-absorptive state'. Therefore, in quantitative terms, the contribution of the post-absorptive period to overall long-term blood glucose control in T1 DM as measured by the percentage HbA_{1c} is greater than that of the post-prandial period.

Physiology teaches that in the fasting state there is a continuous secretion of insulin estimated in the range of 0.1–0.2 mU/kg/minute ($\sim$0.5–1.0 U/hour). If fasting is prolonged over 14–16 hours, the rate of endogenous insulin secretion decreases to prevent hypoglycaemia and indirectly favours hormonal and substrate-driven gluconeogenesis. It may seem paradoxical that nature has designed an ongoing insulin secretion in the post-absorptive state of the prolonged fast where the risk is hypoglycaemia. However, in the post-absorptive state, the pivotal role of insulin is not only to restrain endogenous glucose output, primarily from the liver, but mainly to limit lipolysis and excessive flux of free fatty acids to the liver. Because insulin-mediated suppression of lipolysis is a more insulin-sensitive process than insulin-mediated suppression of endogenous glucose output (11), if insulin secretion in the post-absorptive state decreases below the physiological needs, the first effect is exaggerated lipolysis, enhanced flux of free fatty acids to the liver and hepatic release of ketone bodies. If insulin deficiency progresses, then endogenous glucose production also increases and hyperglycaemia ultimately develops.

Pathophysiology of basal insulin needs in T1 DM

T1 DM patients lack not only response of insulin to meals, but also continuous insulin secretion in the post-absorptive state. It is quite easy to replace the prandial insulin needs with a bolus of insulin as s.c. injection of a short-acting insulin analogue in T1 DM. However, it remains more difficult to mimic nature in meeting the physiological insulin needs in the fasting state. The night is the longest period of post-absorptive state. Patients with T1 DM have variable insulin requirements at night, i.e. less need for insulin between midnight and 3 a.m. and ~30% greater insulin requirements between 4 a.m. and 7 a.m. (12), primarily because of decreased insulin sensitivity at the liver level (13). An ideal approach to insulin substitution at night should therefore provide variable insulin delivery, i.e. less insulin in the first than the second part of the night.

Approaches to insulin substitution in the post-absorptive state in T1 DM

The gold standard of insulin replacement in the post-absorptive state is CSII by means of an external minipump, which results in a flat, peakless insulin action profile. In addition, variability in insulin absorption is low with CSII, especially with short-acting insulin analogues, which accounts for more reproducible fasting plasma glucose as compared to injection of intermediate- or long-acting insulin preparations. As of today, CSII should be proposed to every single patient with T1 DM for replacement of insulin at night, especially to patients with plasma C-peptide concentration <0.1 nmol/l, in whom attempts to optimize blood glucose with s.c. injection of intermediate- or long-acting insulin preparations have failed.

However, minipumps are expensive. In addition, only a minority of T1 DM patients would agree to long-term use of a minipump for practical reasons. Interestingly, some patients who initially refuse to use the minipump for 24 hours/day ultimately accept a mixed regimen, i.e. multiple pen or syringe injections during the day, and CSII at night. This approach works well because it improves long-term blood glucose control, reduces nocturnal hypoglycaemia and recovers unawareness of hypoglycaemia (7). This regimen should become more popular because the benefits of CSII are demonstrable, especially at night, when minipumps deliver short-acting insulin (analogues), in contrast to NPH or Lente insulin given by syringes or pens. After all, during the day the pump administers prandial boluses of short-acting insulin (analogue), likewise syringes or pens.

More than 95% of T1 DM all over the world use intermediate- and long-acting insulin preparations for s.c. injection, i.e. NPH (and NPL), Ultralente, and mixture of 30% Semilente and 70% Ultralente (Lente). These insulin preparations have three major pharmacokinetic and pharmacodynamic defects. First, in contrast with physiological needs, NPH and Lente exibit an activity profile, with an early peak 4–5 hours after the s.c. injection (15). Second, 5–6 hours after the peak, there is a rapid waning of action. These activity profiles of intermediate-acting insulin contribute to problems of nocturnal blood glucose control in T1 DM. Thus, after the evening injection of NPH or Lente, plasma insulin peaks approximately between midnight and

2 a.m. i.e. at the time at which patients would require less insulin because they are more insulin-sensitive. This contributes to the frequent hypoglycaemia in the early night hours in T1 DM, despite a bedtime snack (15). On the other hand, when T1 DM patients require an increase in plasma insulin to meet the greater hepatic insulin requirements at dawn, the waning of the s.c.-injected intermediate-acting insulin results in increased systemic glucose production (16) and increased fasting blood glucose. Because of the 'hill-like' action profile of NPH and Lente insulin preparations, any attempt to increase plasma insulin bioavailability at dawn simply by increasing the evening insulin dose increases the risk of nocturnal hypoglycaemia, rather than improving nocturnal blood glucose homeostasis. The third pharmacokinetic defect of NPH and Lente is the large variability in absorption after their s.c. injection (9). This has to do with the dissolution process of NPH/Lente insulin crystals in the s.c. tissue into insulin and protamine or zinc. This process is poorly understood and is controlled by unknown factors which are ultimately responsible for the variability in absorption (9).

Nocturnal hypoglycaemia occurs in ~30–40% of patients (15) and causes unawareness of, impaired counterregulation to, and adapted cognitive dysfunction during hypoglycaemia the next day (14). Moreover, sleep appears to impair the counterregulatory hormone response to hypoglycaemia (17), which even further increases the seriousness of this complication. In turn, hypoglycaemia unawareness predisposes to severe hypoglycaemia (18). Nocturnal hypoglycaemia may also contribute to fasting and post-meal hyperglycaemia because of the long-lasting post-hypoglycaemic insulin resistance. Notably, these problems are not due to T1 DM *per se*, but to its treatment with poor surrogate products of basal insulin.

Long-acting insulin analogues

The present candidate long-acting analogues are being developed based on two principles. The first line of research has been to change the isoelectric point (i.e. the pH value at which insulin is least soluble and precipitates) towards neutrality by substituting/adding single amino acids to the molecule of human insulin by means of rDNA technology. The resultant insulin preparation is soluble in acid solution, but precipitates as micro-crystals after injection in the subcutaneous tissue, where the pH is neutral (4). The second principle for protracting a soluble insulin is a modification which promotes the binding to a serum carrier with prolonged half-life, such as albumin (4).

Insulin glargine

Insulin glargine (21A-Gly-30Ba-L-Arg-30Bb-L-Arg-human insulin) (HOE 901, Aventis Pharma) produced by rDNA technology, is a human insulin analogue with prolonged action. It has come to the market in the summer of the year 2000 with the trade name of Lantus®. Insulin glargine results from two modifications of human insulin. First, two positive charges (two arginine molecules) are added at the C-terminus of the B chain. This results in a shift of the isoelectric point from a pH of 5.4 to 6.7±0.2, making the molecule more soluble at slightly acidic pH and less soluble at the physiological pH of s.c. tissue. Because the derivative is formulated at an acidic pH, a second modification is needed to avoid desamidation and dimerization via the acid-sensitive asparagine residue at position 21 in the A chain. The replacement of A21 asparagine by glycine is charge-neutral and associated with good stability of the resulting human insulin analogue. Injected as a clear solution at pH 4.0, insulin glargine forms a microprecipitate at the physiologic, neutral pH of the s.c. space. The stabilization of the insulin hexamer and higher aggregates may influence the nature of the precipitate and the rate of its dissolution and absorption from the site of injection. Consequently, insulin glargine has a delayed and prolonged absorption from the injection site following s.c. administration. The structural changes in the insulin peptide result in an analogue with delayed absorption and a relatively constant basal insulin supply, consistent with that secreted by non-diabetic subjects. Because insulin glargine is formulated as a clear, acidic solution, it cannot be mixed with insulin formulated at a neutral pH, such as regular insulin. Insulin glargine is safe in terms of mitogenic, growth-promoting activity and carcinogenicity (4).

The pharmacokinetics and pharmacodynamics of insulin glargine following bolus s.c. injection have been tested in healthy subjects and patients with both T1 DM and T2 DM (4). In T1 DM, the onset of action using the isoglycaemic clamp technique occurs approximately 90 min after s.c. injection into the internal part of thigh (50 min with NPH), with a duration of action of 24 h, compared to 14 h with NPH (19). Most importantly, the action profile of insulin glargine closely mimics CSII, whereas NPH exhibits a peak action within 3–6 hours, followed by waning (2). Little or no difference exists in the absorption kinetics of insulin glargine from different sites of injection in normal (healthy) subjects (20).

Theoretically, the peakless and prolonged action profile of insulin glargine should therefore result in less frequent hypoglycaemia at night, and the ability to achieve lower fasting blood glucose and, long-term, lower glycosylated haemoglobin. Preliminary data from both short-term (4 weeks) and long-term (16–52 weeks) 'registration'-type studies only in part support these expectations (4,21). Episodes of nocturnal hypoglycaemia were reduced following transfer from once-daily NPH to insulin glargine at the same dose (21). Little or no change in percentage HbA_{1c} has, however, been observed (21). Because the design of the early clinical registration studies fails to define the optimal use of this new insulin analogue, additional studies are necessary to monitor combining insulin glargine once daily with short-acting insulin analogues at meal-time.

A major advantage of insulin glargine over both NPH and Lente insulin is that glargine can be injected without prior need of resuspension in the vial or cartridge, which is a major cause of variability in absorption of the intermediate-acting insulins. Recently, the extent of the poor compliance of T1DM and T2DM patients to accurately re-suspend NPH in cartridges prior to injection has been reported (22). In a series of clamp studies in normal volunteers, it has just been found that after s.c. injection of 0.3 U/kg of NPH, there is up to 50% difference in the time to peak plasma concentration, duration of action and overall activity profile between the properly re-suspended NPH and the non-suspended NPH (Lepore *et al*, personal communication).

The acylated insulin NN304

Another principle for protracting a soluble insulin action is a modification which promotes the binding to serum proteins like albumin. The rationale is that s.c. albumin binding, and consequently increased plasma half-life, will prolong the action profile. The analogue is created by acylation of the ε-amino group of LysB29 with a saturated fatty acid (4). The length of the fatty acid attached to the Lys B29 has a marked effect on the disappearance rate of radiolabelled insulin from the injection site. The highest affinity for albumin and most protracted duration of action was found for LysB29 tetradecanoyl-des (B30) insulin (NN304, Novo Nordisk). Absorption tested in a pig model showed that it was significantly slower than human NPH (4). Intravenous (i.v.) bolus injection of this analogue showed a protracted blood glucose lowering effect compared with human NPH insulin. The intraindividual variation of the absorption from day to day was less for NN304 than for NPH (4). Drugs known to increase the plasma free fatty acid concentration (heparin, β-agonists) and drugs in therapeutic concentration with high affinity for human serum albumin (sulphonylurea, diazepam, valproate) did not significantly influence the NN304 albumin binding (4). Due to the low plasma concentration of NN304, the insulin analogue itself cannot be expected to displace other drugs. Further studies with *in vivo* testing are, however, needed to evaluate if any clinically significant drug levels influence the time/action profile of NN304 in man.

The pharmacokinetics of insulin NN304 has been studied in an euglycaemic glucose clamp trial, comparing NN304 and NPH in healthy subjects (23). Administration of three different doses of NN304 (0.15, 0.3 and 0.6 U/kg) resulted in a proportional increase in the total area under the plasma insulin curve. Compared with NPH, NN304 exhibited a less pronounced peak and maximal concentrations were seen after 4–6 hours. However, NN304 still had a peak and no clear dose–response relationship of NN304 on glucose utilization was demonstrated. Clearly, considerable research is still needed to evaluate the relationship between the attractive pharmacokinetics and dynamics of acylated human insulin as a candidate to replace basal insulin, and its bioavailability in humans.

Models of insulin replacement

At present, there are three models of physiological insulin replacement in T1 DM. These models have in common use of a short-acting insulin analogue at each meal, in doses related to carbohydrate content. The number of daily injections of short-acting analogue is related to the number of meals per day, including snacks. The three models differ regarding substitution of basal insulin. Therefore, lispro (aspart) at mealtime can be combined with basal insulin replaced under the form of either: (a) CSII; (b) multiple daily injections of NPH; or (c) glargine once a day.

Continuous s.c. insulin infusion

It is much easier to maintain long-term near-normoglycaemia in T1 DM patients if basal insulin is replaced by mimicking the physiology of insulin secretion of normal, non-diabetic subjects in the post-absorptive state. This can be best achieved with CSII. As stated earlier, CSII should be presented to T1 DM patients as the gold standard of insulin replacement, particularly as the gold standard of basal insulin substitution, especially when short-acting insulin analogues are used at mealtimes.

Multiple daily insulin injections with NPH as basal insulin

This model is being used extensively (4). Short-acting insulin analogues should be preferred to human regular insulin at mealtime, primarily because of better life-style and also for better post-prandial blood glucose control with a lower risk of hypoglycaemia. However, use of short-acting insulin analogues requires optimization of basal insulin at the same time (4). T1 DM patients who refuse or cannot have access to CSII should use the model of multiple daily injections of NPH. This approach reproduces well what CSII does during the daytime hours, but is less than optimal as compared to CSII at night. For the reasons discussed earlier, the risk for nocturnal hypoglycaemia and fasting hyper-glycaemia are somehow direct consequences of the pharmacokinetic and pharmacodynamic properties of NPH insulin. Specific measures to limit the risk for nocturnal hypoglycaemia with bedtime NPH injection include: (a) NPH doses no greater than 0.20–0.25
U/kg; (b) NPH injection at bed-time, not at dinner time; (c) injection in the internal part of thigh, not the abdomen; (d) administration of a snack with slowly-absorbed carbohydrate (i.e. 20–40 g of bread) if blood glucose is

< 120 mg/dl (in this case, the night NPH dose should not be reduced); (e) if excessive fasting hyperglycaemia persists despite blood glucose at bedtime, < 150 mg/dl and NPH dose up to 0.25 U/kg, 2–3 units of insulin lispro (aspart) should be injected at 3 a.m. rather than increasing the bedtime NPH.

Multiple daily insulin injections with glargine as basal insulin

In this model lispro (aspart) at each meal is combined with s.c. injection of the long-acting insulin analogue glargine once daily. At present there are no studies on intensive treatment of T1 DM using this model, but only registration studies in which, however, the potentials of combination of short- and long-acting insulin analogues have not been examined (4,21). Based on data of pharmacokinetic/pharmacodynamic studies, it is expected that s.c. injection of glargine insulin mimics the effects of CSII at a single rate (Figure 7.2) (19). If so, lower frequency of nocturnal hypoglycaemia and lower fasting blood glucose should occur, as compared to nighttime administration of NPH. Preliminary data indicate this is the case (21). It is also expected that glargine will result in lower variability of day-to-day blood glucose and lower the percentage of HbA_{1c}. Clearly, specific studies addressing these key points are required.

BLOOD GLUCOSE MONITORING

T1 DM patients should regularly check their blood glucose concentration prior to each insulin injection. This is necessary to establish the dose of basal insulin, and also the dose of short-acting insulin analogue to be given with the next meal (in addition to carbohydrate content of the meal and insulin sensitivity). Because the short-acting insulin analogues improve the 2 hour post-meal blood glucose to a greater extent than human regular insulin, patients should check also the 2 hour post-meal blood glucose to titrate the meal dose of lispro (aspart).

BLOOD GLUCOSE TARGETS

Treatment of T1 DM is intensive when long-term blood glucose is near-normal, i.e. fasting, pre-meal, bedtime and 3 a.m. blood glucose between 120–140 mg/dl (6.5–7.7 mmol/l), and 2 hour after meal blood glucose < 160 mg/dl (< 8.8 mmol/l). These blood glucose targets do not aim strictly at normoglycaemia, but at moderate hyperglycaemia. Because our current treatment of T1 DM is so imperfect, we should privilege prevention of hypoglycaemia, not absolute normoglycaemia, as the primary goal, while

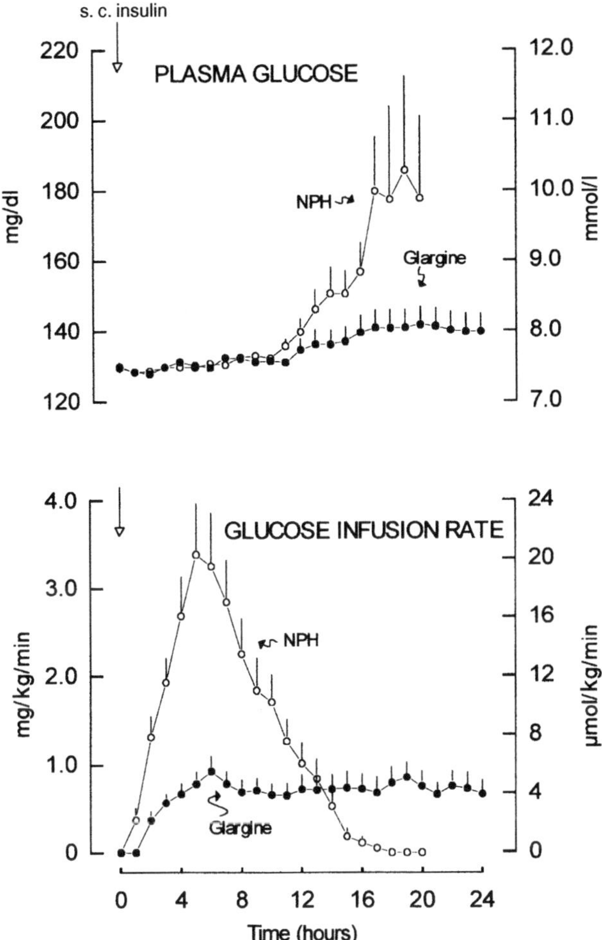

Figure 7.2. Plasma glucose concentration (upper panel) and rates of glucose infusion (lower panel) after a s.c. injection of the long-acting insulin analogue glargine as compared to NPH insulin (0.3 U/kg) in patients with T1 DM. This was a clamp study aiming at maintaining plasma glucose concentration at 130 mg/dl. Glargine maintains plasma glucose concentration at the target longer than NPH, suggesting longer duration of action (upper panel). In addition, in contrast to the peak effect of NPH, glargine is peakless (lower panel). From (19), with permission

aiming at long-term good glycaemic control. The DCCT (2) has shown that with $HbA_{1c} < 7.0\%$, i.e. a slightly greater than normal value, the risk for onset and/or progression of complications appears to be largely, if not fully, prevented. Thus, there seems to be a 'window' of values of HbA_{1c} just above the upper limit of the non-diabetic range at which patients are at the same time protected against onset/progression of complications on the one hand, and against the risk for severe hypoglycaemia, on the other. Until new, safer means of therapy become available, there is no reason to decrease the percentage HbA_{1c} to the normal range, where the risk for hypoglycaemia is greater.

EDUCATION

The time spent with the patient is the most valuable to decrease the percentage HbA_{1c} and frequency of hypoglycaemia. Unfortunately, the patients are many and the real diabetologists only a few. Diabetologists too busy in academia are not the ideal professional people to take care of patients. Nurses, although very important in their job, cannot be fully delegated to assist most of the patients' requirements.

The most important job that a diabetologist should do is to transmit to his/her patient the motivation and the enthusiasm to carry over the burden of intensive therapy (nearly) life-long. The patient should be reassured that he/she can have a normal life-style, can be nearly free of hypoglycaemia and, based on the DCCT data, free of long-term complications. Only if the patient develops a positive attitude toward his/her diabetes, and considers T1 DM not as a disease but a manageable, although sometimes tedious, condition, will the diabetologist have succeeded in his/her job. Understandably, this is particularly important with the youngest patients.

CONCLUSIONS

Insulin replacement in insulin-deficient T1 DM should be physiological. This allows maintenance of long-term near-normolgycaemia with low risk of hypoglycaemia. There are different physiological models of insulin substitution. However, all include the use of a short-acting insulin analogue at each meal (including snacks) and substitution of basal insulin, either in the form of CSII (the gold standard) or multiple NPH injections per day, or injection of insulin glargine once daily. The latter approach appears very attractive from the theoretical point of view, but needs experimental validation in large, long-term clinical trials. With physiological models of insulin substitution, it is possible to achieve glycaemic targets in both intensive and non-intensive therapy. However, to be successful, both intensive and non-intensive therapies require similar efforts by the diabetologist and patient, similar motivation and dedication. When properly performed, both intensive and non-intensive therapy improve blood glucose control, decrease the risk for hypoglycaemia and hypoglycaemia unawareness, and improve life-style.

REFERENCES

1. Reichard P, Nilsson BY, Rosenquist U: The effect of long-term intensified insulin treatment on the development of microvascular complications of diabetes mellitus. *N Engl J Med* 329:304–309, 1993.
2. The Diabetes Control and Complications Trial Research Group: The effect of intensive treatment of diabetes on the development and progression of long-term complications in insulin-dependent diabetes mellitus. *N Engl J Med* 329:977–986, 1993.
3. Dimitriadis GD, Gerich JE: Importance of timing of preprandial subcutaneous insulin administration in the management of diabetes mellitus. *Diabetes Care* 6:374–377, 1983.
4. Bolli GB, Di Marchi RD, Park GD, Pramming S, Koivisto VA: Insulin analogues and their potential in the management of diabetes mellitus. *Diabetologia* 42:1151–1167, 1999.
5. Torlone E, Pampanelli S, Lalli C *et al*: Effects of the short-acting insulin analog [LYS(B28),PRO(B29)] on postprandial blood glucose control in IDDM. *Diabetes Care* 19:945–952, 1996.
6. Pampanelli S, Torlone E, Lalli C *et al*: Improved post-prandial metabolic control after subcutaneous injection of a short-acting insulin analogue in IDDM of short duration with residual pancreatic β-cell function. *Diabet Care* 18:1452–1459, 1995.
7. Del Sindaco P, Ciofetta M, Lalli C *et al*: Use of the short-acting insulin analogue lispro in intensive treatment of IDDM: importance of appropriate replacement of basal insulin and time-interval injection-meal. *Diabet Med* 15:592–600, 1998.
8. Ciofetta M, Lalli C, Del Sindaco P *et al*: Contribution of postprandial vs. interprandial blood glucose to HbA$_{1c}$ in type 1 diabetes on physiologic intensive therapy with lispro insulin at mealtime. *Diabet Care* 22:795–800, 1999.
9. Binder C, Lauritzen T, Faber O, Pramming S: Insulin pharmacokinetics. *Diabet Care* 7:188–199, 1984.
10. Lalli C, Ciofetta M, Del Sindaco P *et al*: Long-term intensive treatment of type 1 diabetes with the short-acting insulin analogue lispro in variable combination with NPH insulin at mealtime. *Diabet Care* 22:468–477, 1999.
11. Nurjhan N, Campbell P, Kennedy F, Miles J, Gerich J: Insulin dose–response characteristics for suppression of glycerol release and conversion to glucose in humans. *Diabetes* 35:1326–1331, 1986.
12. Perriello G, De Feo P, Torlone E *et al*: The dawn phenomenon in type 1 (insulin-dependent) diabetes mellitus: magnitude, frequency, variability, and dependency on glucose counterregulation and insulin sensitivity. *Diabetologia* 34:21–28, 1991.
13. Perriello G, De Feo P, Torlone E, Fanelli C, Brunetti P, Bolli GB: Nocturnal spikes of growth hormone secretion cause the dawn phenomenon in type 1 (insulin-dependent) diabetes mellitus by decreasing hepatic (and extrahepatic) sensitivity to insulin in the absence of insulin waning. *Diabetologia* 33:52–59, 1990.
14. Kanc K, Janssen MMJ, Keulen ETP *et al*: Substitution of night-time continuous subcutaneous insulin infusion therapy for bedtime NPH insulin in a multiple injection regimen improves counterregulatory hormonal responses and warning symptoms of hypoglycaemia in IDDM. *Diabetologia* 41:322–329, 1998.
15. Bolli GB, Perriello G, Fanelli C, De Feo P: Nocturnal blood glucose control in type 1 diabetes mellitus. *Diabet Care* (Suppl 3):71–89, 1993.
16. Koivisto VA, Yki-Järvinen H, Helve E, Karonen S-L, Pelkonen R: Pathogenesis and prevention of the dawn phenomenon in diabetic patients treated with CSII. *Diabetes* 35:78–82, 1986.

17. Jones TW, Porter P, Sherwin RS *et al*: Decreased epinephrine response to hypoglycemia during sleep. *N Engl J Med* 338:1657–1662, 1998.
18. Bolli GB: Hypoglycemia unawareness. *Diabet Metab* 23 (Suppl 3):29–35, 1997.
19. Lepore M, Pampanelli S, Fanelli CG, Porcellati, Brunetti P, Bolli GB: Pharmacokinetics and dynamics of s.c. injection of insulin glargine, NPH and ultralente in T1 DM: comparison with CSII. *Diabetes* 49 (Suppl 1):A9, 2000.
20. Owens DR, Barnett A: *Diabetes: Current Perspectives.* In J Betteridge, Ed. London: Martin Dunitz, 1999.
21. Ratner RE, Hirsch IB, Neifing JL, Garg SK, Mecca TE, Wilson CA, for the USA Study group of Insulin Glargine in type 1 diabetes: Less hypoglycemia with insulin glargine in intensive treatment for type 1 diabetes. *Diabet Care* 23:639–643, 2000.
22. Jehle PM, Micheler C, Jehle DR, Breting D, Boehm BO: Inadequate suspension of neutral protamine Hagedorn (NPH) insulin in pens. *Lancet* 354:1604–1607, 1999.
23. Heinemann L, Sinha K, Weyer C, Loftager M, Hirschberger S, Heise T: Time–action profile of the soluble, fatty acid acylated, long-acting insulin analogue NN304. *Diabet Med* 16:332–338, 1999.

8

Islet Cell Transplantation in Type 1 Diabetes

KONRAD FEDERLIN, MATHIAS BRENDEL and
REINHARD G. BRETZEL
Third Medical Department and Policlinic, Justus-Liebig-University, Giessen, Germany

Long-term studies strongly suggest that tight control of blood glucose achieved by conventional intensive insulin treatment, self-blood glucose monitoring and patient education can significantly prevent the development and retard the progression of chronic complications of type 1 diabetes mellitus (1,2). However, the expense for this benefit was a three-fold increase of the number of severe hypoglycemic episodes, a significant increase in body weight, and dietary and other life-style restrictions affecting the quality of life (3).

By contrast, replacement of a patient's islets of Langerhans, either by pancreas transplantation or by isolated islet transplantation (Figure 8.1), is the only treatment of type 1 diabetes mellitus to achieve an insulin-independent, constant normoglycemic state avoiding hypoglycemic episodes (4,5). The expense of this benefit is the need for immunosuppressive treatment of the recipient, with all its potential risks. Thus, indications for pancreas or islet transplantations at present exist almost exclusively in patients with end-stage renal disease waiting on dialysis for a kidney graft, or in diabetics with an already established kidney graft being, or going to be, obligated to immunosuppression for this reason.

Islet transplantation in principle offers the possibility to alter *in vitro* the islet immunogenicity and antigenicity, to induce an immunotolerant state, or to encapsulate the islets so as to introduce only temporary immunosuppressive treatment of the recipient or to obviate the need for immunosuppression (6).

Diabetes in the New Millennium. Edited by U. Di Mario, F. Leonetti, G. Pugliese, P. Sbraccia and A. Signore.
© 2000 John Wiley & Sons, Ltd.

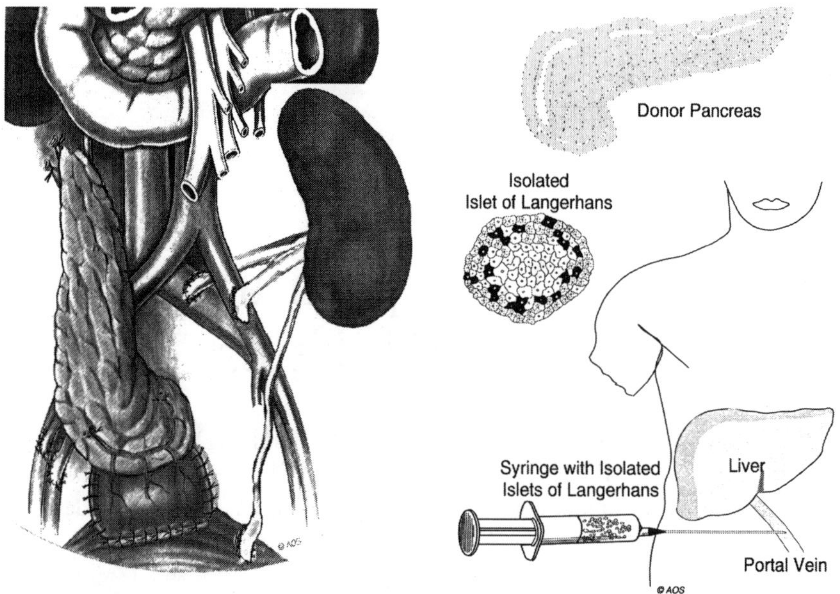

Figure 8.1. Principle of pancreas organ (left) and pancreatic islet (right) transplantation. In the technique shown on the left, the donor pancreas and donor kidney are transplanted into the pelvis. Exocrine secretion into the patient's bladder via a graft of donor duodenum. In the technique shown on the right, islets, yielded through collagenase digestion of the donor pancreas, are transplanted into the liver by percutaneous, transhepatic catheterization of the portal vein under local anesthesia

CURRENT STATUS OF CLINICAL ISLET TRANSPLANTATION

As of December 1995, a total of 270 pancreatic islet transplants in patients with type 1 diabetes mellitus had been reported to the International Islet Transplant Registry (ITR) at our department of Giessen University, Germany, and was published in the *ITR Newsletter* No. 7, 1996 (7). An update by 31 December 1998, shows that for 1990–1998 254 adult islet allografts had been performed in patients with type 1 diabetes and only eight institutions had gained experience of more than 10 cases (Table 8.1).

The number of pre-transplant C-peptide negative (no residual β cell function) patients who ever became insulin-independent for at least more than 7 days post-transplant was 32; the number of those being insulin-independent 1 year after islet transplantation was 17 (8%), with the so far longest insulin-independence follow-up of 45 months. Detailed analyses revealed that achievement of insulin independence was facilitated if islets were isolated from the pancreas with a mean preservation time of less than 8

Table 8.1. Summary of adult islet allografts in patients with type 1 diabetes according to institution and year, 1990–31 December 1998 (data on 1998 incomplete)

Institution (transplantation/isolation)	Year of transplantation									
	90	91	92	93	94	95	96	97	98	$\sum$
Giessen	–	–	1	5	5	12	11	17	6	57
Minneapolis	1	3	5	5	2	10	5	–	–	31
Pittsburgh	7	5	3	3	4	3	–	–	–	25
Milan	4	3	1	4	4	4	–	–	3	23
Miami	4	2	1	1	1	6	2	–	2	19
St Louis	3	3	2	4	2	–	–	–	–	14
Brussels	–	–	–	–	1	3	3	3	?	10
Indianapolis	–	–	–	–	–	–	4	5	1	10
Madrid	–	–	2	1	1	2	2	–	–	8
Oxford	–	1	1	1	1	2	–	1	1	8
Geneva	–	–	–	–	–	–	4	2	–	6
Edmonton	2	–	1	–	1	1	–	–	–	5
Odense/Milan	–	–	–	–	–	5	–	–	–	5
Perugia	1	1	–	–	2	–	–	–	–	4
London (Ontario)/St Louis	2	1	1	–	–	–	–	–	–	4
Stockholm/Giessen	–	–	–	–	–	–	1	2	1	4
Innsbruck/Milan	–	–	–	–	–	2	1	–	–	3
Leicester	–	2	1	–	–	–	–	–	–	3
Los Angeles (UCLA-VA)	–	–	2	–	–	–	1	–	–	3
Paris	3	–	–	–	–	–	–	–	–	3
San Francisco/Los Angeles (UCLA-VA)	–	–	–	1	1	1	–	–	–	3
Charlestown	–	1	–	–	–	–	–	–	–	1
Chicago (NMH)	–	–	–	–	–	–	1	–	–	1
Hamburg (Saar)	–	–	–	1	–	–	–	–	–	1
Lille	–	–	–	–	–	–	–	–	1	1
Omaha	–	–	–	–	1	–	–	–	–	1
Syracuse (NYUMC)	–	–	–	–	–	–	–	1	–	1
Totals	27	22	21	26	26	51	35	31	15	254
Cases transplanted 1974–1989										90
Total										344

UCLA-VA, University of California Los Angeles — Veterans Administration Medical Center; NMH Northwestern Memorial Hospital; NYUMC, New York University Medical Center.

hours; if more than 6000 islet equivalents (number of islets if all had a diameter of 150 μm) per kg body weight of the recipients were transplanted; if islets were transplanted into the liver via the portal vein; and if induction immunosuppression comprised T cell antibodies. Furthermore, analysis for preserved post-transplant β cell function (C-peptide > 0.5 ng/ml) of the graft told us that islet allotransplantation in type 1 diabetics is faced with an approximately 50% failure rate after 3 months (Figure 8.2).

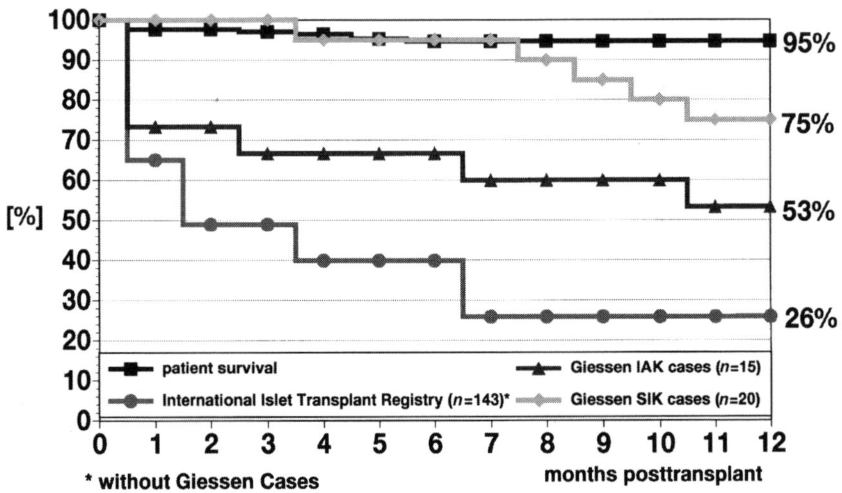

Figure 8.2. One-year patient survival (%) and human pancreatic islet allograft survival (%) in pre-transplant C-peptide-negative type 1 diabetic recipients

Therefore, we implemented into our clinical islet transplant protocol at Giessen University strategies previously shown to promote islet engraftment in experimental models. Using this protocol of refined peritransplant management, we very recently reported a markedly improved 3 months islet cell function rate of 100% for simultaneous islet–kidney (SIK) recipients and 75% for islet-after-kidney (IAK) recipients (8). A follow-up study in our first 37 consecutive cases (SIK, $n=20$ and IAK, $n=17$) illustrates a significantly improved 1 year islet allograft survival of 75% for SIK cases and of 53% for IAK cases, compared to 26% for SIK/IAK cases, reported to the Registry (Figure 8.2). Meanwhile, nine of the 37 (24%) islet recipients transplanted at our center achieved insulin independence, compared to only 8% described in the analysis of the Registry Data.

PERSPECTIVES OF CLINICAL ISLET TRANSPLANTATION

The most appealing aspect of this treatment concept is to transplant islets in non-uremic type 1 diabetic patients long before significant secondary lesions have developed, and this may include also diabetic children (Figure 8.3). We have recently performed for the first time islet transplants alone (ITA) in non-uremic patients with long-standing type 1 diabetes mellitus suffering from hypoglycemia unawareness, defect glucose counterregulation and experiencing recurrent episodes of severe hypoglycemia. We found that intraportal islet

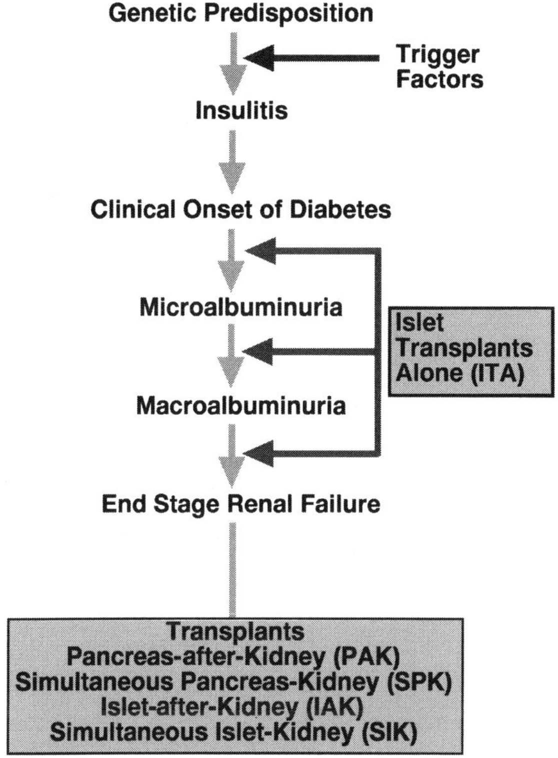

Figure 8.3. Timing of pancreas organ and pancreatic islet transplantation and the perspectives of islet transplants alone (ITA) in the natural course of type 1 diabetes mellitus

transplantation significantly improved the responses of most counterregulatory hormones and (autonomic and neuroglycopenic) hypoglycemia warning symptoms (9).

However, in order to extend the indications for islet transplantations towards the ultimate target group, non-uremic young or adult type 1 diabetic patients, two big hurdles have to be jumped: the allo- and autoimmune destruction of the islet graft and the limited donor tissue supply. Approaches to overcome these obstacles are to encapsulate the islets or to induce immunotolerance by either transient systemic application of anti-CD4/anti-CD45 monoclonal antibodies or cytotoxic T lymphocyte antigen 4–immunoglobulin (CTLA4-Ig), intrathymic transplantation of islets or donor antigens or co-transplantation of donor bone-marrow stem cells, viral or ballistic gene transfer for local expression of immunoregulatory, anti-inflammatory or apoptosis-promoting proteins and cytokines in islets, or provided by co-transplanted bystander cells (Table 8.2). Approaches currently investigated to

Table 8.2. Perspectives of immunotolerance induction methods effective in animal experiments to overcome the problem of islet allograft rejection in man

- Transient systemic application of anti-CD4/anti-CD45 monoclonal antibodies
- Systemic application of CTlA4-Ig
- Intrathymic transplantation of islets or donor antigens
- Co-transplantation of donor bone-marrow stem cells
- Viral and ballistic gene transfer for local expression of immunoregulatory, anti-inflammatory or apoptosis-promoting proteins and cytokines in islets or provided by co-transplanted bystander cells (i.e. myoblasts, Sertoli cells) (e.g. IL-4; IL-10; IL-12; TGF-β; CTLA4-Ig; IL-1 receptor antagonists; TNF-α; FasL; Bcl-2 or A20; HSP and antioxidative enzymes

CTLA4-Ig, cytotoxic T-lymphocyte antigen 4-immunoglobulin; IL, Interleukin; TGF, transforming growth factor; TNF, tumor necrosis factor; FasL, Fas ligand; Bcl-2, B cell lymphoma protein-2; A20, anti-apoptosis protein 20; HSP, heat shock protein.

Table 8.3. Approaches currently under investigation to overcome the problem of limited donor tissue supply

1. Isolation and growth of islet precursor cells (islet 'progenitor' or 'stem cells')
2. Genetic engineering of β cell lines
3. Conditional immortalization of islet cells through genetic engineering ('transgenic cell lines')
4. Removal of somatic cells (e.g. fibroblasts, keratinocytes) from a diabetic patient and transfection of the cells with a new copy of the human preproinsulin gene linked to a promoter ('somatic gene therapy')

overcome the problems with a limited donor tissue supply are the isolation and growth of islet precursor cells, genetic engineering of β cell lines, conditional immortalization of islet cells through genetic engineering (transgenic cell lines) and somatic gene therapy by transfection of cells removed from the patient (e.g. fibroblasts, keratinocytes) with a new copy of the human prepro-insulin gene linked to a promoter (Table 8.3).

REFERENCES

1. The Diabetes Control and Complications Trial Research Group: The effect of intensive treatment of diabetes on the development and progression of long-term complications in insulin-dependent diabetes mellitus. *N Engl J Med* 329:977–986, 1993.
2. Wang PH, Lau J, Chalmers TC: Meta-analysis of effects of intensive blood-glucose control on late complications of type-1 diabetes. *Lancet* 341:1306–1309, 1993.
3. The Diabetes Control and Complications Trial Research Group: Hypoglycemia in the Diabetes Control and Complications Trial. *Diabetes* 46:271–286, 1997.

4. Sutherland DE, Gores PF, Farney AC *et al*: Evolution of kidney, pancreas, and islet transplantation for patients with diabetes at the University of Minnesota. *Am J Surg* 166:456–491, 1993.
5. Bretzel RG, Browatzki CC, Schultz A *et al*: Clinical islet transplantation in diabetes mellitus — report of the Islet Transplant Registry and the Giessen Center experience. *Diabet Stoffw* 2:378–390, 1993.
6. American Diabetes Association: Pancreas transplantation for patients with diabetes mellitus. *Diab Care* 15:1668–1672, 1992.
7. Hering BJ, Brendel MD, Schultz AO, Schultz B, Bretzel RG: Adult islet allografts in patients with type-1 diabetes. *ITR Newsletter* 6:9–15, 1996.
8. Bretzel RG, Brandhorst D, Brandhorst H *et al*: Improved survival of intraportal pancreatic islet cell allografts in patients with type-1 diabetes mellitus by refined peritransplant management. *J Mol Med* 77:140–143, 1999.
9. Meyer C, Hering BJ, Grossmann R *et al*: Improved glucose counterregulation and autonomic symptoms after intraportal islet transplants alone in patients with long-standing type I diabetes mellitus. *Transplantation* 66:233–240, 1998.

9

New Hope from Organ and Tissue Transplantation in Diabetic Patients

ANTONIO SECCHI, LUCA FALQUI, ALBERTO DAVALLI
and GUIDO POZZA

Istituto Scientifico and Università Vita e Salute, San Raffaele,
Milano Università degli Studi di Milano, Milan, Italy

For years transplantation of organs was considered at high risk in diabetic patients, due to the severe conditions of these patients when requiring transplantation: not only were they affected by the consequences of organ failure (liver, kidney, heart) but also micro- or macroangiopathy rendered these patients very sick. Immunosuppression was generally based on drugs, such as high-dose steroids, that enhanced the consequences of late complications of diabetes.

The availability of less toxic and more effective drugs and the increase of clinical expertise made organ transplantation feasible and relatively safe in diabetic patients. Today diabetic patients benefit from organ transplantation like other patients.

New hopes for diabetic patients came from three different approaches in the field of transplantation:

- Pancreas transplantation, aimed at controlling late complications of diabetes, mainly macroangiopathy.
- Islet transplantation aiming at replacing β cell function with a low-invasive method.
- Gene therapy.

Diabetes in the New Millennium. Edited by U. Di Mario, F. Leonetti, G. Pugliese, P. Sbraccia and A. Signore.
© 2000 John Wiley & Sons, Ltd.

EFFECTS OF PANCREAS TRANSPLANTATION ON DIABETIC CARDIOMYOPATHY AND ENDOTHELIAL DYSFUNCTION

The effects of pancreas transplantation on late complications of diabetes were the object of several studies during the last 20 years: nephropathy and neuropathy play positive roles, showing a reversion of already established dysfunctions, while retinopathy does not show further progression, although it does not ameliorate after pancreas transplantation. Despite several investigations performed to evaluate the effects of pancreas transplantation on macroangiopathy, no definitive evidence of a positive effect was available until recently, when long-term studies focused on progression or regression of cardiovascular disease and/or underlying dysfunction, such as endothelial dysfunction, became available.

The impact of tight metabolic control achieved with pancreas transplantation on major determinants of progression of cardiovascular disease was evaluated at three levels: rate of hypertension, diabetic cardiomyopathy and endothelial dysfunction.

Hypertension

When patients affected by arterial hypertension are submitted to kidney or kidney–pancreas transplantation, only 51% of patients with a pancreas transplant are hypertensive at 1 year, *vs.* 81% patients with kidney alone (1). This difference is positively correlated with serum insulin levels and negatively correlated with HbA_{1c}. It is known that insulin resistance and hypertension are frequently associated in diabetic and non-diabetic patients, and a cause–effect relationship was hypothesized. Furthermore, pancreas transplantation has a positive effect on insulin resistance. The positive effects of pancreas transplantation on the rate of hypertension in these patients is probably the consequence of an improvement of insulin sensitivity.

Cardiac function

Diastolic filling more than systolic function is frequently impaired in these patients. The effects of glycometabolic control achieved by pancreas transplantation on left ventricular function were evaluated in uremic IDDM patients in a recent study in 337 uremic IDDM patients, enrolled on a waiting list for kidney–pancreas transplantation: 115 underwent kidney–pancreas transplantation, 34 underwent kidney transplantation alone, whereas 196 patients remained on dialysis (2). Actuarial survival and causes of death were recorded over a period of 7 years. Left ventricular systolic and diastolic function were evaluated with radionuclide ventriculography in a subset of 42 kidney–pancreas (KP) and 26 kidney-alone (KA) recipients (3). The two populations were matched for the most common cardiovascular risk factors. Patients were grouped according to years of follow-up (6 months, 14 KP and nine KA; 2 years, 13 KP and eight KA; 4 years, 15 KP and nine KA). The seven year survival rate was 76.2% for KP, 63.5% for KA and 39.6% for the dialyzed group ($p = 0.001$). The cardiovascular death rate was 7.8% in KP, 14.7% in KA and 16.1% in dialyzed (KP *vs.* dialyzed, $p = 0.05$). The left ventricular ejection fraction was normal in all the patients, with statistically significant higher values in KP transplanted patients with 4 years of graft function ($75.7 \pm 1.8\%$) than in KA with 4 years of graft function ($65.3 \pm 2.8\%$, $p < 0.05$) and IDDM patients ($61.3 \pm 3.7\%$, $p = 0.004$). In patients with 2 and 4 years of graft function, normal diastolic parameters were evident in KP but not in KA and in IDDM (KP *vs.* KA and vs. IDDM: peak filling rate $= 4.46 \pm 0.15$ EDV/s vs. 2.73 ± 0.24 EDV/s, $p < 0.05$, and vs. IDDM $= 3.39 \pm 0.30$ EDV/s, $p = 0.007$; time to peak filling rate $= 141.9 < 7.8$ ms vs. 209.4 ± 13.5 ms, $p < 0.05$ vs. 162.0 ± 7.5 ms; PFR:PER ratio: KP, 1.10 ± 0.04 vs. KA, 0.81 ± 0.08, $p < 0.05$ vs. 0.99 ± 0.16). Diastolic dysfunction was observed in KP and KA patients with 6 months of follow-up, whereas a statistical significant reduction of the rate of diastolic dysfunction was observed 4 years after transplant in KP (pre-transplant, 73%; post-transplant, 26%) but not in KA transplantation (pre-transplant, 88%; post-transplant, 77%) (26). These results were positively correlated with an improvement of glycometabolic and blood pressure control. From these data it appears that normalization of blood glucose metabolism obtained through KP transplant exerts positive effects on survival, cardio-vascular death rate, left ventricular function and blood pressure.

Atherosclerotic risk factors and endothelial dysfunction

The effects of pancreas transplantation on atherosclerotic risk factors, endothelial dysfunction (EDD) and progression of intima-media thickening (IMT) was also evaluated in IDDM patients. Sixty patients submitted to KP treatment and in 30 to KA treatment were studied (4). Atherosclerotic risk factors [i.e. lipid status, fasting and post-methionine load homocysteine (tHcy), von Willebrand factor levels (vwf), D-dimer fragments (ddf), fibrinogen], Doppler-echographic evaluation of IMT, and assessment of endothelial function with flow-mediated dilation (EDD) and nitrates dilation (NDD) of the brachial artery were evaluated. KA, but not KP, showed higher values of HbA$_{1c}$ (KP $= 6.2 \pm 0.1$ vs. KA $= 8.4 \pm 0.5\%$, $p = 0.001$), tHcy (KP $= 13.8 \pm 0.9$ vs. KA $= 19.3 \pm 3.1$ mmol/l, $p = 0.02$), vwf levels (KP $= 173.0 \pm 11.3$ vs. KA $= 247.3 \pm 21.3\%$, $p = 0.003$), ddf (KP $= 0.48 \pm 0.07$ vs. KA $= 0.79 \pm 0.18$ g/ml, $p = 0.06$), fibrinogen (KP $= 369.6 \pm 20.6$ vs. KA $= 905.1 \pm 100.1$ mg/dl, $p = 0.10$) and triglycerides (KP $= 122.7 \pm 8.6$ vs. KA $= 187.0 \pm 30.1$ mg/dl, $p = 0.01$). As regards endothelial function, KP, but not KA, showed a normal EDD (KP $= 6.21 \pm 2.42$ vs. KA $= 0.65 \pm 2.74\%$, $p < 0.01$), while no differences were found for NDD (KP = 9.28 ± 4.3 vs. KA = $5.92 \pm 3.79\%$, not significant). Moreover, IMT was reduced in the KP group rather than in the KA group (KP = 0.743 ± 0.03 vs. KA = 0.865 ± 0.09 mm, $p = 0.04$). From these data it appears that IDDM patients receiving KP treatment have a lower atherosclerotic risk profile than IDDM patients receiving KA treatment. These differences are closely correlated with metabolic control, lower tHcy levels and reduced ddf and vwf levels.

ISLET TRANSPLANTATION IN IDDM PATIENTS

Islet allotransplantation to cure type 1 diabetic patients was proposed by Lacy in the 1970s, who first developed islet isolation procedure.

After 20 years of experimental work, the first islet allotransplantation was performed in 1989 in St Louis (5). After this first attempt several centers started a human islet transplant program. Clinical results, in terms of insulin independence, were not fully satisfying. The registry data showed a low rate of insulin independence at 1 month (13%) that was further reduced at 1 year (8%). Better results were achieved in selected centers, ranging from 30% to 50% insulin independence, although the rate of recurrence of diabetes was still high (6–8). New approaches were proposed to improve these results, mainly focusing at facilitating islet grafting or reducing islet exhaustion.

In order to prevent islet exhaustion due to the stressful condition of recently transplanted islets, which have to tackle hyperglycemia and reduced insulin sensitvity, a protocol including metformin was started in Milan in 1998. The action of metformin on insulin sensivity was supposed to reduce insulin resistance, thus allowing better functional recovery of the islet.

The Milan experience: metformin to prevent islet exhaustion

The first islet graft was performed in Milan in 1989. In this early series of islet allotransplantations in type 1 diabetic patients, evidence of graft function was obtained in five out of six recipients, with reduction of exogenous insulin requirement above 50% of pre-transplantation values in four patients, and complete insulin independence in one patient (7,8). In a more recent experience, seven of 20 type 1 diabetic patients became insulin-independent and two additional patients experienced a 50% decreased exogenous insulin requirement with sustained C-peptide secretion; eight out of nine received islets after a prior kidney graft (8). Three patients showed high C-peptide levels immediately after transplantation, followed by undetectable C-peptide levels, presumably as a consequence of acute rejection. One patient in this cohort did not receive anti-lymphocyte globulin (ALG), due to previous cytomegalovirus uveitis, while anti-thymocyte globulin (ATG) was suspended in another patient for serum sickness. In the last patient, C-peptide secretion was lost concurrently with a steroid-resistant kidney rejection. Functional exhaustion of the transplanted islets was considered responsible for graft failure in a third group of patients (40%), where the post-transplantation increase in C-peptide levels was not accompanied by any metabolic improvement. In these patients, insulin requirement increased after transplantation and C-peptide disappeared in about 4 months. The number of islets transplanted was significantly higher in the successful cases than in patients with presumed functional exhaustion (IEQ 11 137 + 907 vs. 7487 + 025, $p < 0.05$). In addition to the islet mass, another parameter that positively influenced the success of the implantation was the strict metabolic control of the recipients in the early post-surgical period, achieved by intravenous insulin administration to keep glycemic levels constantly below 150 mg/dl. The rationale for this intensive insulin treatment is based on the exquisite susceptibility of human islets to the toxic effects of high glucose concentrations (9).

In our last series of transplantation, we obtained evidence of graft function (post-transplantation C-peptide levels above 1 ng/ml) in all 10 recipients, and insulin independence in about 60% of them. The reasons for these excellent results are probably a new standardized islet isolation procedure and, perhaps, the use in the post-implantation period of a novel adjuvant therapy aimed at reducing insulin resistance in the recipient to diminish the metabolic demand placed on the transplanted islets. To this end, we tested the effect of metformin administration on the function of islet allografts. Metformin is an anti-diabetic drug widely used in patients with type 2 (non-insulin dependent) diabetes and obesity, which acts by increasing the sensitivity of peripheral tissues to the action of insulin, thereby allowing the achievement of normal glucose homeostasis in spite of inadequate insulin secretion. Increasing the sensitivity to insulin of peripheral tissues in patients undergoing islet transplantation might put transplanted islets at partial rest, thereby reducing the risk of their functional exhaustion. Moreover, it has been recently shown that metformin restores normal secretory patterns in islets whose function has been impaired by chronic exposure to elevated free fatty acids or glucose levels. Indeed, our recent results suggest that metformin may contribute to the improvement of the outcome of islet grafts in diabetic recipients, mainly by decreasing the number of grafts lost for functional exhaustion.

'Solitary' islet transplantation

The accumulated experience will help to develop strategies aimed at solving the obstacles, that have been now clearly defined. The appropriate selection of recipients, the availability of non-diabetogenic immunosuppression, and the avoidance of steroids, are expected to improve the long-term survival of islet transplantation in type 1 diabetic patients. Of course, the ultimate aim of islet transplantation remains to cure type 1 diabetic patients before the chronic degenerative complications of diabetes. At the time of diagnosis, most of these patients maintain a significant residual β cell mass that can survive for a prolonged period of time if β cells are kept at rest by intensive insulin treatment (10). Similarly, the survival of residual endogenous β cells should increase following a successful islet graft, early after diagnosis. Obviously the graft should be performed under the cover of an immunosuppressive strategy capable of inhibiting rejection of transplanted islets and autoimmune destruction of residual and transplanted β cells. The goal of a solitary islet graft, performed at the diagnosis of type 1 diabetes and capable of inducing life-long disease remission, appears to be less distant.

Indeed, it has been recently demonstrated that insulin independence can be achieved after solitary islet transplantation in type 1 diabetic patients using steroid-free immunosuppression (11). A series of five patients were transplanted with $> 10\,000$ IE/kg isolated from two or more donors, and were then treated with anti-IL-2 receptor antibodies and ultra-low-dose tacrolimus and sirolimus therapy. The results are impressive, with all five patients attaining immediate and sustained exogenous insulin independence, and all remain off insulin currently, with a median follow-up of about 6 months. Even though, as learned by the case of long-term insulin independence previously reported, it is still early to conclude that such immunosuppressive therapy will consent a real stability of the graft, the outcome of these solitary islet grafts is remarkable.

However, solitary islet transplantation will become a real therapeutic option for all diabetic patients only when strategies aimed at the induction of tolerance will come to fruition. We recently showed that co-administration of mycophenolate mofetil and 1,25-dihydroxyvitamin D_3, an immunomodulator that can downregulate costimulatory molecules on dendritic cells and macrophages, induces tolerance to fully-mismatched islet allografts in mice (12). Tolerance to islet allografts is associated with peri-transplant lymphomono-nuclear cell infiltration, characterized by $CD4^+$ cells with a memory resting phenotype and a reduced proportion of antigen-presenting cells, expressing downregulated costimulatory molecules. Alloreactive T cells from tolerant mice transfer tolerance to islet grafts with an alloantigen-specific active tolerogenic mechanism. Because of the low toxicity profile of mycophenolate mofetil and 1,25-dihydroxyvitamin D_3 we are currently planning to start a clinical trial of solitary islet transplantation in type 1 diabetic patients by utilizing this pharmacologic approach.

GENE THERAPY

Engineered β cell lines

An alternative β cell source for replacement therapy may be provided by xenogeneic (rodent) β cell lines, which are available in large supply, genetically engineered for 'humanized' functions. The genetic manipulation is directed to replace a rodent gene with a human insulin gene, to fine-tune the machinery of insulin secretion for glucose responsiveness in the human physiologic range (13, 14), and to control cell replication by temperature-dependent molecular switches (15). The translation of such a genetic engineering approach into a clinical prospect, however, relies on the development of safe and biocompatible devices to contain and immune-isolate the manipulated cells after transplantation (16). Unfortunately, this issue is still unsolved, despite more than a decade of efforts dedicated to the development of encapsulation technology (17, 18).

Elementary substitutive β cells

A different gene therapy approach is directed to express the human insulin gene in non-endocrine cells, in order to develop 'substitutive β cells'. Pancreatic β cells, however, are unique not only in expressing the insulin gene, but also because they possess additional characteristics which are exquisitely suited for their physiological role. They have an efficient system to translate the preproinsulin mRNA into proinsulin, they efficiently sort the nascent proinsulin into secretory granules (19,20); they contain specific peptidases that cleave proinsulin into insulin and C-peptide with high efficiency (21); and, most importantly, β cells respond to increases in extracellular glucose concentration by promptly activating exocytotic release of insulin and augmenting its synthesis (22,23). A 'substitutive β cell' should ideally contain all these features; it is clear, however, that such a degree of complexity in genetic engineering is beyond present-day capabilities.

Within the boundaries of these limitations, it is conceivable to genetically engineer suitable target cells in order to produce 'elementary β cells', nevertheless capable of the essential function of native β cells — the glucose-regulated release of insulin. The candidate target cell should be autologous, to escape rejection in the absence of immunosuppressive therapy or immune-isolating devices, should be available in large amounts and should be amenable to genetic manipulation.

The hepatocytes represent attractive target cells to be engineered for a glucose-regulated insulin synthesis because they naturally contain the glycolytic enzyme glucokinase which, coupled to the low-affinity membrane glucose transporter (GLUT)-2 confers to β cells the property to 'sense' glucose variations in the physiologic range (13,24). Hepatocytes, however, lack the endocrine cell machinery of granule formation and regulated exocytosis. For this reason, the control of a glucose-regulated release of insulin needs to be exerted at the level of insulin gene transcription. Such control would not have the exquisite sensitivity displayed by the normal pancreas, which responds with a burst of insulin release within 15–30 s after acute elevations in blood glucose. Nevertheless, transcriptional activation could result in secretion of insulin with a 30–60 minute lag period, which is reminiscent of the pattern seen in the clinically-silent phase of prediabetes (25), and which obviously is far better than the negligible insulin production of the diabetic patient. To be proposed for future clinical application, such 'elementary β cells' should produce a sustained basal insulin release coupled to a 10 to 20-fold glucose-induced increment over 1–2 hour lag period. Such a dynamic should be sufficient to control both fasting and post-prandial glucose variations. This hypothesis derives from clinical studies performed in the small number of diabetic patients who became insulin-independent after islet transplantation to the liver. These subjects, who maintain normal fasting and post-prandial blood glucose values and normal glycated hemoglobin, respond to an intravenous glucose challenge with a four- to six-fold increment of insulin secretion, which progressively develops in 1–2 hours post-challenge (26).

Transcriptional regulation of insulin synthesis in engineered hepatocytes

A significant advantage of liver cells to host a transcriptionally controlled insulin synthesis is due to their natural property to modulate endogenous gene expression in response to extracellular carbohydrate levels. An entire set of liver genes, mostly coding for enzymes of the glycolytic and lipolytic metabolic pathways, are induced *in vitro* and *in vivo* by high glucose levels (27,28). This effect is mediated by carbohydrate-responsive DNA regulatory elements (ChoRE, or glucose-responsive elements GlRE), first identified in the promoter of the liver-type pyruvate kinase (L-PK) gene (29), and subsequently described in the regulatory regions of several other genes (30,31). A 230 bp fragment of the L-PK promoter is able to confer glucose-responsive expression to a reporter gene in an hepatocyte-like murine cell line (32). Additionally, experimental evidence suggests that the L-PK promoter is triggered by glucose and fructose metabolism and is rapidly inhibited, via cyclic AMP, by glucagon (33,34). Since glucagon levels sharply increase when blood glucose levels are reduced, such a negative transcriptional effect may provide a safety system to shut off insulin production during hypoglycemia.

Proinsulin processing by non-endocrine cells

Hepatocytes, as all non-endocrine cells, lack the β cell-specific endo-proteases for proinsulin cleavage to insulin. This limitation has been circumvented by introducing a genetic modification into the proinsulin molecule (35). The substitution of two amino acids (a Leu to Arg at the A-chain/C-peptide junction and a Lys to Arg at the B-chain/C-peptide junction) generates the cleavage motifs recognized by the ubiquitous protease furin. By a retrovirus-mediated gene transfer procedure, we induced the synthesis of the furin-sensitive human proinsulin (Fur-HPI) and obtained the release of mature insulin in rodent and human primary cells, as fibroblasts, myocytes and hepatocytes (36). The vector-derived, furin-processed insulin displayed *in vitro* activity comparable to wild-type human insulin. Moreover, the retroviral-derived insulin released by engineered human fibroblasts implants into the peritoneal cavity of immuno-incompetent diabetic mice efficiently reduced blood glucose values. Subsequently, however, insulin levels progressively increased because of transplanted cell proliferation and recipient animals became hypoglycemic, pointing out one of the limitations of the *ex vivo* approach.

Liver-directed gene therapy

Liver-directed gene therapy is currently considered for correction of several inherited and acquired disorders (37). Explorative studies aimed at IDDM gene therapy demonstrated that human proinsulin synthesis can be induced in cultured hepatocytes by disparate gene transfer tools (48,36). The *ex vivo* approach is limited by the surgical risk of segmental liver harvesting, by a labor-intensive procedure for transduction of hepatocytes in culture and, most importantly, by poor grafting ($\leqslant 7\%$) of transplanted hepatocytes (38). These limitations make the *ex vivo* procedure unsuitable for IDDM gene therapy. The feasibility of an *in vivo* approach has been explored in a single study, by intraportal injection of a retroviral vector to express rat proinsulin in rat livers. However, because of the absence of proinsulin processing, and possibly because of low transduction efficiency, mature insulin was not detected in the blood and metabolic effects in the diabetic recipients were mainly limited to the prevention of lethal acute ketosis (39).

In recent years however, *in vivo* gene transfer to liver cells has been successfully accomplished using adeno- (40), lenti- (41) and adeno-associated viral vectors [rAAVv, recently reviewed by Ferry and Heard (49)]. These vectors can accommodate from 4.7 kb (in the case of rAAVv) to ~30 kb (for AdVv) of foreign DNA, which may contain the therapeutic gene and other DNA elements for transcriptional and post-transcriptional control. Indeed, a number of ubiquitous, tissue-specific or regulatable promoters have been included into rAAVv, to obtain distinct levels of production of transgenic proteins (42–44). Hepatic gene transfer by rAAVv produced therapeutic amounts of human factor IX in mice for up to 17 months (45,46) and sub-therapeutic levels of canine factor IX in hemophilic dogs, for at least 8 months. Very recently, Thulè and Liu (47) have reported the results of initial studies, in which they have been able to modulate blood glucose levels in diabetic rats by *in vivo* gene transfer of an AdV-expressing insulin under the transcriptional control of a glucose responsive promoter.

CONCLUSIONS

Despite major hurdles to be overcome, a gene therapy approach to insulin-dependent diabetes is now conceivable, either in the form of transplantation of murine β cells with humanized functions into immunoprotective devices or as a viral vector-mediated gene transfer into non-endocrine cells to develop the elementary β cell function of glucose-regulated insulin production. In these coming years, continuous improvements in microencapsulation and in gene transfer technologies, coupled to extensive studies in appropriate animal models, will allow evaluation of the effectiveness of these strategies, hopefully opening the way to the clinical application.

REFERENCES

1.	La Rocca E, Secchi A, Gianotti L *et al*: Kidney and pancreas transplantation improves hypertension in type I diabetic patients. 7th Congress of the European Society for Organ Transplantation, ESOT 1995; Vienna, October 3–7, 1995, *Abstract Book* 362, 1995.
2.	La Rocca E, Fiorina P, Astorri E *et al*: Patients' survival and cardiovascular events after kidney–pancreas transplantation: comparison with kidney transplantation alone in uremic IDDM patients. *Cell Transplant* (in press).
3.	Fiorina P *et al*: Reversal of left ventricular diastolic dysfunction after kidney–pancreas transplantation in uremic IDDM patients. *Acta Diabetol* (in press).
4.	Fiorina P *et al*: Effects of kidney pancreas transplantation on athersoclerotic risk factors and endothelial dysfunction in IDDM patients. *Diabetes* (in press).
5.	Schard DW, Lacy PE, Santiago JV *et al*: Results of our first nine intraportalislet allograft in IDD patients. *Transplantation* 51:76–85, 1991.
6.	Bretzel RG, Brandhorst D, Brandhorst H *et al*: Improved survival of inraportal pancreatic islet cell allografts in patients with IDDM by refined peritransplant management. *J Mol Med* 77:140–143, 1999.
7.	Socci C, Falqui L, Davalli AM *et al*: Fresh human islet transplantation to replace pancreatic endocrine function in type 1 diabetic patients. *Acta Diabetol* 28:151–157, 1991.
8.	Secchi A, Socci C, Maffi P *et al*: Islet transplantation in IDDM patients. *Diabetologia* 40:225–231, 1997.
9.	Davalli AM, Ricordi C, Socci C *et al*: Abnormal sensitivity to glucose of human islets cultured in a high glucose medium: partial reversibility after an additional culture in a normal glucose medium. *J Clin Endocrinol Metab* 72:202–208, 1991.
10.	Mirouze J, Selam JL, Pham TC, Mendoza E: Remission of diabetes during conventional insulin therapy or therapy controlled by use of an artificial pancreas. *Semin Hôp* 55:354–359, 1979.
11.	Shapiro AMJ, Lakey JRT, Ryan E *et al*: Insulin independence after solitary islet transplantation in type 1 diabetic patients using steroid-free immunosuppression. *Transplantation* 69 (Suppl 1), 2000.
12.	Gregori S, Casorati M, Amuchastegui S *et al*: Transplantation tolerance by 1,25dihydroxyvitamin D_3 induced T cell costimulation blockade. 17th Congresso Italiano di Immunologia, Ferrara, 7–10 June 2000.

13. Newgard CB: Cellular engineering and gene therapy strategies for insulin replacement in diabetes. *Diabetes* 43:341–350, 1994.

14. Clark SA, Quaade C, Constandy H *et al*: Novel insulinoma cell lines produced by iterative engineering of GLUT-2, glucokinase and human insulin expression. *Diabetes* 46:958–967, 1997.

15. Efrat S, Leiser M, Surana M, Tal M, Fusco-Demane D, Fleisher N: Murine insulinoma cell line with normal glucose-regulated insulin secretion. *Diabetes* 42:901–907, 1993.

16. Lanza RP, Sullivan SJ, Chick WL: Islet transplantation with immunoisolation. *Diabetes* 41:1503–1510, 1992.

17. Siebers U, Horcher A, Bretzel RG, Federlin K, Zekorn T: Alginate-based microcapsules for immunoprotected islet transplantation. *Ann NY Acad Sci* 831:304–312, 1997.

18. De-Vos P, De-Haan BJ, Wolters GH, Strubbe JH, Van-Schilfgaarde R: Improved biocompatibility but limited graft survival after purification of alginate for microencapsulation of pancreatic islets. *Diabetologia* 40:262–270, 1997.

19. Orci L, Ravazzola M, Amherdt M *et al*: Conversion of proinsulin to insulin occurs coordinately with acidification of maturing secretory vescicles. *J Cell Biol* 103:2273–2281, 1986.

20. Orci L, Ravazzola M, Storch M-J, Anderson RGW, Vassalli J-D, Perrelet A: Proteolytic maturation of insulin is a post-Golgi event which occurs in acidifying clathrin-coated secretory vescicles. *Cell* 49:865–868, 1987.

21. Smeekens SP, Montag, AG, Thomas G *et al*: Proinsulin processing by the subtilisin-related preprotein convertases furin, PC2 and PC3. *Proc Natl Acad Sci USA* 89:8822–8826, 1992.

22. Nielsen DA, Welsh M, Casadaban MJ, and Steiner DF: Control of insulin gene expression in pancreatic β-cells and in an insulin-producing cell line. *J Biol Chem* 260:13585–13589, 1985.

23. Boam DSW, Clark AR, and Docherty K: Positive and negative regulation of the human insulin gene by multiple *trans*-acting factors. *J Biol Chem* 265:8285–8296, 1990.

24. German MS: Glucose sensing in pancreatic islet beta cells: the key role of glucokinase and the glycolytic intermediates. *Proc Natl Acad Sci USA* 90:1781–1785, 1993.

25. Srikanta G, Ganda OP, Gleason RE, Jackson RA, Soeldner JS, and Eisenbarth GS: Pre-type 1 diabetes: linear loss of beta cell response to intravenous glucose. *Diabetes* 33:717–720, 1984.

26. Luzi L, Hering B, Socci C *et al*: Metabolic effects of successful intraportal islet transplantation in insulin-dependent diabetes mellitus. *J Clin Invest* 97:2611–2618, 1996.

27. Vaulont S, and Kahn A: Transcriptional control of metabolic regulation genes by carbohydrates. *FASEB J* 8:28–35, 1994.

28. Towle H: Metabolic regulation of gene transcription in mammals. *J Biol Chem* 270:23235–23238, 1995.

29. Bergot MO, Diaz-Guerra M-JM, Puzenat N, Raymondjean M, Kahn A: *Cis*-regulation of the L-type pyruvate kinase gene promoter by glucose, insulin and cyclic AMP. *Nucleic Acids Research* 20:1871–1878, 1992.

30. Shih H, Towle HC: Definition of the carbohydrate response element of the rat S14 gene. Evidence for a common factor required for carbohydrate regulation of hepatic genes. *J Biol Chem* 267:13222–13228, 1992.

31. Shih H, Towle HC: Definition of the carbohydrate response element of the rat S14 gene. Context of the CACGTG motif determinates the specificity of carbohydrate regulation. *J Biol Chem* 269:9380–9387, 1994.

32. Chen R, Doiron B, and Kahn A: Glucose responsiveness of a reporter gene transduced into hepatocytic cells using a retroviral vector. *FEBS Lett* 365:223–226, 1995.

33. Noguchi T, Inoue H, Tanaka T: Transcriptional and post-transcriptional regulation of L-type pyruvate kinase in diabetic rat liver by insulin and dietary fructose. *J Biol Chem* 260:14393–14397, 1985.

34. Munnich A, Lyonnet S, Chauvet D, Van Schaftingen E, Kahn A: Differential effects of glucose and fructose on liver L-type pyruvate kinase gene expression *in vivo*. *J Biol Chem* 262:17065–17071, 1987.

35. Groskreutz DJ, Sliwkowski MX, Gorman CM: Genetically engineered proinsulin constitutively processed and secreted as mature, active insulin. *J Biol Chem* 269:6241–6245, 1994.

36. Falqui L, Martinenghi S, Severini GM: Reversal of diabetes in mice by implantation of human fibroblasts gentically engineered to release mature human insulin. *Human Gene Ther* 10:1753–1762, 1999.

37. Kay MA, Woo SLC: Gene therapy for metabolic disorders. *Trends Genet* 10:253–257, 1994.

38. De-Roos WK, Von-Geusau BA, Bouwman E, Van-Dierendonck JH, Borel-Rinkes IH, Terpstra OT: Monitoring engraftment of transplanted hepatocytes in recipient liver with 5-bromo-2′-deoxyuridine. *Transplantation* 63:513–518, 1997.

39. Kolodka TM, Finegold M, Moss L, Woo SLC: Gene therapy for diabetes mellitus in rats by hepatic expression of insulin. *Proc Natl Acad Sci USA* 92:3293–3297, 1995.

40. Schneider G, Morral N, Parks RJ *et al*: Genomic DNA transfer with a high-capacity adenovirus vector results in improved *in vivo* gene expression and decreased toxicity. *Nature Genet* 18:180–183, 1998.

41. Kafri T, Blomer U, Peterson DA, Gage FH, Verma IM: Sustained expression of genes delivered directly into liver and muscle by lentiviral vectors. *Nature Genet* 17:314–317, 1997.

42. Rendahl KG, Leff ST, Otten GR *et al*: Regulation of gene expression *in vivo* following transduction of two separate rAAV vectors. *Nature Biotechol* 16:757–751, 1998.

43. Xiao X, Samulski RJ: Efficient long-term gene transfer into muscle tissue of immunocompetent mice by adeno-associated viral vector. *J Virology* 70:8090–8108, 1996.

44. Ye X, Rivera VM, Zoltick P *et al*: Regulated delivery of therapeutic proteins after *in vivo* somatic cell gene transfer. *Science* 283:88–91, 1999.

45. Wang L, Takabe K, Bidlingmaier SM, Ill CR, Verma IM: Sustained correction of bleeding disorder in hemophilia B mice by gene therapy. *Proc Natl Acad Sci* 96:3906–3910, 1999.

46. Snyder RO, Miao C, Meuse L *et al*: Correction of hemophilia B in canine and murine models using recombinant adeno-associated viral vectors. *Nature Med* 5:64–70, 1999.

47. Thulè PM, Liu J-M: Glucose regulated hepatic production of human insulin ameliorates hyperglycemia in streptozotocin treated rats. American Society of Gene Therapy, 2nd Meeting, Washington, DC. *Abstract* 939, 237a, 1999.

48. Lu D. *et al*: Regulatable production of insulin from primary-cultured hepatocytes: insulin production is up-regulated by glucagon and cAMP and down-regulated by insulin. *Gene Ther* 5:888–895, 1998.

49. Ferry N, Heard JM: Liver-directed gene transfer vectors. *Hum Gene Ther* 9:1975–1981, 1998.

10

Insulin Resistance vs. Insulin Deficiency: Which Comes First? The Old Question Revisited

ANDRÉ J. SCHEEN & PIERRE J. LEFÈBVRE

Division of Diabetes, Nutrition and Metabolic Disorders,
Department of Medicine, CHU Sart Tilman, Liège, Belgium

Type 2 diabetes is a popular topic in biomedical science because of its high prevalence (markedly increasing with industrialization and aging), severe morbidity and excessive mortality (due to both micro- and macro-angiopathy), and undefined pathophysiological aspects. It can be defined as a heterogeneous condition caused by genetic (polygenic in most instances) and environmental (acquired due to 'Westernization') factors, which is usually expressed late in life and is characterized by a progressive deterioration of the metabolic state (1). It has been postulated that various environmental factors (physical inactivity, and increased fat and caloric intake) operate on susceptible genotype(s) ('diabetogenic' genes) to promote the development of type 2 diabetes (2,3). Over the last decade, major advances have been made in our understanding of the pathophysiology and molecular biology of the disease [review in (3)], but the answer to the old question of which form insulin resistance or insulin deficiency plays a primary role in the development of the disease still remains a matter of controversy (4–6). In addition, there is clearly a difference in perception of the relative importance of these two defects in the pathophysiology of type 2 diabetes when one carefully examines two recent parallel reports, the World Health Organization (WHO) report on *Definition, diagnosis and classification of diabetes mellitus and its complications'* (7) and the American Diabetes Association (ADA) *'Report of the Expert Committee on the Diagnosis and Classification of Diabetes Mellitus*' (8). In the WHO report, the definition of type 2 diabetes reads: 'The type named type 2 includes the common major form of diabetes, which results from defect(s) in *insulin secretion*, almost always with a major contribution from insulin resistance'. On the other hand, in the ADA report, the definition of type 2 diabetes reads: 'Type 2 diabetes... is a term used for individuals who have *insulin resistance* and usually have relative (rather than absolute) insulin deficiency'. Even if the difference may appear subtle, it is essential indeed, and, as most recently pointed out by Skyler (9), the perception clearly depends from which side of the Atlantic Ocean one views the disease!

In this concise review, we will summarize the relative roles of insulin resistance and insulin deficiency in the pathophysiology of type 2 diabetes and analyse the pros and cons of a primary role of each of these two endocrine/metabolic abnormalities in the pathogenesis of the most common form of type 2 diabetes.

TYPE 2 DIABETES, A HETEROGENEOUS DISEASE

Several lines of evidence indicate that great heterogeneity exists within the diabetes phenotype (6). These include both genetic and pathophysiological arguments. The former especially include the facts that more than 60 different genetic syndromes are associated with impaired glucose tolerance, and that within maturity-onset diabetes of the young (MODY) an increasing number of genetic defects have been recently reported (10). The latter include the common observations of physiological heterogeneity in patterns of body weight and insulin response among type 2 diabetic patients (1,3).

Epidemiological studies have shown a great between-subject heterogeneity among insulin sensitivity and insulin secretion indices, even within a normal non-diabetic population (3). Those subjects with low insulin sensitivity are characterized by high insulin secretion, whereas those with high insulin sensitivity are characterized by low insulin secretion. The relationship between insulin secretion and insulin sensitivity is best represented by an hyperbolic curve and subjects with normal glucose tolerance are distributed along this curve. A similar hyperbolic curve is found in obese non-diabetic subjects with the only difference of a left-shifted distribution of insulin sensitivity and a right-shifted distribution of insulin secretion. So most obese subjects are characterized by low insulin sensitivity, which is compensated for by a high insulin secretory response in order to maintain normal glucose tolerance. In contrast, most subjects with type 2 diabetes are characterized by the coexistence of low insulin sensitivity and relatively low insulin secretion rate regarding insulin resistance. Consequently, they are below the normal hyperbolic curve and unable to maintain normal glucose tolerance (11).

However, among type 2 diabetic patients, some individuals appear to be essentially insulin-resistant, whereas others seem to be particularly insulin deficient, a finding which emphasizes again the great heterogeneity of the disease (1,3).

ROLE OF INSULIN RESISTANCE IN TYPE 2 DIABETES

Even if insulin exerts numerous different effects, so far insulin sensitivity has been considered mainly in the context of glucose metabolism, especially at the liver and muscle sites, the two most important organs, apart from the pancreas, involved in the pathogenesis of type 2 diabetes (12,13). The presence of insulin resistance *in vivo* can be evidenced during various dynamic tests, such as an oral glucose tolerance test (OGTT), an intravenous glucose tolerance test (IVGTT) and a euglycaemic hyperinsulinaemic clamp (13–15). At present, the basic defect responsible for insulin resistance in subjects prone to develop type 2 diabetes is unknown and multiple (probably secondary) factors may explain decreased insulin action in overweight patients with frank hyperglycaemia (3,4). Insulin action results from a complex sequence of extracellular and intracellular events so that prereceptor, receptor and postreceptor defects all may contribute to insulin resistance (12). Although diabetologists have traditionally tended to focus their attention on intracellular defects involving glucose metabolism, a number of other explanations are equally plausible [review in (3)]. Even if it is true that most individuals with impaired glucose tolerance are insulin-resistant, it is unclear whether insulin resistance in these subjects is directly genetic (the search for candidate genes linked to insulin resistance has yet to prove fruitful) or merely secondary to obesity or other factors, such as decreased physical fitness, inappropriate diet, etc. (5). Despite these uncertainties, the weight of current evidence supports the view that insulin resistance is very important in the aetiology of typical type 2 diabetes [review in (4)].

A vast majority of type 2 diabetic patients are overweight and obesity undoubtedly plays a major role in the development of the disease (1,15). Excess fat mass, especially visceral adiposity, is associated with an increased release of free fatty acids (FFA), which may trigger a reduction in insulin sensitivity at both the hepatic and the muscular levels. In the liver, this results in an increased glucose output (essentially due to enhanced gluconeogenesis), a decreased insulin extraction and an increased VLDL production, while in the skeletal muscle this results in a reduction in glucose oxidation and glucose storage as glycogen (1). Conversely, weight reduction in severely obese diabetic patients results in marked reduction of insulin resistance and remarkable improvement of glycaemic control (16).

ROLE OF INSULIN DEFICIENCY IN TYPE 2 DIABETES

B cell function in type 2 diabetes has been the subject of intense investigation for several decades, and considerable progress has been made during the recent years in the knowledge of the physiology and pathophysiology of insulin secretion (17). However, given the number of variables that could contribute to a disordered insulin secretory response, it is obvious that a precise definition of the sequence of events that leads to this disorder in a given patient with common type 2 diabetes remains, in most cases, an elusive goal.

Three main mechanisms have been proposed during the last 10 years to explain the B cell deficiency observed in some subjects prone to develop type 2 diabetes (1). First, a genetic defect may be present, although such a defect has not yet been detected in subjects with common type 2 diabetes associated with obesity, in contrast to what was reported in some particular forms of MODY (mutation of the glucokinase gene in MODY 3, for instance) (10,18). Second, *in utero* malnutrition may lead to insufficient B cell development and later partial insulin secretory defect. This hypothesis has been called the 'thrifty phenotype hypothesis' (19). And third, unfavourable metabolic environment may also play a deleterious role, especially increased glucose levels, which may induce glucotoxicity, and a chronic increase in FFA levels, which may induce lipotoxicity, both processes contributing to alter insulin secretion (3). Several early markers of B cell dysfunction have been described, such as impaired glucose-induced and glucose-potentiated insulin secretion, secretion of proinsulin-enriched material and alteration in the pulsatility of insulin secretion (17). To some extent, the natural history of the obese subjects developing type 2 diabetes after a prolonged phase of compensatory hyperinsulinism may be explained by the 'overworked B cell' hypothesis, an hypothesis supported by observations in various animal models (20).

TYPE 2 DIABETES, A PROGRESSIVE DISEASE RESULTING FROM A DYNAMIC INTERACTION BETWEEN INSULIN ACTION AND INSULIN SECRETION

Subjects with type 2 diabetes are characterized by both tissue insulin resistance and impaired insulin secretion. The development of diabetes requires the presence of these two fundamental defects, which disrupt the delicate balance by which insulin-target tissues communicate with the B cells and *vice versa*. Numerous observations underscore the important interplay between insulin resistance and insulin secretion [review in (1,3)]. Both abnormalities must be looked at in concert and the relative importance of these two factors can be estimated with the aid of a theoretical mathematical model of glucose

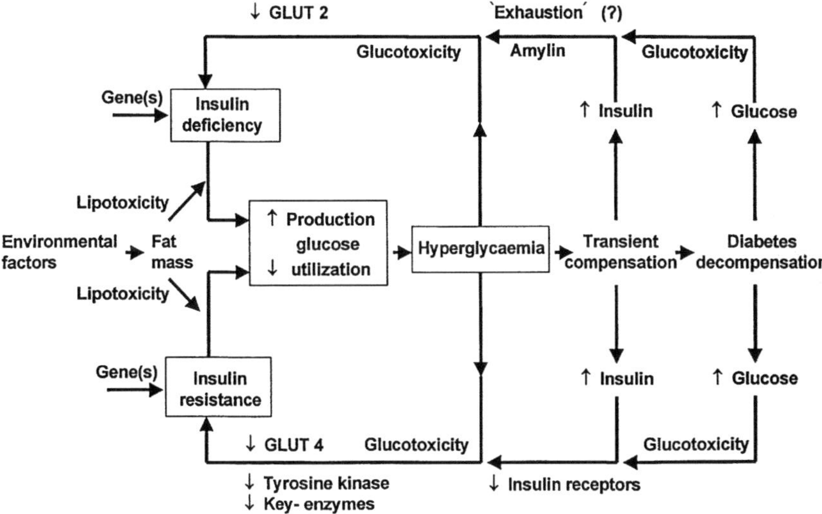

Figure 10.1. Vicious circle perpetuating and aggravating type 2 diabetes, whatever the priming defect in insulin secretion or in insulin action

metabolism (21). Insulin resistance alone is, in most instances, insufficient to cause overt glucose intolerance (22). To observe the development of frank diabetes mellitus, a defect in insulin secretion must be superimposed on insulin resistance (1,3,5,6,9).

Once it develops, either from insulin deficiency or from insulin resistance, hyperglycaemia will exacerbate both defects, thereby closing a pathological feedback loop (Figure 10.1). There appears to be a counterproductive interplay between B-cell inadequacy and insulin resistance: a primary B cell defect could result in hypoinsulinaemia and subsequent postreceptor insulin resistance, while insulin resistance and hyperglycaemia could exhaust B cells and make them unresponsive to glucose. A vicious circle can therefore be envisioned, in which B cell function and insulin resistance both deteriorate with time (1,3). Recent data from the UK Prospective Diabetes Study demonstrated that in newly diagnosed type 2 diabetes, the progressive deterioration of blood glucose control over the next 10 years can essentially be explained by a linear decrease of B cell insulin secretory capability (23). Even though our understanding of the mechanisms leading to the appearance and the progression of type 2 diabetes is incomplete, the counterproductive interplay between insulin resistance and insulin deficiency and the concept of glucose (and lipid) toxicity have important clinical and therapeutical implications (16).

Type 2 diabetes occurs as a late phenomenon in obese subjects and is preceded by years of normal glucose tolerance or impaired glucose tolerance

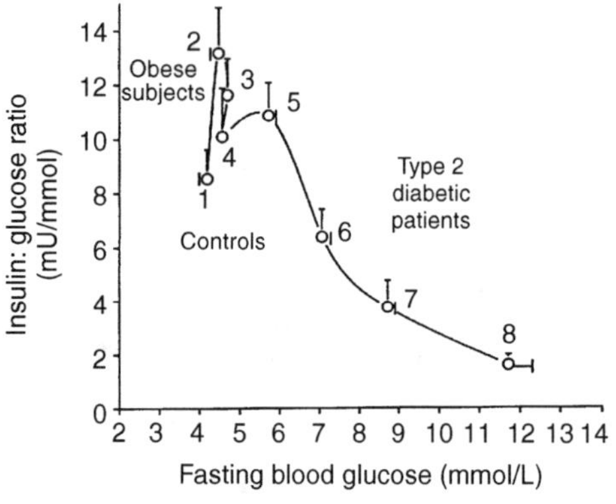

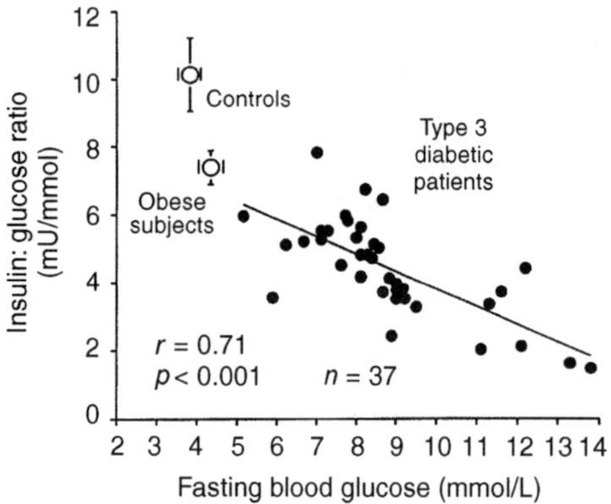

Figure 10.2. Relationship between the insulin response evaluated during an oral glucose tolerance test (upper panel) or the insulin-stimulated glucose disposal measured during a euglycaemic insulin clamp (lower panel) and fasting blood glucose levels. In the upper panel, insulin response is evaluated by dividing the $AUC_{0-180\,min}$ of plasma insulin levels by that of blood glucose concentrations in lean controls (1), obese subjects with normal (2) or impaired (3) glucose tolerance, and in obese subjects with type 2 diabetes of progressively increased severity (4–8) (mean $\pm$ SEM of 12–30 subjects). In the lower panel, glucose MCR is measured during an insulin clamp (insulin delivery rate, 100 mU/ kg/h) in 15 lean controls and 16 non-diabetic obese subjects (mean $\pm$ SEM), and in 37 overweight type 2 diabetic patients. Reproduced from (13), by permission of Karger, Basel

(IGT) as suggested by several cross-sectional studies (1,3,24). The progression from IGT to diabetes occurs when the B cell becomes unable to maintain its previously high rate of insulin secretion in response to glucose. We studied the insulin response to glucose during an OGTT in various groups of obese subjects in function of fasting blood glucose levels (Figure 10.2), as well as the metabolic clearance rate of glucose measured during a euglycaemic

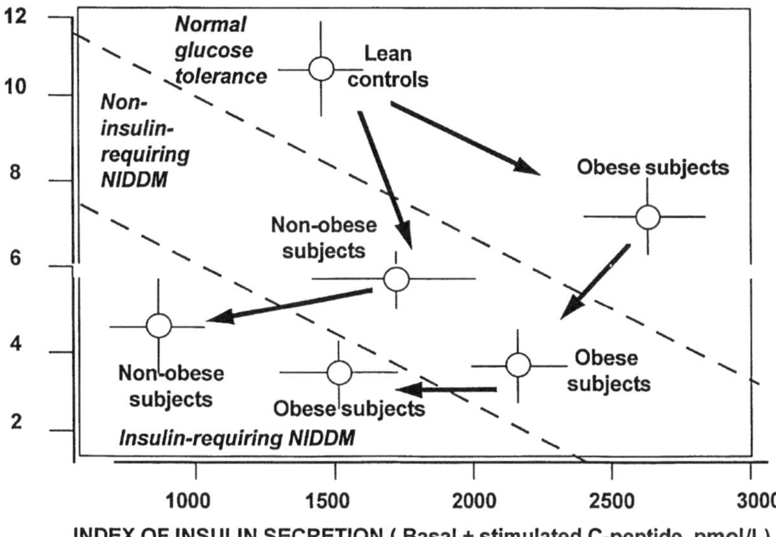

Figure 10.3. Hypothetical scheme of the natural history of type 2 diabetes mellitus: changes in insulin secretion and insulin sensitivity in six groups of subjects, three without obesity ('lean') and three with obesity ('obese'). The upper broken line separates non-diabetic subjects (with normal glucose tolerance) and non-insulin-requiring diabetic patients, while the lower broken line separates non-insulin-requiring and insulin-requiring diabetic patients. Results are expressed as mean ± SEM. Reproduced from (11), by permission of *Acta Clinica Belgica*

hyperinsulinaemic clamp in obese subjects with various fasting plasma glucose levels (Figure 10.2, bottom panel) (13). Obese non-diabetic subjects were characterized by a significant reduction in glucose utilization during the clamp, which appears, however, to be compensated for by an increased insulin response during the OGTT. In contrast, as basal hyperglycaemia increased, there was a progressive decline in glucose metabolic clearance rate and simultaneously a dramatic decrease in insulin response during the OGTT. Longitudinal studies confirmed that this evolution occurs along the natural history of obesity (25). During the first years of obesity, the subjects are normoglycaemic but hyperinsulinaemic. Afterwards they become hyperglycaemic at a time when hyperinsulinaemia is not maintained any more.

We have had the opportunity to evaluate insulin secretion using plasma C-peptide levels in the fasting condition and after the intravenous injection of 1 mg glucagon, and insulin sensitivity by measuring the metabolic clearance rate of glucose during a euglycaemic hyperinsulinaemic glucose clamp in six groups of about 15 subjects each (Figure 10.3) (11). These subjects were separated according to the presence or not of obesity (three groups of lean subjects and three groups of obese subjects) and according to the presence or not of diabetes (two groups with normal glucose tolerance, two groups with non-insulin-requiring type 2 diabetes, and two groups with insulin-requiring diabetes, one group of lean subjects and one group of obese subjects in each category). Obese patients with normal glucose tolerance are characterized by a significant reduction in insulin sensitivity, which is almost fully compensated for by an appropriate increase in insulin secretion. Obese patients with non-insulin-requiring diabetes showed an even lower insulin sensitivity associated with a partial defect in insulin secretion. Finally, obese patients with insulin-requiring type 2 diabetes were characterized by a marked reduction in insulin secretion without further worsening of insulin resistance. Thus, such cross-sectional observations suggest that type 2 diabetes occurs when obese subjects are not able to maintain hyperinsulinaemia any more to compensate for decreased insulin sensitivity, and the late progression to an insulin-requiring state is best explained by an exhaustion of insulin secretion in the face of persistent insulin resistance. A quite similar evolution was noticed in non-obese subjects, with the landmark difference, however, of a significantly reduced insulin secretion when compared to that of obese patients.

WHAT IS THE PRIMARY DEFECT, INSULIN RESISTANCE OR INSULIN DEFICIENCY ?

Despite extensive efforts, it is currently not known which defect, of insulin action or insulin secretion, comes first in the most 'common' form of type 2 diabetes (Figure 10.1) (1,3,4,5). Studies of candidate genes for insulin secretion and insulin sensitivity have explained little about disease susceptibility, so that research has moved recently from a focus on candidate genes to a search for novel genes, using a variety of methods in families and sib pairs with type 2 diabetes (18).

A number of investigators have examined insulin secretion and insulin sensitivity in first-degree relatives of type 2 diabetic patients with the assumption that disturbances observed at this stage are genetic in origin and thus may lead to the primary defect of the disease [review in (3) and)5)]. About half of the numerous studies testing B cell function reported a defect in insulin secretion, while two-thirds of the less numerous studies assessing insulin action reported the presence of insulin resistance. It is noteworthy that in most of the studies demonstrating a decrease in insulin secretion, insulin resistance was not measured, so that it is not possible to define whether both defects were present simultaneously in these subjects. Furthermore, several studies reported a significant increase in insulin secretion as the major abnormality. As reviewed by DeFronzo (3), taken collectively, these studies indicate that insulin resistance is the earliest identifiable metabolic/endocrine abnormality in the first-degree relatives of type 2 diabetic subjects in high-risk populations, such as Native Americans and Pima Indians, whereas both impaired insulin secretion and insulin resistance have been described in first-degree relatives of type 2 diabetic patients of European ancestry.

Studies that have examined identical-twin pairs who were discordant for type 2 diabetes provided support for both impairment of insulin secretion and impairment of insulin action as early genetic lesions for type 2 diabetes. Similarly, both insulin resistance and impaired insulin secretion appear to be important precursors of eventual progression to overt type 2 diabetes in women with gestational diabetes [review in (3) and (5)]. Consequently, these two models do not bring convincing support in favour of one or the other hypothesis.

In absence of a definite answer and keeping in mind that type 2 diabetes is a heterogeneous disease, we will list below some major arguments in favour of the hypothesis of either insulin resistance or insulin deficiency as the primary defect in type 2 diabetes.

Insulin resistance

Insulin resistance is a universal finding in patients with established type 2 diabetes (1,13), and is also present in patients at risk to develop the disease (3,25). The view that insulin resistance is the primary genetic factor predisposing to the development of type 2 diabetes arose mainly from cross-sectional observations of individuals with varying degrees of glucose tolerance. It has repeatedly been demonstrated that as 2 hour plasma glucose values from OGTTs increased, 2 hour plasma insulin levels increased up to plasma glucose values of approximately 200 mg/dl. These data were generally interpreted to indicate that because individuals with impaired glucose tolerance had increased 2 hour plasma insulin levels, they must be insulin-resistant, and because they were secreting more than a normal amount of insulin, they did not have impaired insulin secretion. The decrease in 2 hour plasma insulin responses, which occurred at plasma glucose levels above 200 mg/dl, was viewed largely as an acquired defect caused by 'β-cell exhaustion' (Figure 10.2). It was inferred that, because insulin resistance apparently preceded impaired insulin secretion, insulin resistance was the genetic defect and reduced insulin responses were the acquired defect. Such results provide conclusive evidence that insulin resistance is an early (inherited?) defect that may initiate the diabetic condition.

Prospective studies have demonstrated that insulin resistance and hyper-insulinaemia precede the development of impaired glucose tolerance and predict the later development of type 2 diabetes [(25); review in (3)]. In high-risk ethnic populations (e.g. Native Americans, Pima Indians, Mexican-Americans and Pacific Islanders), which have a high prevalence of diabetes, insulin secretion is enhanced and both fasting and glucose-stimulated plasma insulin levels are elevated during the earliest stages of the natural history of type 2 diabetes, compared with age- and weight-matched non-diabetic control subjects (3). Most of the available evidence suggests that, at least in such populations, insulin resistance is the primary genetic disturbance and that augmented B cell function represents a compensatory adaptation to offset the defect in insulin action (3,26) (Figure 10.1). However, primary search for candidates genes involved in insulin action (glucose transporter family, insulin receptor, insulin receptor substrate, glycogen synthase, etc.) has failed, up until now, to find any consistent association with type 2 diabetes (18).

Insulin deficiency

More than 30 years ago, impaired β-cell function was proposed to be the primary genetic abnormality predisposing to the development of type 2 diabetes (27). The bases for this theory were the findings that insulin secretion was under genetic control, and was reduced in normal glucose-tolerant individuals who have a first-degree relative with type 2 diabetes. As already discussed, the latter finding has been confirmed in several subsequent studies.

There appears to be growing support for the primacy of insulin deficiency in the pathogenesis of IGT (22) or type 2 diabetes (5,6). This is particularly the case in certain subgroups, especially in subjects with older age (>60 years at age of onset), with less or no excess weight and of European ancestry (in this group, however, it is important to first exclude late-onset type 1 diabetes because positive islet cell and/or GAD antibodies are not rare) (3). It is important to recognize that there are well-described type 2 diabetic populations in whom insulin sensitivity is normal at the onset of diabetes, whereas insulin secretion is severely impaired: this profile is much more frequent in lean than in obese patients (28,29). So, as an alternative hypothesis, a genetic defect in insulin secretion may be seen as the earliest event in the development of type 2 diabetes, at least in some patients (21,27,30).

Some observations showed that subjects with type 2 diabetes have lower insulin concentrations than previously appreciated by classical radio immuno-assays because of the presence of proinsulin and inactive split products [review in (1)]. Moreover, most studies which emphasized the exaggerated insulin response did not take into account the kinetics of insulin secretion (5): indeed, in most subjects, deficient insulin response can be evidenced in the early phase (e.g. within the first 30 min of an OGTT) (22), while late insulin response is increased because of the stimulatory effect of exaggerated glucose excursion. So, patients with impaired glucose tolerance were characterized by the presence of a significant defect in early glucose-stimulated insulin secretion. Moreover, impaired early insulin release during OGTT can cause increased late plasma insulin levels, and thus 2 hour hyperinsulinaemia may be the consequence of impaired insulin secretion, and is not necessarily indicative of early insulin resistance (5,6). Finally, as already mentioned, abnormalities in both the amount and pattern of insulin secretion have been demonstrated in normoglycaemic relatives of patients with type 2 diabetes, indicating that B cell dysfunction may be the primary defect (5,6). A plausible sequence of events, starting with a defect in insulin secretion and leading to the emergence of insulin resistance, can also be described on the basis on the information currently available (Figure 10.1).

Thus, while most investigators agree that insulin secretion and insulin action must both be impaired for the development of overt diabetes, there is no consensus as to which comes first (3–6). Owing to increasing evidence of heterogeneity of the disease (28,29), it is highly probable that each defect will prove to be primary in some forms of type 2 diabetes. The answer will most certainly be provided by genetic analysis. Indeed, genetic research of type 2 diabetes is undergoing rapid development, and many studies are in progress, especially using genome-wide scans which may lead to new genes. However, despite exciting developments, the genetic susceptibility of type 2 diabetes still remains an enigma (18).

CONCLUSIONS

The development of type 2 diabetes requires the presence of two fundamental defects, i.e. insulin resistance and impaired insulin secretion, which disrupt the delicate balance by which insulin target tissues communicate with the B cells and *vice versa*. Thus, type 2 diabetes is a heterogenous disorder characterized by impaired insulin secretion, diminished peripheral (muscular) insulin action, and increased hepatic glucose production, all defects being present in variable proportions in different individuals, but also prone to changes in a given individual with the progression of the disease. Considerable controversy has arisen about the primary genetic disturbance(s) responsible for impaired glucose homeostasis in patients with type 2 diabetes, and powerful arguments can be generated in favour of either diminished insulin secretion or insulin resistance. Even though we are not yet able to pinpoint the primary defect in most patients with type 2 diabetes, there appears to be a counterproductive interplay between B cell inadequacy and insulin resistance, which leads to a vicious circle that perpetuates and aggravates the metabolic disorder. On clinical and epidemiological grounds, it would appear that insulin resistance is most commonly an early defect in the sequence of events leading to type 2 diabetes in overweight people. In such patients, once the pancreas cannot secrete enough insulin, due to genetic or acquired defects of the B cells, glucose tolerance deteriorates rapidly and a frank diabetic state ensues. Emphasis should be placed upon developing an approach to the therapy of type 2 diabetes which is firmly based upon recent knowledge of the metabolic defects characteristic of the disease and adapted to the main endocrine/metabolic characteristics of each individual patient.

REFERENCES

1. Scheen AJ, Lefèbvre PJ. Pathophysiology of type 2 diabetes. In: Kuhlmann J, Puls W, Eds. *Handbook of Experimental Pharmacology, Oral Antidiabetics*. Berlin: Springer Verlag, pp. 7–42, 1996.
2. Kahn C: Insulin action, diabetogenes, and the cause of type II diabetes. *Diabetes* 43:1066–1084, 1994.
3. DeFronzo RA: Pathogenesis of type 2 diabetes: metabolic and molecular implications for identifying diabetes genes. *Diabet Rev* 5:177–269, 1997.
4. Ferrannini E: Insulin resistance vs. insulin deficiency in non-insulin-dependent diabetes mellitus: problems and prospects. *Endocr Rev* 19:477–490, 1998.
5. Gerich J: The genetic basis of type 2 diabetes mellitus: impaired insulin secretion vs. impaired insulin sensitivity. *Endocr Rev* 19:491–503, 1998.
6. Gerich JE: Is insulin resistance the principal cause of type 2 diabetes? *Diabet Obes Metab* 1:257–263, 1999.
7. World Health Organization, Department of Non-Communicable Disease Surveillance: Definition, diagnosis and classification of diabetes mellitus and its complications. *Report of a WHO Consultation. Part 1: Diagnosis and Classification of Diabetes Mellitus*. Geneva: WHO, 1999.
8. The Expert Committee on the Diagnosis and Classification of Diabetes Mellitus: Report on the Expert Committee on the Diagnosis and Classification of Diabetes Mellitus. *Diabet Care* 20:1183–1197, 1997.
9. Skyler JS: Type 2 diabetes: insulin secretion *vs* insulin action. *Int Diabet Monitor* 12 (3):1–3, 2000.
10. Froguel Ph, Vaxillaire M, Velho G: Genetic and metabolic heterogeneity of maturity-onset diabetes of the young. *Diabet Rev* 5:123–130, 1997.
11. Scheen AJ: From obesity to diabetes. Why, when and who? *Acta Clin Belg* 55:9–15, 2000.
12. Scheen AJ, Lefèbvre PJ: Insulin action in man. *Diabet Metab* 22: 105–110, 1996.
13. Scheen AJ, Lefèbvre PJ: Assessment of insulin resistance *in vivo*. Application to the study of type 2 diabetes. *Horm Res* 38:19–27, 1992.
14. Scheen AJ, Castillo MJ, Paquot N, Lefèbvre PJ: How to measure insulin action *in vivo*. *Diabet Metab Rev* 10:151–88, 1994.
15. Scheen AJ, Paquot N, Letiexhe MR, Paolisso G, Castillo MJ, Lefèbvre PJ: Glucose metabolism in obese subjects: lessons from OGTT, IVGTT and clamp studies. *Int J Obesity* 19 (Suppl 3):S14–S20, 1995.
16. Scheen AJ, Lefèbvre PJ: Management of the obese diabetic patient. *Diabet Rev* 7:77–93, 1999.
17. Polonsky KS. Lilly Lecture 1994: The beta-cell in diabetes: from molecular genetics to clinical research. *Diabetes* 44:705–717, 1995.
18. Elbein SC: An update on the genetic basis of type 2 diabetes. *Curr Opin Endocrinol Diabet* 5:116–125, 1998.
19. Hales CN: The pathogenesis of NIDDM. *Diabetologia* 37 (Suppl 2):S162–S168, 1994.

20. Leahy JL: Impaired β-cell function with chronic hyperglycemia: 'overworked β-cell' hypothesis. *Diabet Rev* 4:298–319, 1996.
21. Turner RC, Matthews DR, Clark A, O'Rahilly S, Rudenski AS, Levy J: Pathogenesis of NIDDM — a disease of deficient insulin secretion. *Baillière's Clin Endocrinol Metab* 2:327–342, 1988.
22. O'Rahilly S, Hattersley A, Vaag A, Gray H: Insulin resistance as the major cause of impaired glucose tolerance: a self-fulfilling prophesy? *Lancet* 344:585–589, 1994.
23. UKPDS Group: UK Prospective Diabetes Study 16: overview of six years' therapy of type 2 diabetes — a progressive disease. *Diabetes* 44:1249–1258, 1995.
24. Felber JP, Acheson KJ, Tappy L: *From Obesity to Diabetes.* Wiley, Chichester, p. 302, 1993.
25. Martin BC, Warram JH, Krolewski AS, Bergman RN, Soeldner JS, Kahn CR: Role of glucose and insulin resistance in development of type 2 diabetes mellitus: results of a 25-year follow-up study. *Lancet* 340:925–929, 1992.
26. Saad MF, Knowler WC, Pettitt DJ, Nelson RG, Charles MA, Bennett PH: A two-step model for development of non-insulin-dependent diabetes. *Am J Med* 90:229–235, 1991.
27. Cerasi E, Luft R: 'What is inherited — what is added' hypothesis for the pathogenesis of diabetes mellitus. *Diabetes* 16:615–627, 1967.
28. Banerji MA, Lebovitz HE: Insulin-sensitive and insulin-resistant variants in NIDDM. *Diabetes* 38:784–792, 1989.
29. Arner P, Pollare T, Lithell H: Different aetiologies of type 2 (non-insulin-dependent) diabetes mellitus in obese and non-obese subjects. *Diabetologia* 34:483–487, 1991.
30. Polonsky KS, Sturis J, Bell GI: Non-insulin-dependent diabetes mellitus: a genetically programmed failure of the beta cell to compensate for insulin resistance. *N Engl J Med* 334:777–783, 1996.

11

Pathophysiological Mechanisms of Type 2 Diabetes

WERNER WALDHÄUSL

Division of Endocrinology and Metabolism, Department of Medicine III,
University of Vienna, Allgemeines Krankenhaus, Vienna, Austria

The hyperglycaemic syndrome, type 2 (non-insulin-dependent) diabetes mellitus, is a disease that has been known since ancient times. It is non-communicable but to a large extent acquirable and is characterized by multiple abnormalities in insulin action and release, which are almost inseparable. The incidence of the disease is strongly associated with increasing age, body weight and calorie/fat intake as well as with lifestyle and ethnic origin. The prevalence of type 2 diabetes varies widely between countries and populations within a country. The disease approaches epidemic levels in the industrialized world. Around 5–7% of adults in the USA are affected (up from 2.3% in 1975) and their treatment accounts for about 12% of the national health care costs (1). In China in 1980 the overall prevalence of type 2 diabetes was about 1% but with the country's economic development it has since risen by three-fold in defined areas. The prevalence is even higher among male Chinese living outside China in Hong Kong (5%), Singapore (9%), Taiwan (13%) and Mauritius (17%) (2). In Europe the trend is equally depressing, with 4.7% for men and 5.6% for women aged 18–70 years in Germany. The former East Germany saw a 7.9-fold increase in prevalence from 0.44% in 1960 to 3.68% in 1989 (3). The same trend can be seen in the number of patients with impaired glucose tolerance (IGT) who progress to type 2 diabetes, the range being from 2% (Denmark) to 14.3% (The Netherlands) (4).

Clearly, therefore, the prevalence of type 2 diabetes in a population depends not only on genetic predisposition but is also largely influenced by the lifestyle

Diabetes in the New Millennium. Edited by U. Di Mario, F. Leonetti, G. Pugliese, P. Sbraccia and A. Signore.
© 2000 John Wiley & Sons, Ltd.

which seems to inevitably result from urbanization and industrialization. With an estimated increase in overall prevalence of 50%, meaning that 213 million people will be affected by the year 2010, we can expect an epidemic of type 2 diabetes in the coming decades (2). This will be accompanied by a proportional rise in macroangiopathic and microangiopathic multimorbidity among those people and a consequent major increase in health care expenditure.

The diagnosis of type 2 diabetes has changed since it became obvious that it is more than the mere description of a hyperglycaemic patient who survives without prompt insulin treatment that is required. Definitions of type 2 diabetes include: a 2 hour blood glucose value of 200 mg/dl or more in response to a 75 g oral glucose tolerance test, a random sample of plasma glucose in excess of 200 mg/dl, or a fasting plasma glucose in excess of 126 mg/dl. In addition, the term 'impaired fasting plasma glucose' (110 to 125 mg/dl) has been coined to identify people who are at high risk of developing the disease and its associated late complications (5). Clinically, glucose intolerance and type 2 diabetes have, independently of obesity, been linked to hypertension and they have been related selectively to insulin resistance of glucose but not of lipid and potassium metabolism (6).

The aetiology of the diabetic phenotypes of type 2 diabetes is complex. The development of such phenotypes seems to depend on both a polygenic background and strong environmental influences, such as weight gain and physical inactivity, as well as inappropriate nutrition which mediates insulin resistance and reduction in insulin secretion. It is therefore obvious that the risk of developing clinically manifest type 2 diabetes can be reduced by foregoing excess calorie intake and engaging in more physical activity.

Heritability of type 2 diabetes is suggested by familial clustering of insulin resistance among Mexican American subjects with a parental history of diabetes (7) and by the population-based observation of a difference in concordance between monozygotic (0.63) and dizygotic twin pairs (0.43; $p < 0.01$) with either type 2 diabetes or impaired glucose tolerance (8). Surprisingly, so far all attempts to identify the genes responsible at large for the associated defects of insulin secretion and sensitivity have failed.

Although by definition the genetic burden in a given population remains constant within the lifespan of one generation, environmental factors such as life-style, food habits and migration can change. Thus, type 2 diabetes has spread in step with 'cocacolonisation', industrialization and urbanization (2). This development challenges the metabolic characteristics of 'primitive' man, which are more suitable for rural life, as evident from the low prevalence of type 2 diabetes in rural populations.

Insulin resistance in type 2 diabetes seems to have been a useful trait ('thrifty genotype') for the survival of primitive man when food was inadequate because it would have prevented the excessive uptake of glucose by muscles for energy (9). In addition, adult type 2 diabetes has been linked to the intrauterine environment in that mothers in a poor nutritional state during pregnancy have been found to give birth to babies of low birth weight (10), which in turn is associated with subsequent development of type 2 diabetes in the offspring.

It is of note that both insulin resistance and hyperinsulinaemia have even been described as independent risk factors for the development of myocardial infarction and atherosclerosis (11). Potentially, these states could be caused by a partial loss of insulin's ability to augment endothelial NO production (12).

POINTS OF CONCERN

Maintenance of normoglycaemia in humans depends on appropriate insulin secretion and action, as well as on an adequate endogenous glucose (substrate) supply. The major endocrine and metabolic defects in type 2 diabetes include declining insulin release, a rise in hepatic glucose production, a reduction in glucose uptake by skeletal muscle, and a loss of insulin sensitivity in tissues that are the target of insulin action (i.e. insulin resistance). Even after decades of research it is still a matter of debate which defect comes first. This failure to solve the riddle of the primary metabolic defect in type 2 diabetes could lie in systematic errors in our approach to analysing the factors controlling glucose homeostasis (13).

The first such error arises from the frequent misunderstanding by many clinicians of the term 'insulin action' by equating it only to insulin availability, without appreciating that insulin action is a functional entity that depends inseparably on both insulin availability and the insulin sensitivity of target tissues. The contribution of these two components to insulin action can differ widely between patients, and likewise between healthy subjects, while the blood glucose concentration, which is determined by insulin action, can remain constant if changes in insulin availability and those in insulin sensitivity compensate for each other. This interaction between insulin sensitivity and insulin release follows a hyperbolic function and is consistent with a regulated feedback loop control system. Thus, β-cell function varies in a given person, not only with actual blood glucose concentration but also in a quantitative manner with any change in insulin sensitivity (14). This explains the wide range of plasma insulin concentrations found in type 2 diabetic patients, which can be both normal and increased in the fasting/postabsorptive state, but also in the stimulated state (11).

Second, it is difficult to establish which of the two major defects, impaired insulin secretion or loss of insulin sensitivity, dominates in type 2 diabetes. This is because these functions are interdependent and inseparable *in vivo*. To avoid pitfalls we have to remember, on the one hand, that any development of hyperinsulinaemia without insulin resistance results in hypoglycaemia and, on the other hand, isolated increases in insulin resistance without compensatory hyperinsulinaemia end in hyperglycaemia due to functional/'relative' insulin deficiency. This interdependence between insulin resistance and sensitivity implies that any loss in insulin sensitivity has to be counteracted by an increase in insulin release, as long as this is possible. These actions are inseparable. Any relative defect in insulin secretion will, however, be followed by hyperglycaemia and the associated insulin resistance mediated by 'glucose toxicity' (15).

Third, part of the difficulty in identifying the primary metabolic defect in type 2 diabetes could also be our inability to define the level of glycaemia that characterizes the disease precisely in absolute terms beyond conventions. In addition, diagnostic procedures might not be sufficiently sensitive to determine small deviations in insulin sensitivity and secretion definitively.

The fourth possibility is that we are failing to search in detail for metabolic/ endocrine factors that cause strictly simultaneous deterioration in insulin release and the sensitivity of tissues to insulin. A major role here is perhaps to be assigned to inappropriate diet, leading to high concentrations of plasma free fatty acids or an excessive calorie supply resulting in loss of insulin sensitivity and an associated insulin secretion defect (16,17).

Finally we could also be misled in our search for the origin of the disease if the causal role of genetic factors is overemphasized. The importance of genetic factors has to be balanced against the ability of type 2 diabetes to become epidemic within the time of one generation. A 7.8-fold (East Germany) and three-fold (USA) rise in the prevalence of the disease within 29 years and 25 years, respectively, cannot be explained by a change in genetic background, only by environmental effect(s). In other words, more than two-thirds of the prevalence of type 2 diabetes in the industrialized world probably relates to non-genetic factors, and thus to this extent the disease must be preventable.

It is not my wish to belittle the genetic background of type 2 diabetes, only to indicate that non-genetic environmental factors must have a far greater role in the clinical manifestation of this debilitating disease than is commonly accepted. Nobody would doubt such a statement if it were made of an epidemic of an infectious disease like tuberculosis, which also requires some genetic disposition but does not occur without any exposure to tubercle bacilli. Just four generations ago, tuberculosis exterminated in excess of 50% of the populations who adopted an urban lifestyle with the conditions that prevailed in the late nineteenth century. Obviously, from this example there is something to be learnt about the interdependence between modern lifestyle attributes and the manifestation of type 2 diabetes.

PATHOPHYSIOLOGY

Genetic background

Heritability of type 2 diabetes and abnormal glucose tolerance has recently been estimated in a population-based twin study as 26% and 61%, respectively

(8). So far all attempts to successfully identify the genes responsible for the defects of insulin secretion and sensitivity in type 2 diabetes at large have failed, although several monogenic forms of diabetes exhibiting severe insulin deficiency have been identified. Among these maturity-onset diabetes of the young, type II (MODY II) is associated with mutations in the glucokinase gene on chromosome 7p (18). This is of note because the enzyme glucokinase is critical for glucose sensing by the pancreatic β cell and serves as a rate-limiting step for glucose metabolism by the islets (11,19). Defects in alleles of the insulin receptor gene found in patients with severe insulin resistance in leprechaunism and type A insulin resistance in acanthosis nigricans are also of major interest. These two mutations affect the major components dominating insulin secretion, insulin action and insulin sensitivity. Although important, these mutations account, however, only for less than 1% of the common form of type 2 diabetes (11) and cannot explain the high prevalence of the disease. Thus, less pronounced genetic defects need to predominate and latently impair prevailing glycaemia in those prone to develop type 2 diabetes, which could then be precipitated by the additional influence of detrimental environmental factors.

Interaction of insulin release and sensitivity

In the basal/postabsorptive state, fasting plasma insulin concentration has to vary in response to prevailing overall insulin sensitivity of target tissues, otherwise ('normal') insulin action on carbohydrate metabolism cannot be maintained. It follows that any loss in this interdependence between insulin concentration and target tissue sensitivity will inevitably result in blood glucose fluctuations. Thus, hyperglycaemia can result either from a loss of appropriate insulin release for a given state of insulin sensitivity or, conversely, from an insufficient insulin sensitivity of target tissues at a constant plasma insulin concentration. The interpretation of prevailing plasma insulin concentration in the age group over 50 years that is susceptible to type 2 diabetes is also rendered difficult because normal ageing itself reduces mass and amplitude of rapid insulin pulses (20). The inherent ability of both the pancreatic β cell and insulin sensitivity to adapt to change in metabolic environment accentuated the debate over the proportion that each contributes to the development of type 2 diabetes. Against this background both insulin resistance (11,15) and impaired insulin secretion (21) are championed as the predecessors to type 2 diabetes.

Insulin secretion

β Cells release insulin after glucose has been taken up by GLUT-2 transporters and glucokinase has mediated phosphorylation of the glucose (19). Insulin is released in a pulsatile fashion in both the basal and stimulated state to guarantee optimal insulin action. This pulsation is largely lost in type 2 diabetic patients and in their prediabetic offspring. As insulin secretion is regulated by prevailing blood glucose concentration, it is of no surprise that the absolute postabsorptive/fasting plasma insulin concentrations in response to hyperglycaemia in type 2 diabetes have been found to be either normal or increased. Prevailing insulin deficiency and a defect in the ability of the pancreatic β cell to release insulin is, however, unmasked in the majority of type 2 diabetic patients when plasma insulin concentration is related to that of associated blood glucose. Such dysfunction applies in part also to stimulated plasma insulin concentration in response to oral or intravenous glucose, which in absolute terms is impaired in about 50% of the patients (11) if the early insulin response at 30 min is calculated [for review, see (22)]. Hyperinsulinaemia, stimulated by glucose in an insulin resistant state, has been found to be associated not only with prevailing glycaemia but also to a greater than normal decrease in splanchnic insulin trapping (23).

Although it has been stated that hyperinsulinaemia always precedes the development of diabetes (11,15), this contention clearly depends on the definition of the plasma glucose concentration that is regarded to be diagnostic for type 2 diabetes. The higher the plasma glucose concentration, the more and earlier hyperinsulinaemia will be found in the natural course of the disease. Hypoinsulinaemia has, however, not only been assigned the primary defect in MODY (which is characterized by an early age of onset and mutations of the glucokinase gene) but also to type 2 diabetes at large (21) and particularly for stimulated insulin release (23). In this context, it has been observed that early (first-phase) insulin deficiency, after a stimulus has been given, can result in hyperglycaemia followed by late hyperinsulinaemia (11,13). After correction for excess plasma proinsulin by using highly specific antibodies for insulin and/ or C peptide, these observations could even more frequently relate to stimulated insulin deficiency.

Apart from such quantitative defects in insulin secretion, type 2 diabetes is also characterized by qualitative changes in insulin release. These start with a loss of the normal oscillatory pattern of insulin secretion and end with the progressive failure of insulin release in response to stimulation by glucose (23,24), but less so in response to that of amino acids (25). This sequence of events, though, does not exclude insulin deficiency in the presence of absolute hyperinsulinaemia, which commonly remains inappropriately low compared with non-diabetic subjects and prevailing plasma glucose concentration. This applies in particular once fasting plasma glucose concentration exceeds 120 mg/dl and the early phase of insulin secretion is lost. A similar pattern is also seen in the as-yet non-diabetic offspring of type 2 diabetic parents. Such offspring who are predisposed to develop type 2 diabetes have disorderly and non-stationary insulin secretion and spontaneous irregularity of high-frequency insulin oscillations (26). In addition, the early phase of insulin secretion, in response to both an oral and an intravenous glucose load, tends to be reduced in type 2 diabetic patients with fasting glycaemia.

A major role in the control of insulin release is to be assigned to plasma free fatty acids, which stimulate insulin secretion in the short term but reduce it by 60% after a prolonged 24 hour lipid infusion. This results in failure to compensate appropriately for insulin resistance induced by free fatty acids. This 'Jekyll and Hyde' character of fatty acids means that at any given time insulin secretion will not only be governed by the prevailing plasma concentrations of glucose and amino acids, but also by that of free fatty acids and their qualitative nature (16). In addition, chronic hyperglycaemia seems to be detrimental to the β cells and to impair insulin release by glucose toxicity (15).

In this context, a decisive part is played by glucokinase and its associated glucose-sensing mechanism. This mechanism depends on appropriate physiologic glucose transport and phosphorylation, which are the limiting steps for induction of a physiologic insulin response to a glucose signal. Furthermore, impairment of β-cell function has also been ascribed to islet amyloid polypeptide (IAPP). It not only suppresses insulin action but also is a component of pancreatic islet amyloid, which has been found in excess in the islets of more than 50% of type 2 diabetic patients (27).

Insulin resistance

Insulin resistance (11,28) is a biological state in which a given amount of insulin produces a subnormal metabolic response not only of glucose but also of all other target systems of insulin action including lipolysis. Such impaired insulin sensitivity has been found in states of central (android) obesity, type 2 diabetes, in response to extreme plasma concentrations of triglycerides in familial lipoprotein lipase deficiency (29) and also secondary to TNFα and augmented stress hormone exposure (30). Major locations of insulin resistance are, in decreasing order of magnitude of insulin sensitivity, adipose tissue (lipolysis, lipogenesis and triglyceride storage), liver (glucose production) and peripheral/skeletal muscle (glucose uptake).

Insulin resistance can be quantified by a variety of tests without (hyperglycaemic clamp) and with maintenance of normoglycaemia (euglycaemic hyperinsulinaemic clamp). By measuring glucose disposal and endogenous glucose production, such clamp study permits the muscle (glucose uptake) and hepatic (glucose production, HGP) insulin sensitivity to be estimated simultaneously. To estimate insulin sensitivity in a given test situation, insulin-mediated glucose disposal/production is related to prevailing insulinaemia. In type 2 diabetes such analysis of muscle glucose uptake shows both reduced insulin sensitivity, as reflected by a rightward shift of the

Table 11.1. Insulin sensitivity of different metabolic processes expressed as ED_{50} of insulin (range of means, $\mu U/ml$) in healthy subjects and type 2 diabetic patients. n, number of groups studied (32)

Metabolic process	Healthy subjects (n)	Type 2 diabetic patients (n)
Lipolysis (adipose tissue)	7–17 (6)	22–44 (2)
Glucose production (liver)	26 (2)	66 (1)
Glucose uptake (muscle)	58–60 (2)	118–130 (2)

dose–response curve, and impaired insulin responsiveness, shown by a reduced maximum/plateau in response.

Because skeletal muscle is by volume the major target tissue of insulin action, which controls glycogen synthesis by alleviation of glucose transport and activation of glycogen synthase (31), peripheral muscle must be the major site of glucose uptake reducing insulin resistance (11). Once there is build-up of overall insulin resistance at this final site, compensatory mechanisms of carbohydrate metabolism start to fail and to be largely exhausted. This results in overt hyperglycaemia, with fasting blood glucose concentration exceeding 110 mg/dl, the threshold in the diagnosis of diabetes that has been newly recommended by the ADA for defining an increased risk.

Of note, relative insulin sensitivity is greatest, in falling order of magnitude, for lipolysis, but smaller for glucose production and glucose uptake (32). This sequence of events applies both to healthy subjects and to type 2 diabetic patients (Table 11.1). From these data it is apparent that any insulin resistant state is characterized by an early rise in plasma free fatty acid concentration. This is only subsequently followed by a rise in glucose production and a fall in glucose uptake, which is the least sensitive component of the metabolic response to insulin resistance. The importance of HGP as a main feature of insulin resistance and contributor to hyperglycaemia in type 2 diabetes is also apparent from the observation that hepatic glucose production is commonly completely suppressed during an hyperinsulinaemic euglycaemic clamp. From the above it is clear that the prevailing rate of lipolysis must have a major role in the control of overall insulin sensitivity. Lipolysis-mediated fluctuations in free fatty acids catalyse the degree of insulin resistance in liver and muscle. In addition, increased concentration of plasma free fatty acids causes pronounced accumulation of the end products of the hexosamine biosynthetic pathway and thereby further promote insulin resistance (33). Simultaneously, increased free fatty acid concentration augments insulin release by the pancreatic β cells in the short term (16) and thus contribute to compensatory hyperinsulinaemia (Figure 11.1).

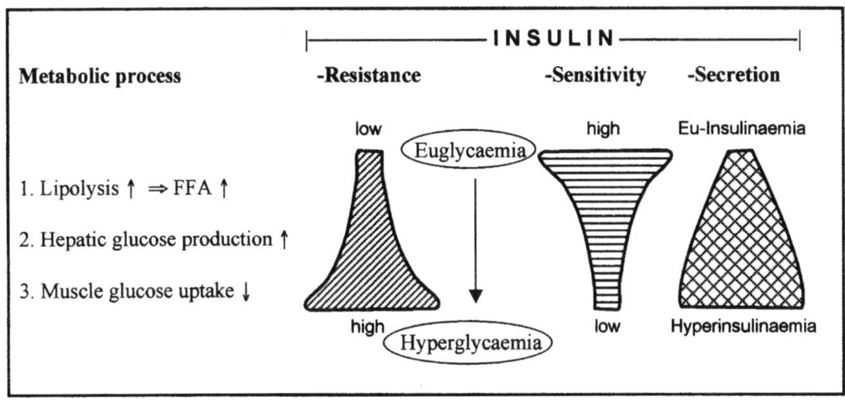

Figure 11.1. Sequential development of hyperglycaemia (arrow) in response to metabolic changes (lipolysis, hepatic glucose production, glucose uptake, insulin resistance) and of augmented insulin secretion secondary to reduced insulin action in the early stages of type 2 diabetes mellitus

In the early phase of type 2 diabetes and insulin resistance, the sequence of events described results in a higher than normal plasma concentration of insulin at a blood glucose concentration that is still normal. Such hyperinsulinaemia also applies to obesity (23,34), where insulin resistance is a major pathogenetic factor. This condition seems to precede the onset of type 2 diabetes by 10–20 years and thereby is to some extent a predictor of the disease (35). Whether it is in reality depends, however, heavily on the criteria used for the diagnosis of diabetes, so that hyperinsulinaemia might be a more marked predictor if a higher diagnostic threshold of blood glucose is applied.

Available data suggest that neither reduced insulin binding nor decreased insulin receptor number are responsible for impaired insulin action in type 2 diabetes but rather the existence of a major post-receptor defect (11). Such a defect would go along with the observed substantial reduction in muscle glycogen synthesis (36) and glucose-6-phosphorylation (37). This associated impaired stimulation of the glycogen synthase-1 gene by insulin in patients with type 2 diabetes is, however, acquired (38) and most likely secondary to both glucotoxicity and lipotoxicity.

It is of note that these phenomena can be triggered by treatment with lipid, which not only inhibits skeletal muscle glucose disposal but also glucose transport/phosphorylation and glycogen synthesis in humans (39,40). Conversely, reduction of plasma free fatty acids improves muscle glucose disposal (41).

These findings are in line with an inverse correlation between intracellular lipid content in skeletal muscle and insulin sensitivity in rats (42) and humans

(43). Reduction by increased plasma free fatty acids of intramuscular glucose phosphorylation has even been observed at a physiological concentration of 0.35 mmol/l (44).

CONCLUSION

From these data it is apparent that any non-physiological rise in the concentration of plasma free fatty acids due either to increased lipolysis or excess exogenous fat supply will deteriorate glucose homeostasis. This effect is mediated by an impairment in glucose phosphorylation and glycogen synthesis in skeletal muscle caused by fatty acids. It is likely that the deterioration of glucose-induced insulin secretion, which also requires cellular glucose entry and phosphorylation, is caused by the same mechanism, both in the early phase of type 2 diabetes and in particular after years of exposure to high concentrations of plasma free fatty acids (16). Such coincidence of free fatty acid (lipotoxicity) mediating impairment of glucose transport and phosphorylation, both in the β cell and skeletal muscle disposal, could well explain the inseparable coexistence of reduced insulin sensitivity and abnormal insulin release in the metabolic obesity/type 2 diabetes mellitus syndrome (17).

REFERENCES

1. Fujimoto WY: Background and recruitment data for the U.S. diabetic prevention program. *Diabet Care* 23 (Suppl. 2):B11–B13, 2000.
2. Zimmet PZ: Diabetes epidemiology as a tool to trigger diabetes research and care. *Diabetologia* 42:499–518, 1999.
3. Evidenzbasierte Diabetes-Leitlinien DDG: Epidemiologie und Verlauf des Diabetes mellitus in Deutschland. W.A.Scherbaum, K.W.Lauterbach, R.Renner. *Deutsche Diabet Gesellsch* 1:2000.
4. Alberti KGMM: The clinical implications of impaired glucose tolerance. *Diabet Med* 13:927–937, 1996.
5. Mahler RJ and Adler ML: Type 2 diabetes mellitus: update on diagnosis, pathophysiology and treatment. *J Clin Endocrinol Metab* 84:1165–1171, 1999.
6. Ferrannini E, Buzzigoli G, Bonadonna R, Giorico MA, Oleggini M, Graziadei L, Pedrinelli R, Brandi L, Bevilacqua S: Insulin resistance in essential hypertension. *N Engl J Med* 317:350–357, 1987.
7. Haffner SM, Miettinen H, Gaskil SP, Stern MP: Decreased insulin secretion and increased insulin resistance are independently related to the 7-year risk of non-insulin-dependent diabetes mellitus in Mexican Americans. *Diabetes* 44:1386–1391, 1995.
8. Poulsen P, Ohm Kyvik K, Vaag A, Beck-Nielsen H: Heritability of type 2 (non-insulin-dependent) diabetes mellitus and abnormal glucose tolerance—a population-based twin study. *Diabetologia* 42:139–145, 1999.
9. Neel JV: Diabetes mellitus: a 'thrifty' genotype rendered detrimental by 'progress'? *Am J Hum Genet* 14:353–362, 1962.

10. Barker DJP: Editorial. Foetal and infant origins of adult disease. *Br Med J* 301:111, 1990.
11. DeFronzo RA: Pathogenesis of type 2 diabetes: metabolic and molecular implications for identifying diabetes genes. *Diabet Rev* 5:177–269, 1997.
12. King GL, Wakasaki H: Theoretical mechanisms by which hyperglycaemia and insulin resistance could cause cardiovascular diseases in diabetes. *Diabet Care* 22 (Suppl. 3):C31–C37, 1999.
13. Cerasi E: Insulin deficiency or insulin resistance in the pathogenesis of NIDDM: is a divorce possible? *Diabetologia* 38:992–997, 1995.
14. Kahn SE, Prigeon RL, McCulloch DK, Boyko EJ, Bergman RN, Schwartz MW, Neifing JL, War WK, Bear JC, Palmer JP, Porte D Jr: Quantification of the relationship between insulin sensitivity and -cell function in human subjects. *Diabetes* 42:1663–1672, 1993.
15. Yki-Järvinen H: Pathogenesis of non-insulin-dependent diabetes mellitus. *Lancet* 343: 91–95, 1994.
16. McGarry JD, Dobbins RL: Fatty acids, lipotoxicity and insulin secretion. *Diabetologia* 42:128–138, 1999.
17. Waldhäusl WK, Roden M: Effects of free fatty acids on glucose transport/phosphorylation in skeletal muscle in humans. *Curr Opin Endocrinol and Diabet* 2000 (in press).
18. Froguel P, Vaxillaire M, Sun F, Velho G, Zouali H, Butel MO, Lesage S, Vionnet N, Clement K, Fougerousse F, Tanizawa Y, Weissenbach J, Beckmann JS, Lathrop GM, Passa P, Permutt MA, Cohen D: Close linkage of glucokinase locus on chromosome 7p to early-onset non-insulin-dependent diabetes mellitus. *Nature* 356:162–164, 1992.
19. Matschinsky FM: Banting lecture 1995. A lesson in metabolic regulation inspired by the glucokinase glucose sensor paradigm. *Diabetes* 45:223–241, 1996.
20. Meneilly GS, Veldhuis JD, Elahi D: Disruption of the pulsatile and entropic modes of insulin release during an unvarying glucose stimulus in elderly individuals. *J Clin Endocrinol Metab* 84:1938–1943, 1999.
21. Gerich JE: The genetic basis of type 2 diabetes mellitus: impaired insulin secretion vs. impaired insulin sensitivity. *Endocr Rev* 19:491–503, 1998.
22. Hales CN: The pathogenesis of NIDDM. *Diabetologia* 37 (Suppl 2):S162–S168, 1994.
23. Waldhäusl W, Bratusch-Marrain P, Gasic S, Korn A, Nowotny P: Insulin production rate, hepatic insulin retention and splanchnic carbohydrate metabolism after oral glucose ingestion in hyperinsulinaemic type 2 (non-insulin-dependent) diabetes mellitus. *Diabetologia* 23:6–15, 1982.
24. Weyer Ch, Bogardus C, Mott DM, Pratley RE: The natural history of insulin secretory dysfunction and insulin resistance in the pathogenesis of type 2 diabetes mellitus. *J Clin Invest* 104:787–794, 1999.
25. Ratheiser K, Reitgruber W, Komjati M, Bratusch-Marrain P, Vierhapper H, Waldhusl W: Quantitative and qualitative differences in basal and glucose- and arginine-stimulated insulin secretion in healthy subjects and different stages of NIDDM. *Acta Diabetol Latina* 27:197–213, 1990.
26. Schmitz O, Porksen N, Nyholm B, Skjaerbaek C, Butler P, Veldhuis J, Pincus SM: Disorderly and non-stationary insulin secretion in relatives of patients with NIDDM. *Am J Physiol* 272:E218–E226, 1997.
27. Westermark P, Johnson KH, O'Brien TD, Betsholtz C: Islet amyloid polypeptide—a novel controversy in diabetes research. *Diabetologia* 35:297–303, 1992.

28. Reaven GM: Role of insulin resistance in human disease. *Diabetes* 37:1595–1607, 1988.
29. Mingrone G, Henriksen FL, Greco AV, Krogh LN, Capristo E, Gastaldelli A, Castagneto M, Ferrannini E, Gasbarrini G: Triglyceride-induced diabetes associated with familial lipoprotein lipase deficiency. *Diabetes* 48:1258–1263, 1999.
30. Waldhäusl W, Gasic S, Bratusch-Marrain P, Komjati M, Korn A: Effect of stress hormones on splanchnic substrate and insulin disposal following glucose ingestion in healthy man. *Diabetes* 36:127–135, 1987.
31. Azpiazu I, Manchester J, Skurat AV, Roach PJ, Lawrence JC Jr: Control of glycogen synthesis is shared between glucose transport and glycogen synthase in skeletal muscle fibers. *Am J Physiol Endocrinol Metab* 278:E234–E243, 2000.
32. Stummvoll M, Jacobs S: Multiple sites of insulin resistance: muscle liver and adipose tissue. *Exp Clin Endocrinol Diabetes* 107:107–110, 1999.
33. Hawkins M, Barzilai N, Liu R, Chen W, Rossetti L: Role of the glucosamine pathway in fat-induced insulin resistance. *J Clin Invest* 99:2173–2182, 1997.
34. Haffner SM, Stern MP, Hazuda HP, Pugh JA, Patterson JK: Hyperinsulinaemia in a population at high risk for non-insulin-dependent diabetes mellitus. *N Engl J Med* 315:220–224, 1986.
35. Haffner SM, Stern MP, Dunn J, Mabley M, Blackwell J, Bergman RN: Diminished insulin sensitivity and increased insulin response in non-obese, non-diabetic Mexican Americans. *Metabolism* 39:842–847, 1990.
36. Cline GW, Petersen KF, Krssak M, Shen J, Hundal RS, Trajanoski Z, Inzucchi S, Dresner A, Rothman DL, Shulman GI: Impaired glucose transport as a cause of decreased insulin-stimulated muscle glycogen synthesis in type 2 diabetes. *N Engl J Med* 341:240–246, 1999.
37. Roden M, Shulman GI: Applications of NMR spectroscopy to study muscle glycogen metabolism in man. *Ann Rev Med* 50:277–290, 1999.
38. Huang X, Vaag A, Hansson M, Wenig J, Laurila E, Groop L: Impaired insulin-stimulated expression of the glycogen synthase gene in skeletal muscle of type 2 diabetic patients is acquired rather than inherited. *J Clin Endocrinol Metab* 85:1584–1590, 2000.
39. Boden G, Chen X, Ruiz J, White JV, Rossetti L: Mechanisms of fatty acid-induced inhibition of glucose uptake. *J Clin Invest* 93:2438–2446, 1994.
40. Roden M, Price TB, Perseghin G, Petersen KF, Rothman DL, Cline GW, Shulman GI: Mechanism of free fatty acid induced insulin resistance in humans. *J Clin Invest* 97:2859–2865, 1996.
41. Piatti PM, Monti LD, Davis SD, Conti M, Brown MD, Pozza G, Alberti KGMM: Effects of an acute decrease in non-esterified fatty acids levels on muscle glucose utilisation and forearm indirect calorimetry in lean NIDDM patients. *Diabetologia* 39:103–112, 1996.
42. Pan DA, Lillioja S, Kriketos AD, Milner MR, Baur LA, Bogardus C, Jenkins AB, Storlien LH: Skeletal muscle triglyceride levels are inversely related to insulin action. *Diabetes* 46:983–988, 1997.
43. Krssak M, Falk Petersen K, Dresner A, DiPietro L, Vogel SM, Rothman DL, Roden M, Shulman GI: Intramyocellular lipid concentrations are correlated with insulin sensitivity in man: a ^{1}H NMR spectroscopy study. *Diabetologia* 42:113–116, 1999.
44. Roden, M., Krssak M, Stingl H, Gruber St, Hofer A, Fürnsinn C, Moser E, Waldhäusl W: Rapid impairment of skeletal muscle glucose transport/phosphorylation by free fatty acids in man. *Diabetes* 48:358–364, 1999.

12

Molecular Basis of Insulin Resistance

MASSIMO FEDERICI and RENATO LAURO
Department of Internal Medicine, University of Rome Tor Vergata, Rome, Italy

The emerging role of insulin resistance in the pathophysiology of diseases such as obesity, atherosclerosis and hypertension in addition to type 2 and type 1 diabetes is attracting the interest of many researchers from various areas of internal medicine. Nevertheless, the exact role and pathogenesis of insulin resistance are far from a resolution (1).

Insulin resistance may be defined as an impairment in insulin action due to both genetic and non-genetic factors. This impairment, at a cellular level, leads to a reduction in insulin ability to exert its pleiotropic and powerful metabolic effects (2).

The events after insulin binds to its receptor are now more known than ever but again, we still have not identified all the key molecular mechanisms leading to the development of insulin resistance.

Another paradigm that has been changing regards the sites of insulin resistance. As insulin resistance has been historically related to an impairment of glucose and lipid metabolism, the attention of clinicians and researchers had always focused on the principal sites of glucose/lipid metabolism: muscle (skeletal and cardiac), adipose tissue and liver. Despite their central role recently, outstanding acquisitions have spread the sites of insulin action to at least two other fundamental tissues: islets of Langerhans (the source of insulin itself) and vasculature (both endothelial and smooth muscle cells) (3,4).

Insulin resistance is a complex biological phenomenon and each insulin resistant patient hides several diverse defects that produce the impairment of

Diabetes in the New Millennium. Edited by U. Di Mario, F. Leonetti, G. Pugliese, P. Sbraccia and A. Signore.
© 2000 John Wiley & Sons, Ltd.

insulin action. Only the definition of the whole of these defects will lead us to a complete and definitive understanding of insulin resistance and its relationships with other pathologies. Then we will be able to classify each patient in different classes and degrees of insulin resistant states. Finally, these efforts will allow us to prevent and cure diabetes and the other insulin resistant related diseases. In this chapter we focus on the state of the art of knowledge about molecular mechanisms of insulin resistance, considering lessons from both animal and human studies.

INSULIN SIGNAL TRANSMISSION PATHWAY: THE ROLE OF PROTEIN–PROTEIN INTERACTIONS

Insulin binding to its tyrosine kinase receptor is followed by phosphorylation of insulin receptor substrates. The phosphorylation events result in protein–protein interactions, which transmit and compartmentalize insulin signal in order to exert hormone final effects as glucose uptake, glycogen and protein synthesis or tissue-specific gene expression (2).

Many studies have contributed to define the factors that modify insulin signaling to determine insulin resistance. There is a consensus that genetic and non-genetic factors may modulate insulin signaling through alteration of expression, conformational properties or polymorphic variants of proteins involved in insulin signaling (2). Here we analyze, in a separate context, genetic and metabolic alterations contributing to the impairment of insulin action known as insulin resistance.

Genetic variants and their significance in insulin signaling

The first substrate to be identified for insulin was the insulin receptor (IR) itself. The receptor possesses an intrinsic tyrosine kinase activity that is essential for transmission of insulin signal (2). Mutations in IR have been described in patients characterized by extreme insulin-resistance syndromes, as type A syndrome and leprechaunism, but are very rare. Genomic scanning of patients with type 2 diabetes or obesity suggests that IR mutations do not have a significant role in the genetics of insulin resistance states (5).

The second substrate to be identified was insulin receptor substrate-1 (IRS-1) the first of several IR substrates (IRS-1/2/3/4, Shc and GAB-1) that function as docking proteins which transmit the signal through a serine/threonine kinases-related pathway. The IRS proteins seem to be highly polymorphic (2). IRS-1 polymorphisms are significantly associated with type 2 diabetes compared to controls in both Caucasian and Japanese patients (6–8). Among variants (G972R, S892G, G819R, R1221C in Caucasians and in Japanese type 2 diabetic patients, also P190R, M209T and S809F variants) the glycine to arginine substitution at codon 972 of IRS-1 gene (G972R) is the most commonly studied. In Caucasian patients the prevalence of this variant is 5.8% in normal vs. 10.7% in type 2 diabetic patients. Carriers of this variant have decreased fasting insulin and c-peptide levels (7). Obese carriers show decreased insulin sensitivity to an oral glucose tolerance test (7). Several *in vitro* studies have been performed to analyze the functional properties of this variant. The variant reduces the binding of p85 subunit of PI3-kinase to IRS-1, causing a 30–50% reduction in insulin-induced IRS-1-associated PI3-kinase activity (9,10). Since this amino acid substitution lies in proximity of the IRS-1/ PI3-kinase interacting domain, it has been suggested that G972R interferes with the ability of IRS-1 to dock with the SH2 domains of PI3-kinase to activate this fundamental enzyme fully. The presence of this G972R IRS-1 variant in muscle cells impairs glucose transport and glycogen synthesis (11). But the most surprising effects are in pancreatic β cells. Two studies analyzing human islets from carriers of this variant and rat β cells transfected with G972R IRS-1 cDNA showed that this variant greatly impairs glucose-induced insulin secretion, while reducing insulin's ability to transduce a pro-survival effect to β cells (10,12). Thus, a new role for IRS-1 is emerging in controlling secretion and survival of human differentiated β cells.

The second substrate for IR is IRS-2, which appears to be higher polymorphically in prevalence than IRS-1 in humans. In fact three variants have been identified (G1057D, G879S and L647V), with a prevalence of 31% in type 2 diabetes vs. 32% in control patients. In spite of an emerging role for IRS-2 in coordinating insulin and IGF action, no association with type 2 diabetes or insulin resistance *per se* has been identified (13).

Thus, among insulin receptor substrates only IRS-1 appears to be associated with type 2 diabetes and insulin resistance. A further interesting association between G972R IRS-1 variant and coronary heart disease comes from a recent study (14) but this requires further investigation.

The IRS proteins recruit PI3-kinase to transmit insulin metabolic signals (GLUT4 translocation and glycogen synthesis), through their interaction with the p85 regulatory subunit of this key enzyme. The p85α subunit then interacts with the catalytic p110 subunit to exert full effects through its lipid kinase activity (2). Since PI-3 kinase appears to be an essential component of insulin signaling, genomic scanning was performed to define the presence of polymorphism in p85 or p110 subunit. Only one study localized a variant (M326I) in a region between the SH2 and SH3 domains of the p85 subunit (15). This variant is common in its heterozygous form in a Caucasian population (31%) and less common in the homozygous form (2%). Despite an association between the homozygous state and reduced insulin sensitivity, a clear functional role of this variant is still lacking. Nevertheless, since PI-3 kinase is a key signaling component of the tyrosine kinase-related pathway in many tissues, as vascular and inflammatory cells, an evaluation for the role of this variant in insulin resistance states, such as in atherosclerosis or hypertension, would be interesting.

Another potential interesting class of genes are represented by peroxisome proliferator-activated receptor (PPAR), in particular PPAR-γ, which is a nuclear receptor that appears to be involved in the regulation of adipocyte differentiation and monocyte/smooth muscle/endothelial cells activation. The interest in PPAR-γ is increased when it was shown that its synthetic ligands, the thiazolidinediones, act as insulin sensitizers.

Four polymorphisms within PPAR-γ have been described. A P12A mutation at the extreme amino-terminus of PPAR-γ is most common, and its effect on weight gain and insulin sensitivity is discussed (16). A P115Q mutation was identified in four extremely obese patients with no effects on insulin sensitivity (16). This mutation occurs in the proximity of an important phosphorylation site, resulting in constitutively activating PPAR-γ. This leads to increased adipogenesis but normal insulin sensitivity. *In vitro* studies showed a clear effect of this mutation in accelerating adipogenic differentiation. It was speculated that this may simultaneously sensitize the whole body to insulin action. Two new mutations have been found in patients suffering from severe insulin resistance, diabetes and hypertension, but not obesity (16). Overall, the data suggest that PPAR-γ promotes fat storage and insulin sensitivity, but additional studies are needed to fully evaluate the intersection between insulin resistance and PPAR-γ activation. Despite the fact that all of these findings on PPAR-γ need to be confirmed, PPAR-γ appears to be a promising prospect as a gene linking obesity, insulin resistance and coronary heart disease.

Lessons from transgenic models

Targeted disruption and transgenic expression of genes related to insulin signaling as IR, IRS-1 and IRS-2 had provided clues to understand the temporal and molecular events leading to the development of insulin resistance and its related diseases. The first model to be produced was the IR knockout (KO), which taught us the essential role of IR in mediating insulin action but also showed that the syndrome most resembling IR KO in humans, leprechaunism, has a really distinct and unrelated phenotype with respect to mouse model (17). A recent approach in this sense had demonstrated that the disruption of just one gene may determine mild insulin resistance and glucose intolerance, as in the case of IRS-1 (KO) or the muscle IR (MIRKO) or even diabetes, as in the case of IRS-2 (KO) (18–20). However, IRS-2 does not play any diabetogenic role in humans, while the most common IRS-1 polymorphism in Caucasians seems to be related to a phenotype different from mouse model of IRS-1 ablation.

Animal models may also provide fundamental help in defining tissue-specific roles in glucose metabolism, since ablation of IR in both muscle and adipose tissues does not cause diabetes but only results in insulin resistance (21).

However, emerging evidence for an important role of genetic background in these mice led to the consideration of the influence of distinct mice strains on the phenotype determined by knock-out genes (22). Again this reminds us that insulin resistance disorders are polygenic in their nature and that several diverse mutations may be necessary to determine the type 2 diabetes or obesity phenotype.

Metabolic factors leading to insulin resistance

Several observations have provided evidence for a role of genotype–phenotype interaction in the development of insulin resistance (2). In the second part of this chapter we discuss the principal acquired factors that reduce the insulin receptor's ability to transmit the signal through its intracellular substrate. Again, we will emphasize those mechanisms that have been provided for a functional explanation of their role.

Several studies have provided some evidence for a reduction of IR expression and tyrosine kinase activity in tissues from type 2 diabetic or obese subjects. While obesity-associated defects regarding IR seem to be fully restored by weight loss (which restores insulin sensitivity), this is not the case in type 2 diabetics. Hence, these data suggest the existence of post-receptor defects in type 2 diabetes (2).

Studies on animal models of obesity have in fact shown a clear negative correlation between levels of hyperinsulinemia and the number of active IRs. The amount of IRs and their function were restored after metabolic compensation (2). Thus, hyperinsulinemia determines a downregulation of IR that is normalized by metabolic compensation.

Another finding concerns the potential alteration in receptor assembly observed in diverse states of insulin resistance. In fact, in type 2 diabetes the expression of insulin/IGF-1 hybrid receptors, which are sensitive to IGF-1, is enhanced, and not insulin at physiological hormone concentrations (23). Thus, increased levels of hybrid receptors would subtract active IR to insulin to exert its metabolic effects. The augmentation of insulin/IGF-1 hybrid receptors has been confirmed in animal models of pluri-metabolic syndrome in the macro- and micro-vessels potentially linking this receptor to the development of vascular complications (4).

The sites of post-receptor insulin signaling are still under investigation. Several studies have indicated a potential explanation in reduced tyrosine-phosphorylation of IRS-1 and PI3-kinase activity. On the contrary, IRS-2 level and function in some cases seem to be enhanced or at least normal, with a full activation of PI3-kinase but still in the presence of insulin resistance (2). These findings would suggest that over-activation of IRS-2 is not able to compensate for a reduction in IRS-1 activation.

Other alterations in the insulin signaling cascade involve the action of counterregulatory hormones such as GH, cortisol or epinephrine, which antagonize insulin action, reducing IRS-1 and PI3-kinase activation (2). A similar mechanism is thought to be involved in TNFα-induced insulin resistance. TNFα is a cytokine secreted by inflammatory activated cells and also by adipose tissue in positive correlation to body mass index. Weight loss reduces its level of expression. TNFα acting through a putative serine kinase determines a serine-phosphorylation of IR and IRS-1, which impairs PI3-kinase activity and downstream signaling (2). Interestingly counter-regulatory hormones and TNFα action might be responsible for enhanced insulin resistance associated with inflammatory states.

A major determinant of insulin resistance is glucose toxicity, a phenomenon related to the hyperglycemic states observed in insulin-resistant subjects in both fasting and non-fasting states. In particular, glucose toxicity is responsible for insulin resistance observed in type 1 diabetic subjects, especially under metabolic derangement. The glucose-toxic effect has been related to increased protein kinase C (PKC) activity, and enhanced O-linked protein glycosylation mediated by the hexosamine pathway (2). Furthermore, the free fatty acids (FFAs) might represent a new category of metabolic effectors of insulin resistance (24–27). The PKCs belong to a family of serine kinases with numerous substrates, including IR, IRS proteins, protein kinase B (PKB/Akt) and others. PKCs are also considered among substrates of IR. While the exact function of PKC upon insulin stimulation remains elusive, it is well established that hyperglycemia-related enhancement in diacylglycerol level leads to PKC activation in a glucose-dependent manner. PKC inhibitors seem to block the glucose-toxic effect on glucose transport; moreover, the serine phosphorylation of IR, which is considered a plausible cause for PKC-induced insulin resistance, is blocked by PKC inhibitors (2). A member of the PKC family, PKCβ, has a role in hyperglycemia-related microvascular complications and diabetic cardiomyopathy (2). Recently, outstanding observations related the increased flux of glucose through the hexosamine pathway to the development of hyperglycemia-related insulin resistance. The hexosamine pathway metabolizes glucose, increasing tissue concentrations of UDP-GlcNAc. The same effect is seen in treating cells or animals with glucosamine, which bypasses the rate-limiting enzyme in the hexosamine pathway, glutamine-fructose-1,6-diphosphate aminotransferase. Moreover, treating hypoinsulinemic hyperglycemic rats with glucosamine does not further reduce insulin sensitivity. This suggests a common mechanism for glucosamine- and hyperglycemia-induced insulin resistance. Two studies have provided a potential explanation. In the first, enhanced O-linked glycosylation of IRS proteins and PI3-kinase lead to insulin resistance (28). In fact, the overall effect of increased activity of the hexosamine pathway leads to protein O-glycosylation on serine and threonine residues. This would implicate a putative competition for serine/threonine residues among kinase cascades and the hexosamine pathway. In the second, insulin/IGF-1 hybrid receptors were increased in both partially pancreatectomized hyperglycemic and glucosamine-infused rats. The receptors appeared to have increased O-glycosylated residues in hyperglycemic and glucosamine-infused animals with respect to controls (29).

Since vascular cells such as smooth muscle and endothelial cells seem to be very susceptible to hexosamine metabolites, this pathway might have a role in hyperglycemia-induced vascular complications.

Interestingly, free fatty acids also activate the hexosamine pathway, inducing insulin resistance (24). Recent studies have suggested that FFA elevations would impair IRS-1-associated PI3-kinase activity in muscle, but no molecular evidence for a role of O-glycosylation was provided in that study (25). Two other studies have suggested that insulin resistance associated with FFA was determined by increased activity of PKCθ, which leads to reduced IRS/PI3-kinase/Akt activity through serine phosphorylation, or ceramide inhibition of Akt phosphorylation, respectively (26,27).

CONCLUSIONS

Insulin resistance is a key phenomenon in the development of diseases such as type 2 diabetes or obesity, and may have a role in the pathogenesis of vascular alterations as hypertension and atherosclerosis. The new concepts that have emerged in these two last decades of intense research have established a role for both genetic and metabolic factors in determining insulin resistance. The principal defect observed in humans concerns the IRS-1/PI3-kinase pathway, both at genetic (but not with a major unique role) and at an acquired (metabolic) level. The IRS-1/PI3-kinase pathway is reduced by about 50% in type 2 diabetic and obese subjects, but this may only partially explain the complexity of insulin-resistant states.

Insulin resistance derives from a defect in insulin action at multiple levels in various tissues. From this point of view, while we have always considered muscle, fat and liver as the primary source of insulin resistance, their overall role has been reconsidered after lessons from animal models of insulin resistance. Now other tissues are emerging as plausible important sites for insulin action: the vascular tissues and the pancreatic β cells. The next decade will certainly develop further knowledge about insulin resistance in these tissues.

However, even if the inheritable nature of insulin resistance is certain, we are still far from the identification of all the major susceptibility genes. On the contrary, we have identified several acquired factors (FFA, hexosamines, hyperglycemia *per se*, TNFα) on which we may act through treatment to improve insulin sensitivity in patients.

The next decade's challenge is the identification of the whole genetic determinants of insulin resistance in order to classify the various subtypes of insulin resistance that lead to development of type 2 diabetes, obesity, hypertension and coronary heart disease.

REFERENCES

1. Kahn CR *et al*: Genetics of non-insulin-dependent (type-II) diabetes mellitus. *Ann Rev Med* 47:509–531, 1996.
2. Virkamaki A *et al*: Protein–protein interaction in insulin signaling and the molecular mechanisms of insulin resistance. *J Clin Invest* 103:931–43, 1999.
3. Kulkarni RN *et al*: Tissue-specific knockout of the insulin receptor in pancreatic beta cells creates an insulin secretory defect similar to that in type 2 diabetes. *Cell* 96:329–339, 1999.
4. Jiang ZY *et al*: Characterization of selective resistance to insulin signaling in the vasculature of obese Zucker (fa/fa) rats. *J Clin Invest* 104:447–457, 1999.
5. Moller DE: Insulin resistance — mechanisms, syndromes, and implications. *N Engl J Med* 325:938–948, 1991.
6. Imai Y *et al*: Variant sequences of insulin receptor substrate-1 in patients with noninsulin-dependent diabetes mellitus. *J Clin Endocrinol Metab* 79:1655–1658, 1994.
7. Clausen JO *et al*: Insulin resistance: interactions between obesity and a common variant of insulin receptor substrate-1. *Lancet* 346:397–402, 1995.
8. Ura S *et al*: Molecular scanning of the insulin receptor substrate-1 (IRS-1) gene in Japanese patients with NIDDM: identification of five novel polymorphisms. *Diabetologia* 39:600–608, 1996.
9. Almind K *et al*: A common amino acid polymorphism in insulin receptor substrate-1 causes impaired insulin signaling. Evidence from transfection studies. *J Clin Invest* 97:2569–2575, 1996.
10. Porzio O *et al*: The Gly972->Arg amino acid polymorphism in IRS-1 impairs insulin secretion in pancreatic beta cells. *J Clin Invest.* 104:357–64, 1999.
11. Hribal ML *et al*: The Gly->Arg972 amino acid polymorphism in insulin receptor substrate-1 affects glucose metabolism in skeletal muscle cells. *J Clin Endocrinol Metab* 85:2004–2013.
12. Federici M *et al*: The common Gly->Arg972 polymorphism in insulin receptor substrate-1 (IRS-1) impairs human pancreatic β-cell secretion and survival. *Diabetes* 49(Suppl.1): A198, 2000.
13. Almind K *et al*: Search for variants of the gene-promoter and the potential phosphotyrosine encoding sequence of the insulin receptor substrate-2 gene: evaluation of their relation with alterations in insulin secretion and insulin sensitivity. *Diabetologia* 42:1244–1249, 1999.
14. Baroni MG *et al*: A common mutation of the insulin receptor substrate-1 gene is a risk factor for coronary artery disease. *Arterioscler Thromb Vasc Biol* 19:2975–2980, 1999.

15. Baynes KC *et al*: Natural variants of human p85 alpha phosphoinositide 3-kinase in severe insulin resistance: a novel variant with impaired insulin-stimulated lipid kinase activity. *Diabetologia* 43:321–331, 2000.
16. Kersten S *et al*: Roles of PPARs in health and disease. *Nature* 405: 421–484, 2000.
17. Accili D *et al*: Early neonatal death in mice homozygous for a null allele of the insulin receptor gene. *Nature Genet* 1:106–109, 1996.
18. Araki E *et al*: Alternative pathway of insulin signalling in mice with targeted disruption of the IRS-1 gene. *Nature* 372:186–190, 1994.
19. Bruning JC *et al*: A muscle-specific insulin receptor knockout exhibits features of the metabolic syndrome of NIDDM without altering glucose tolerance. *Mol Cell* 2:559–569, 1998.
20. Withers DJ *et al*: Disruption of IRS-2 causes type 2 diabetes in mice. *Nature* Feb 26;391(6670):900–904, 1998.
21. Lauro D *et al*: Impaired glucose tolerance in mice with a targeted impairment of insulin action in muscle and adipose tissue. *Nature Genet* 20:294–298, 1998.
22. Kido Y *et al*: *Diabetes* 49: 589–596, 2000.
23. Federici M *et al*: Increased expression of insulin/insulin-like growth factor-I hybrid receptors in skeletal muscle of noninsulin-dependent diabetes mellitus subjects. *J Clin Invest*. 98:2887–2893, 1996.
24. Hawkins M *et al*: Role of the glucosamine pathway in fat-induced insulin resistance. *J Clin Invest* 99:2173–2182, 1997.
25. Dresner A *et al*: Effects of free fatty acids on glucose transport and IRS-1-associated phosphatidylinositol 3-kinase activity. *J Clin Invest* 103:253–259, 1999.
26. Griffin ME *et al*: Free fatty acid-induced insulin resistance is associated with activation of protein kinase C theta and alterations in the insulin signaling cascade. *Diabetes* 48:1270–1274, 1999.
27. Schmitz-Peiffer C *et al*: Ceramide generation is sufficient to account for the inhibition of the insulin-stimulated PKB pathway in C2C12 skeletal muscle cells pretreated with palmitate. *J Biol Chem* 274:24 202–24 210, 1999.
28. Patti ME *et al*: Activation of the hexosamine pathway by glucosamine *in vivo* induces insulin resistance of early postreceptor insulin signaling events in skeletal muscle. *Diabetes* 48:1562–151, 1999.
29. Federici M: Evidence for glucose/hexosamine *in vivo* regulation of insulin/IGF-I hybrid receptor assembly. *Diabetes* 48:2277–2285, 1999.

13

Role of Membrane Glycoprotein PC-1 in the Etiology of Insulin Resistance

IRA D. GOLDFINE[1], BETTY MADDUX[1], PAOLO SBRACCIA[2] and LUCIA FRITTITTA[3]

[1]University of California at San Francisco, CA, USA; [2]University of Rome "Tor Vergata", Italy; [3]University of Catania, Italy

PC-1 content is elevated in muscle and fat of insulin resistant, non-diabetic and diabetic subjects and plays a role in this pathological process. PC-1 binds to the connecting domain of the insulin receptor (IR) α subunit, and when either overexpressed or in the Q allele form, prevents insulin from activating the β subunit tyrosine kinase domain. These data indicate, therefore, that PC-1 may play a role in states of insulin resistance.

BACKGROUND

Membrane glycoprotein PC-1 and insulin resistance

Two lines of evidence suggest that PC-1 has a role in decreased IR function and insulin resistance. First, we have found that PC-1 is elevated in fibroblasts, muscle and fat of patients with insulin resistance, and in muscle of streptozotocin-treated diabetic rats. Also, the Q allele of PC-1 (a variant that has an amino acid change in one somatomedin B-like domain) has an enhanced inhibitory effect on the IR and is strongly associated with clinical insulin resistance. Second, we have observed that overexpression of PC-1 in cultured cells reduces IR tyrosine kinase activity (see below).

Diabetes in the New Millennium. Edited by U. Di Mario, F. Leonetti, G. Pugliese, P. Sbraccia and A. Signore.
© 2000 John Wiley & Sons, Ltd.

Characteristics of membrane glycoprotein PC-1

PC-1 is a class II transmembrane glycoprotein that is located both on plasma membranes and in the endoplasmic reticulum (Figure 13.1). PC-1 is the same protein as liver nucleotide pyrophosphatase/alkaline phosphodiesterase I (1–9). In addition to muscle tissue (*see below*), PC-1 has been reported to be expressed in plasma and intracellular membranes of plasma cells, placenta, the distal convoluted tubule of the kidney, ducts of the salivary gland, epididymis, proximal part of the *vas deferens*, chondrocytes and dermal fibroblasts (7). PC-1 exists as a homodimer of 230–260 kDa; the reduced form of the protein has a molecular size of 115–135 kDa, depending on the cell type. Human PC-1 is predicted to have 873 amino acids.

PC-1 is inserted into the plasma membrane, such that there is a small cytoplasmic amino terminus and a much larger extracellular carboxyl terminus (3,4,9) (Figure 13.1). The extracellular domain of PC-1 has an enzymatic activity that cleaves sugar–phosphate, phosphosulphate, pyrophosphate and phosphodiesterase linkages. The active enzyme site for phosphodiesterase and pyrophosphatase contains a key threonine residue. We have shown that mutation of this residue does not impair the ability of PC-1 to inhibit IR function (10). It has been suggested that PC-1 may have threonine-specific protein kinase activity (11), although it does not have sequence homology to the known threonine kinases; recently, the existence of this protein kinase activity has been questioned (9).

The physiological function of PC-1 is unknown. It has been proposed that PC-1 may belong to an enzyme cascade system working in concert with other ecto-enzymes that hydrolyze nucleotides and nucleic acids to nucleosides, which are then taken up by cells via a nucleoside transporter (7–9). This pathway would allow the salvage of nucleotides from the extracellular fluid, and also allow the uptake of nucleosides by cells that are unable to synthesize purines by the *de novo* pathway. In addition, there is evidence that PC-1 plays a role in bone and cartilage metabolism (9,12).

PC-1 has: (a) an EF-hand domain (two alpha helices, "E" and "F", joined by a Cd^{+2}-binding loop) which binds Ca^{+2} and stabilizes the structure of the molecule; (b) an ATP binding site; (c) a phosphodiesterase site that has a critical threonine; (d) a proteolytic cleavage site that allows PC-1 to be shed by cells; and (e) two somatomedin B-like domains that are part of a cysteine-rich domain (Figure 13.1). The phosphodiesterase activity of PC-1 is not involved in the inhibition of IR function (10). Proteolytic cleavage of PC-1 may represent a degradation mechanism for this protein and alterations in cleavage may cause elevations of cellular PC-1 content.

The gene for PC-1 is in the chromosomal region 6q22–q23. Two groups have found linkages between this region and diabetes. Duggirala *et al* (13) have found that a type 2 diabetes marker, DGS290, is located near the PC-1 gene in

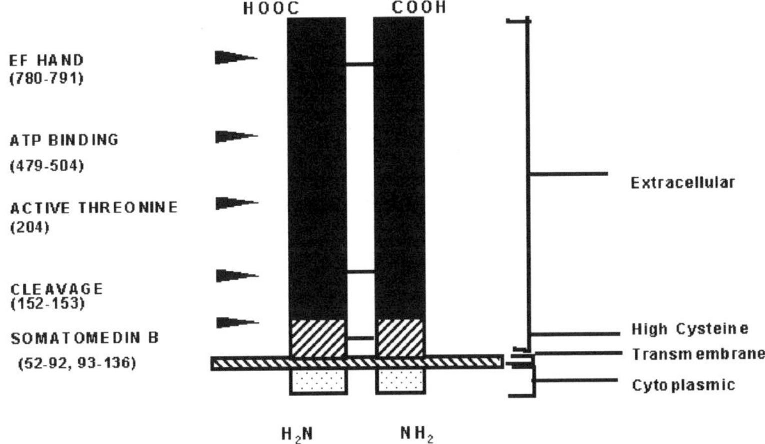

Figure 13.1. Structure of membrane glycoprotein PC-1

Mexican-Americans. Temple *et al* (14) have found that a gene for neonatal diabetes is localized to 6q22-q23. Neonatal diabetes is usually transient but predisposes to type 2 diabetes later in life.

PC-1 is closely related to two other phosphodiesterase proteins: 1) PD-1 α (also known as autotaxin), and PD-1β (also known as gp103RB[13–6])[14–17]. PD-1α is a tumor motility protein and PD-1β is a brain phosphodiesterase. The PD-1α gene is on chromosome 8q24.1, and the PD-1β gene is on chromosome 6q22. Since this latter location is near the gene for PC-1, it is likely that this close proximity reflects gene duplication. Both PD-1α and PD-1β have domains similar to those of PC-1. PD-1α, like PC-1, has a proteolytic cleavage site and circulates; this appears not to be the case for PD-1β (9).

PC-1 is controlled by genetic and other regulatory systems. PC-1 is upregulated by glucocorticoids (18), agents that raise cyclic AMP (19), PKC (19), growth factors such as FGF (20,21) and cytokines including interleukin-1β (22). The glucocorticoid effect may be through a GRE-like sequence in the PC-1 promoter. The finding that PC-1 is regulated by glucocorticoids and other factors provides an explanation as to why PC-1 content is elevated with loss of glycemic control and may be elevated in stress and infection. Bollen and colleagues (23) have recently reported in rodent liver that PC-1 is absent in rapidly growing cells; fetal mouse liver, regenerating mouse liver and rat-cultured HTC cells. In these conditions where PC-1 protein was not present, PC-1 mRNA was decreased. However, this decrease in PC-1 was not due to decreased PC-1 gene transcription. Rather, they suggested that PC-1 expression is controlled by a putative mRNA stabilizing protein.

Elevated tissue content of PC-1 as a cause of insulin resistance

Studies in muscle and adipose tissue

To determine whether PC-1 plays a role in both the insulin resistance and the impaired IR tyrosine kinase activity in lean, insulin-resistant subjects, we established a collaborative project with Dr Riccardo Vigneri, University of Catania, Italy. Very recently, we have measured PC-1 content in healthy, non-diabetic, non-obese subjects (seven females, five males; 36 ± 4 years; body mass index, $23.4\pm1\,\mathrm{kg/m^2}$; fasting blood glucose $91\pm2\,\mathrm{mg/dl}$) (unpublished data). All patients had a biopsy of the external oblique muscle. In this group, there was a wide range of insulin sensitivity. There was significant inverse correlation between PC-1 content in muscle, and insulin sensitivity as measured by the insulin clamp ($r=0.82$; $p<0.01$). In a similar group of patients (24), there was the same correlation between adipose tissue, PC-1 content and insulin sensitivity (data not shown).

Studies in fibroblasts from type 2 diabetes patients

Our initial investigation of PC-1 began when we studied skin fibroblasts derived from a 42 year-old woman (MW) who had type 2 diabetes mellitus with resistance to insulin (24,25). In her cultured cells, insulin action was impaired as measured by a variety of parameters, including IR autophosphorylation, IRS-1 phosphorylation, and biological functions including glucose and amino acid transport (Figure 13.2). IR tyrosine kinase activity, but not IGF-I R tyrosine kinase activity, was impaired (Figure 13.3). The IR content and insulin binding to her fibroblasts were normal, and, when purified, the IR had normal tyrosine kinase activity. Her fibroblasts had an elevated level of PC-1. Measurement of PC-1 enzyme activity, PC-1 Western blot analysis, and ELISA with antibodies specific for PC-1 indicated that there was an approximate 5–10-fold increase in PC-1 content when extracts from the patient's cells were compared to those from controls. Moreover, when we carried out Northern blot analysis of her PC-1 mRNA, there was an approximate 5–10-fold increase in the major mRNA species for PC-1. We next determined whether an elevation in PC-1 was unique to patient MW or was present in the cells of others. Accordingly, we studied PC-1 content in fibroblasts from nine additional insulin-resistant type 2 patients (24). Seven of the nine patients had elevated PC-1. In these patients with increased PC-1, IR tyrosine kinase activity was studied and found to be decreased in fibroblasts. These studies suggested, therefore, that in fibroblasts from type 2 diabetic patients, elevations in PC-1 play a role in insulin resistance.

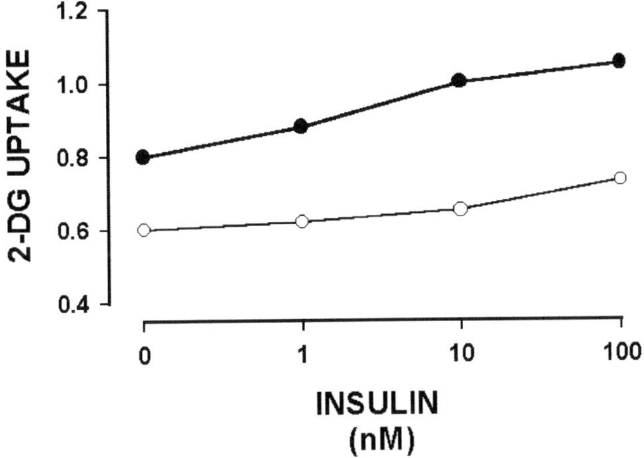

Figure 13.2. *Impaired insulin action in fibroblasts from patient MW.* Cells were incubated 1 h with insulin and 30 min with [³H] 2-deoxy-D-glucose (2-DG). Uptake was measured and expressed as fmol/mg protein

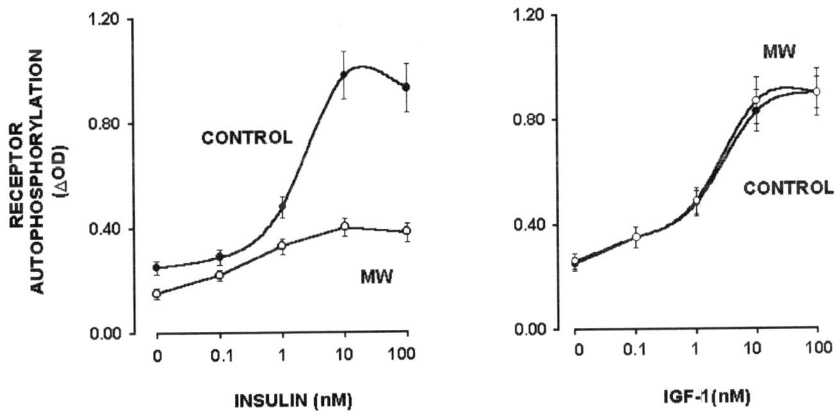

Figure 13.3. Stimulation of IR but not IGF-I-Rβ subunit autophosphorylation in fibroblasts from patient (MW) and a sex-matched and age-matched control. Fibroblasts were grown in multiwell plates and stimulated with insulin or IGF-1 for 5 min. Cells were washed thrice, then solubilized in buffer containing 50 mM Hepes (pH 7.6), 1% Triton-X100, 1 mM PMSF, and 2 mM sodium orthovanadate for 1 hour at 4°C. Receptors were captured on ELISA plates coated with either an insulin antibody (MA20) or an anti-IGF-1 antibody (α-IR3). After 2 hours at 22°C, ELISA plates were washed and probed with an anti-phosphotyrosine kinase antibody and activity measured

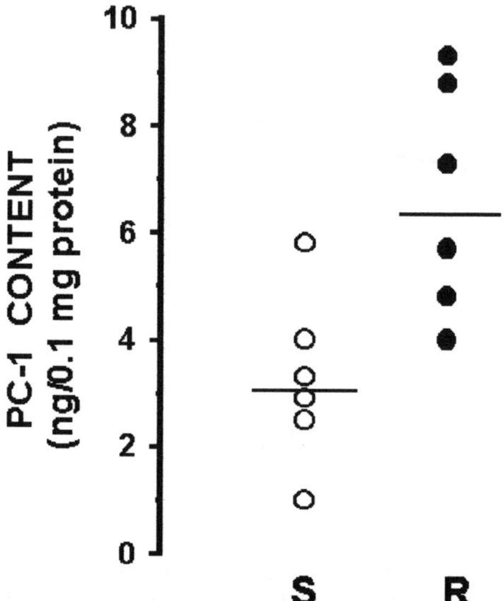

Figure 13.4.   PC-1 content in insulin-sensitive (o) and insulin-resistant individuals

Studies in fibroblasts from insulin-resistant non-diabetic subjects

We then studied PC-1 in skin fibroblasts from 12 non-diabetic subjects (26). On the basis of the insulin clamp, the subjects were divided into an insulin-sensitive group of six and an insulin-resistant group of six. The insulin-resistant subjects had higher fibroblast PC-1 levels (Figure 13.4), and decreased maximal

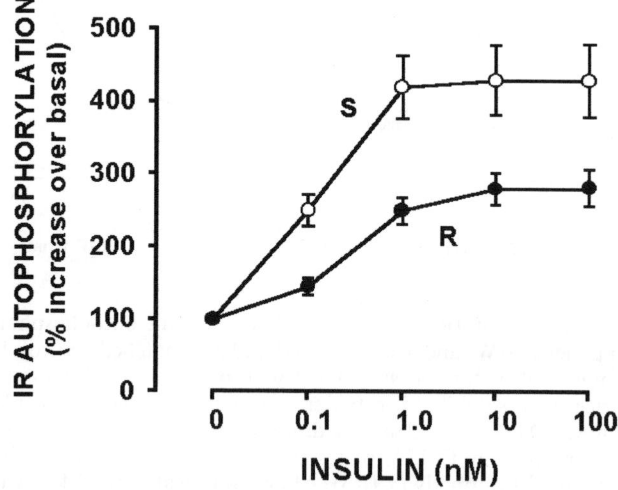

Figure 13.5.   IR autophosphorylation in insulin-sensitive (S) and insulin-resistant (R) subjects

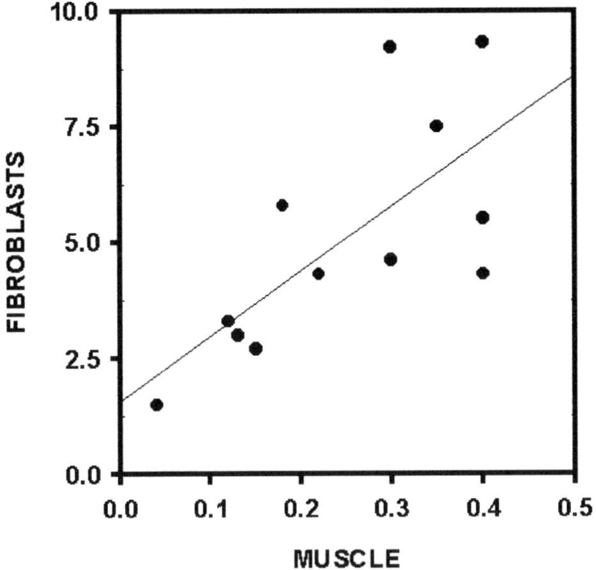

Figure 13.6. Correlation of muscle and fibroblasts PC-1 content in 12 non-diabetic subjects. Results are expressed per 100 µg protein

responsiveness of IR tyrosine kinase activity (Figure 13.5). Moreover, since the fibroblasts were grown for multiple passages in culture, the alterations in PC-1 content did not reflect the metabolic status of the subjects at the time the sample was obtained. When muscle biopsies and cultured fibroblasts from the same patients were compared, fibroblast PC-1 levels correlated with muscle PC-1 levels (Figure 13.6). Thus, PC-1 expression is under similar regulation across tissue types, and is intrinsically upregulated in insulin-resistant subjects. Therefore, cultured fibroblasts can be used to study the mechanisms of PC-1 overexpression.

In vitro studies of PC-1 overexpression

Transfection of PC-1 cDNA and overexpression of PC-1 protein decreases IR but not IGF-I R autophosphorylation in cultured cells

Our studies in fibroblasts that had naturally occurring elevations in PC-1 content demonstrated a correlation between PC-1 content and IR signaling. To demonstrate causality, we next carried out studies with MCF-7 cells, a human breast carcinoma cell line that had previously been used to investigate insulin action. MCF-7 cells were then transfected with an expression plasmid containing PC-1 cDNA (24,27). Control cells had a PC-1 content of 20–30 ng/0.1 mg

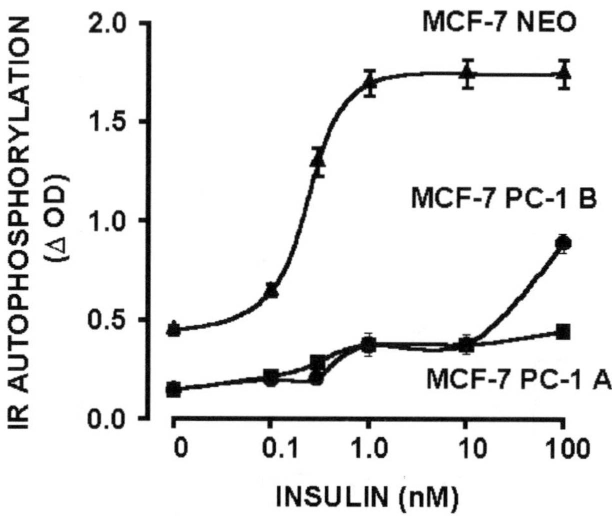

Figure 13.7. PC-1 transfection inhibits IR tyrosine kinase activity. Effect of a 5 min incubation with insulin on IR tyrosine kinase activity in MCF-7 NEO control, and two separate clones of MCF-7-PC-1 cells

protein, and this level was increased to 250–400 in transfected cells. Overexpression of PC-1 did not alter IR binding. However, with PC-1 overexpression, there was marked inhibition of insulin-stimulated tyrosine kinase activity in whole cells (Figure 13.7).

In contrast to the IR, PC-1 overexpression did not influence the IGF-I R (24,27). We then studied the effect of PC-1 overexpression on insulin-regulated biological functions in MCF-7 cells. For example, when [³H] thymidine incorporation and p70 S6 kinase were studied, the effect of insulin was blunted and insulin stimulation of leucine incorporation into protein, and glucose transport were also blunted (unpublished data).

Studies in HTC-IRα subunit mutant

The IR has a tyrosine kinase regulatory site in the IRα subunit located in residues 485–599. When these residues are deleted, the mutant molecule can bind insulin (26,28), but the hormone loses its ability to activate the β subunit tyrosine kinase domain. We next studied rat HTC cells overexpressing PC-1 that were cotransfected and overexpressed either the wild-type IR (HTC-IR) or this mutant (HTC-IR Δ485–599) (Figure 13.8). In HTC-IR cells, as in MCF-7 cells, PC-1 overexpression inhibited IR autophosphorylation. In HTC-IR Δ485–599 cells, IR autophosphorylation was not stimulated by insulin. PC-1 overexpression did not influence IR autophosphorylation in this cell line. We

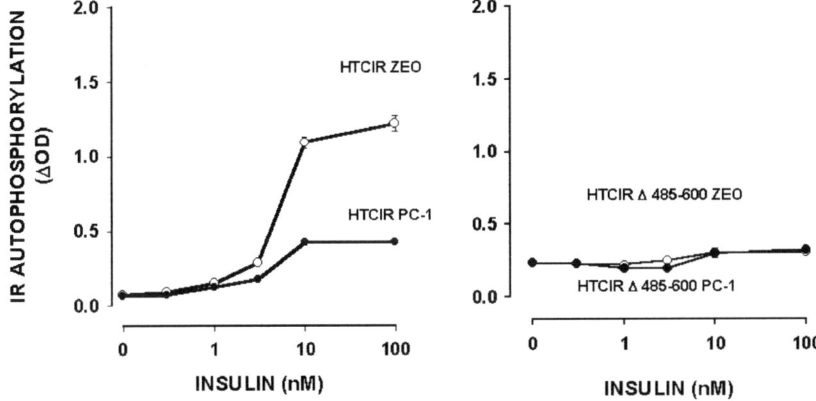

Figure 13.8. Effect of PC-1 overexpression on IR autophosphorylation in HTC-IR ZEO and HTC IR Δ485–599 ZEO cells. HTC cell lines treated as in Figure 3. (A) HTC-IR ZEO compared to HTC-IR PC-1. (B) HTC-IR (Δ485–599) ZEO compared to HTC-IR (Δ485–599) PC-1. Results are the mean ± SD of triplicate determinations from a representative of three experiments. ZEO = selectable marker control.

next studied whether PC-1 associated with the wild-type IR and the mutated IR (Δ485–599) in HTC cells. There was enhanced association of PC-1 with the IR in HTC-IR PC-1 cells, but no association detected in HTC-IR Δ485–599 cells (Figure 13.8).

Q allele

We have recently described a polymorphism for PC-1 that correlates with insulin resistance (29). Overlapping cosmid clones containing the PC-1 gene were isolated by screening with a human full-length PC-1 cDNA, and cosmids were digested with four different base cutter enzymes, blotted and hybridized to oligonucleotides designed on the cDNA sequence. Positive fragments were cloned and sequenced. The human PC-1 gene has 25 exons. Exon amplimers, obtained using specific oligonucleotides as primers, were analysed in 200 unrelated subjects with single-strand conformation polymorphism. In exon 4 at amino acid 121 there was a *Q for K polymorphism* that was associated with insulin resistance. In insulin-resistant subjects the KQ allele frequency was 27.5% as compared to the Q allele frequency in insulin-sensitive subjects (11.1%). When fibroblasts of individuals with the KQ allele were compared to those of the KK allele, IR tyrosine kinase activity was significantly reduced. To our knowledge, this is the first instance in which a common polymorphism of a gene involved in regulating insulin action has been associated with insulin resistance.

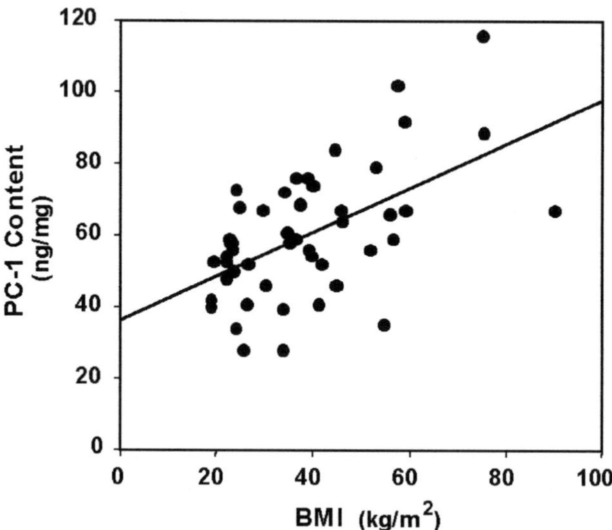

Figure 13.9. Relationship between skeletal muscle PC-1 content and body mass index. PC-1 content was determined by radio-immunoassay

PC-1 in obesity

In addition, we have studied PC-1 content in muscle from obese and insulin-resistant individuals (30). In a collaborative study with Lynis Dohm at East Carolina University, we studied rectus abdominus muscle from individuals with a wide range of obesity, as determined by increased body mass index (BMI) (Figure 13.9). There was a highly significant correlation between PC-1 content and obesity. Moreover, there was a very strong correlation between PC-1 content and the ability of insulin to stimulate glucose transport in isolated muscle strips (30).

Studies of PC-1 in other laboratories

Other laboratories have published studies on PC-1 and insulin resistance. Teno *et al* (31) have published that there is an increase in membrane glycoprotein PC-1 in the fibroblasts from non-insulin-dependent diabetes mellitus patients with insulin resistance. Shao *et al* have reported that PC-1 content is elevated in muscle from women with gestational diabetes (32). In these latter two studies, the elevated PC-1 content was associated with decreased IR tyrosine kinase activity. Stefanovic *et al* (33) have reported that PC-1 is increased in lymphocytes from type 2 diabetic patients, and this increase is reversed by metformin treatment.

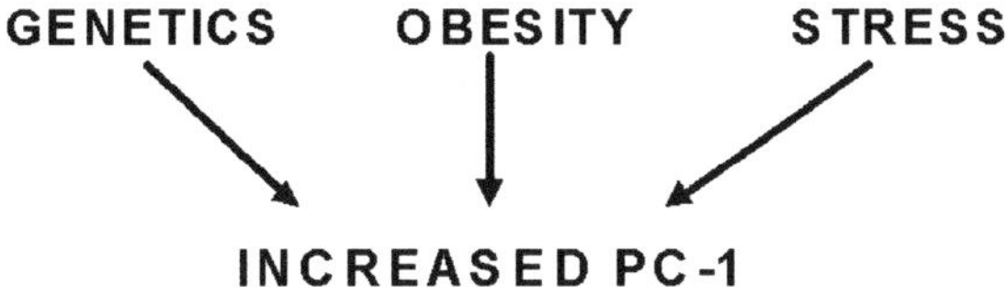

Figure 13.10. Factors that may influence PC-1 content in key insulin-sensitive tissues

Recently, Sakoda *et al* (34) have published data concerning both cell culture and animal studies of PC-1. They reported that very diabetic rats (blood glucose 500 mg/dl) that had lost approximately 30% of body weight did not have elevations of muscle PC-1. Since we observed a rise in PC-1 in less diabetic animals, it is likely that in their studies, PC-1 did not increase because the animals were very diabetic and thus catabolic. In addition, they reported studies in which they infected mouse 3T3-L1 cells with an adenovirus construct containing the human PC-1 coding sequence, and concluded from their observations that PC-1 overexpression does not inhibit IR function in mouse and human tissues. There are several explanations for their negative results. Most importantly, they did not measure the IR directly. Rather, after stimulating the cells with a single high concentration of insulin they measured the IR with a non-specific anti-phosphotyrosine antibody that could detect other tyrosine phosphorylated proteins, such as the IGF-I R, that are not influenced by PC-1. In fact, we observe that 3T3 cells infected by a PC-1 adenovirus construct show decreased IR autophosphorylation when anti-IR antibodies are employed. Thus, it is very likely that in the study of Sakoda *et al*, PC-1 effects on the IR were masked by the detection of other tyrosine phosphorylated receptors, such as the IGF-I R that are highly expressed in 3T3 cells.

Multifactorial regulation of PC-1

These data indicate that multiple factors may influence PC-1 content in key insulin sensitive tissues (Figure 13.10). These factors include genetic influences, obesity and stress.

SIGNIFICANCE OF THESE FINDINGS AND FUTURE RESEARCH

Insulin resistance is a feature of both type 1 and type 2 diabetes. In type 1 diabetes, insulin resistance occurs secondary to hyperglycemia, stress and infection. Under these conditions, insulin resistance causes poor glycemic control, predisposing to ketoacidosis. In other individuals, primary insulin resistance can lead to the onset of type 2 diabetes. In both types of diabetes, the cause(s) of insulin resistance are largely unknown. We have observed that membrane glycoprotein PC-1 is overexpressed in tissues of individuals with various forms of insulin resistance. Since PC-1 overexpression inhibits insulin receptor function, PC-1 may be a common factor in the causes of several types of insulin resistance. Additional studies are needed to investigate the direct interactions of PC-1 with the insulin receptor. These studies will help reveal the mechanism(s) causing certain forms of insulin resistance. Moreover, these studies should lead to new pharmacological therapies that would interrupt IR–PC-1 interactions and reverse insulin resistance and diabetes mellitus.

REFERENCES

1. Driel IR, Goding JW: Plasma cell membrane glycoprotein PC-1. *J Biol Chem* 262:4882, 1987.
2. Harahap R, Goding JW: Distribution of PC-1 in non-lymphoid tissues. *J Immunol* 141:2317, 1988.
3. Buckley MF, Loveland KA, McKinstry WJ, Garson OM, Goding JR: Plasma cell membrane glycoprotein PC-1 cDNA cloning of the human molecule, amino acid sequence, and chromosomal location. *J Biol Chem* 265:29,17506, 1990.
4. Rebbe NF, Tong BD, Finley EM, and Hickma S: Identification of nucleotide pyrophosphatase/alkaline phosphodiesterase I activity associated with the mouse plasma cell differentiation antigen PC-1. *Proc Natl Acad Sci USA* 88:5192, 1991.
5. Funakoshi I *et al*: Molecular cloning of human nucleotide pyrophosphatase. *Arch Biochem Biophys* 295:180, 1992.
6. Uriarte M, Stalmans W, Hickman S, Bollen M: Phosphorylation and nucleotide-dependent dephosphorylation of hepatic polypeptides related to the plasma cell differentiation antigen PC-1. *Biochem J* 293:93, 1993.
7. Rebbe NF, Tong BD, Hickman S: Expression of nucleotide pyrophosphatase and alkaline phosphodiesterase I activities of PC-1, the murine plasma cell antigen. *Mol Immunol* 30:87, 1993.
8. Yoshida H, Fukui S, Yamashina I: Substrate specificity of a nucleotide pyrophosphatase responsible for the breakdown of 3′-phosphoadenosine 5′-phosphosulfate (PAPS) from human placenta. *J Biochem* 93:1641, 1983.
9. Goding JW, Terkeltaub R, Maurice M, Deterre P, Sali A, Belli S: Ecto-phosphodiesterase/pyrophosphatase of lymphocytes and non-lymphoid cells: structure and function of the PC-1 family. *Immunol Rev* 161:11–26, 1998.
10. Grupe A, Alleman J, Goldfine ID, Sadick M, Stewart T: Inhibition of insulin receptor phosphorylation by PC-1 is not mediated by the hydrolysis of adenosine triphosphate or the generation of adenosine. *J Biol Chem* 270:22 085–22 088, 1995.
11. Oda Y, Kuo M-D, Huang SS, Huang JS: The plasma cell membrane glycoprotein, PC-1, is a threonine specific protein kinase stimulated by acidic fibroblast growth factor. *J Biol Chem* 266:16 791, 1991.
12. Johnson K, Moffa A, Chen Y, Pritzker K, *et al*: Matrix vesicle plasma cell membrane glycoprotein-1 regulates mineralization by murine osteoblastic MC3T3 cells. *J Bone Min Res* 14:883–892, 1999.

13. Duggirala R, Blangero J, Mitchell B, O'Connell P, Stern M: Evidence for linkage between fasting and 2-hr plasma glucose levels and regions on chromosomes 6 and 11 in Mexican Americans. Abstract (#839) presented at the 58th Scientific Sessions of the American Diabetes Association, San Francisco, CA, 8–11 June, 1996.

14. Temple IK, Gardner RJ, Robinson DO *et al*: Further evidence for an imprinted gene for neonatal diabetes localized to chromosome 6q22–q23. *Human Mol Genet* 5:1117–1121, 1996.

15. Kawagoe H, Soma O, Goji J *et al*: Molecular cloning and chromosomal assignment of the human brain-type phosphodiesterase I/nucleotide pyrophosphotase gene (PDNP2). *Genomics* 30:380–384, 1995.

16. Murata J, Lee HY, Clair T *et al*: DNA cloning of the human tumor motility-stimulating protein, autotaxin, reveals a homology with phosphodiesterase. *J Biol Chem* 269:30 479–30 484, 1994.

17. Deisler H, Lottspeich F, Rajewsky MF: Affinity purification and cDNA cloning of rat neural differentiation and tumor cell surface antigen gp130 RB13–6 reveals relationship to human and murine PC-1. *J Biol Chem* 270:9849–9855, 1995.

18. Rousseau GG, Amar-Costesec A, Verhaegen M, Granner DK: Glucocorticoid hormones increase the activity of plasma membrane alkaline phosphodiesterase I in rat hepatoma cells. *Proc Natl Acad Sci USA* 77(2):1005–1009, 1980.

19. Deterre P, Gelman L, Gary-Gouy H *et al*: Coordinated regulation in human T cells of nucleotide-hydrolyzing ecto-enzymatic activities, including $CD_3 8$ and PC-1. *J Immunol* 157:1381–1388, 1996.

20. Uriarte M, Stalmans W, Hickman S, Bollen M: Regulation of purified hepatic PC-1 (phosphodiesterase-I/nucleotide pyrophosphatase) by threonine auto(de) phosphorylation and by binding of acidic fibroblast growth factor. *Biochem J* 306:271–277, 1995.

21. Solan JL, Deftos LJ, Goding JW, Terkeltaub RA: Expression of the nucleoside triphosphate pyrophosphohydrolase PC-1 is induced by basic fibroblast growth factor (bFGF) and modulated by activation of the protein kinase A and C pathways in osteoblast-like osteosarcoma cells. *J Bone Min Res* 11:183–193.

22. Lotz M, Rosen F, McCabe G *et al*: Interleukin 1β suppresses transforming growth factor-induced inorganic pyrophosphate (PPi) production and expression of the PPi-generating enzyme PC-1 in human chondrocytes. *Proc Natl Acad Sci USA* 92:10 364–10 368, 1995.

23. Stefan C, Stalmans W, Bollen M: Growth-related expression of the ectonucleotide pyrophosphatase PC-1 in rat liver. *Hepatology* 28:1497–1503, 1998.

24. Maddux BA, Sbraccia P, Kumakura S *et al*: Membrane glycoprotein PC-1 and insulin resistance in non-insulin-dependent diabetes. *Nature* 373:448–451, 1995.

25. Sbraccia P, Goodman PA, Maddux BA, Chen Y-DI, Reaven GM, Goldfine ID: Production of an inhibitor of insulin receptor tyrosine kinase in fibroblasts from a patient with insulin resistance and NIDDM. *Diabetes* 40:295, 1991.

26. Frittitta L, Spampinato D, Solini A, Nosadini R, Goldfine ID *et al*: Elevated PC-1 content in cultured skin fibroblasts correlates with decreased *in vivo* and *in vitro* insulin action in nondiabetic subjects. Evidence that PC-1 may be an intrinsic factor in impaired insulin receptor signaling. *Diabetes* 47:1095–1100, 1998.

27. Maddux BA, Goldfine ID: PC-1 inhibition of insulin receptor function occurs via direct interaction with the receptor alpha subunit. *Diabetes*, 49:13–19, 2000.

28. Sung CK, Wong KY, Yip CC, Hawley DM, Goldfine ID: Deletion of residues 485–599 from the human insulin receptor abolishes antireceptor antibody binding and influences tyrosine kinase activation. *Mol Endocrinol* 8:315–324, 1993.

29. Pizzuti A, Frittitta L, Argiolas A *et al*: Brief genetics report: a polymorphism (K121Q) of the human glycoprotein PC-1 gene coding region is strongly associated with insulin resistance. *Diabetes* 48:1881–1884, 1999.
30. Youngren JF, Maddux BA, Sasson S *et al*: Skeletal muscle content of membrane glycoprotein PC-1 in obesity: relationship to muscle glucose transport. *Diabet* 45:1324–1328, 1996.
31. Teno S, Kanno H, Oga S, Kumakura S *et al*: Increased activity of membrane glycoprotein PC-1 in the fibroblasts from non-insulin-dependent diabetes mellitus patients with insulin resistance. *Diabetes Res Clin Pract* 45:25–30, 1999.
32. Shao J-H, Catalano PM, Huston L *et al*: Impaired insulin receptor tyrosine kinase activity and overexpression of PC-1 in skeletal muscle from obese women with gestational diabetes mellitus. *Diabetes* 48:A53, 1999.
33. Stefanovic V, Antic S, Mitic-Zlatkovic M, Vlahovic P: Reversal of increased lymphocyte alkaline phosphodiesterase I (PC-1) expression in NIDDM patients treated with metformin. *Diabet Metab Res Rev*, 1999 (in press).
34. Sakoda H, Ogihara T, Anai M *et al*: No correlation of plasma cell 1 overexpression with insulin resistance in diabetic rats and 3T3-L1 adipocytes. *Diabetes* 48:1365–1371, 1999.

14

Insulin and Its Receptor in Growth Promotion

RICCARDO VIGNERI[1] and ANTONINO BELFIORE[2]

[1]Cattedra di Endocrinologia, Istituto di Medicina Interna, Malattie Endocrine e del Metabolismo, University of Catania, Ospedale Garibaldi, Catania, Italy;
[2]Cattedra di Endocrinologia e Malattie del Metabolismo, Dipartimento di Medicina Sperimentale e Clinica, University of Catanzaro 'Magna Graecia', Policlinico Mater Domini, Catanzaro, Italy

A large body of evidence suggests that insulin, in addition to its well known metabolic effect, also has growth-promoting activity and can act as a growth factor, both *in vitro* and *in vivo*. However, the physiological relevance and the mechanisms of growth stimulation by insulin have long been unclear. One key question is whether the growth effect observed in cells exposed to insulin is mediated by the insulin receptor (IR) or by the closely related type I receptor for IGF-1 (IGF-1-R). This issue has been difficult to study because of the many structural and functional similarities between the two ligands and their cognate receptors.

Both the IR and IGF-1-R belong to a supergene family of molecules with tyrosine kinase activity which includes both growth factor receptors and oncogenic proteins (1,2). Both are tetrameric glycoproteins composed by two extracellular ligand binding domains (α subunits) connected by disulphide bonds to two cytoplasmic domains with tyrosine-kinase activity (β subunits). The tyrosine-kinase activity of these receptors (which is ligand-stimulated) appears to be tightly linked with some of the major mechanisms that control cell growth (2).

Recent studies in different models (engineered cells, transgenic mice) have now partially clarified the mechanisms by which insulin and its receptor are directly involved in cell growth regulation.

Diabetes in the New Millennium. Edited by U. Di Mario, F. Leonetti, G. Pugliese, P. Sbraccia and A. Signore.
© 2000 John Wiley & Sons, Ltd.

INSULIN STIMULATES MITOGENESIS THROUGH
THE INSULIN RECEPTOR

Insulin has long been used to support optimal growth of cell cultures in a defined medium. In culture media, however, insulin has been used at high concentration and in some cells, such as rat aortic smooth muscle cells, insulin is approximately 100-fold less potent than IGF-1. Since 1:100 is the affinity ratio between insulin and IGF-1 binding to the IGF-1-R, these data may suggest that insulin acts via the IGF-1-R. However, in different normal or transformed cell lines, evidence is available that insulin stimulates mitogenesis through its own receptor. For instance, in rat hepatoma cells (H-35) and in embryonal carcinoma cells (F9), low insulin concentrations (that would only minimally interact with the IGF-1-R) induced a growth response, suggesting that insulin acted via its own receptor.

Using breast cancer cells in culture, we showed that insulin induces a dose-dependent growth response starting at concentrations as low as 0.1–1.0 nM, unable to interact substantially with the IGF-1-R (3). This proliferative response to insulin was not inhibited by the monoclonal antibody αIR3 (which blocks the IGF-1-R), while it was reproduced by exposing cells to a monoclonal antibody that specifically binds and activates the IR (3).

At least two cell lines (Chinese hamster ovary cells, CHO-K1, and LB cells, a murine T cell lymphoma) have been reported to be dependent on physiological concentrations of insulin for growth. When incubated without insulin in serum-free medium for 48–72 hours, CHO-K1 cells accumulate in G_1; they enter phase S following exposure to insulin but not to similar concentrations of IGF-1 or IGF-2 (4). Insulin is also a limiting factor for the malignant growth of LB cells, since in the absence of insulin cell growth it is almost completely abolished (5). These results are not peculiar to cancer cell lines, since similar findings have been obtained in normal human diploid fibroblasts. Furthermore, NIH-3T3 fibroblasts transfected with the human IR cDNA became quiescent when cultured in serum-free medium, while they underwent active mitogenesis in response to insulin, with loss of contact inhibition and foci formation (6). These data could not be reproduced with exposure to IGF-1 (6).

Finally, R-cells (3T3-like fibroblasts generated from mouse embryos with a targeted disruption of the IGF-1-R gene), when transfected with and overexpressing the IR, become able to grow in serum-free medium supplemented with either insulin or IGF-2, but not with IGF-1 (7).

In the animal model the mitogenic role of insulin has been studied in breast cancer. MCF-7 breast cancer cells do not form tumors in diabetic nude mice, while they do form tumors in 100% diabetic nude mice treated with insulin (8). Conversely, alloxan- and streptozotocin-induced diabetes prevents, and can reverse, chemically-induced breast cancer in the rat (9). Since insulin stimulates glucose uptake and metabolism, this might be a mechanism for insulin stimulation of neoplastic cell growth. Heuson and Legros studied the role of insulin and glucose on thymidine incorporation into DMBA-induced tumor explants and concluded that the insulin-induced stimulation of thymidine incorporation was not the simple consequence of enhanced glucose uptake, although glucose was rate-limiting (10).

INSULIN ANALOGS AND MITOGENESIS

Prolonged IR activation by insulin analogs and mitogenesis

Substitutions of one or more amino acid residues of the insulin molecule by recombinant DNA technology created insulin analogs with different chemical and pharmacological characteristics, which will interact differently with the insulin receptor. So far, more than 300 insulin analogs have been produced. The study of these analogs has provided new insights on the role of insulin as a growth factor (11). Glucose metabolism stimulation (a major metabolic effect of insulin) and mitogenesis have been separately assessed for each analog and expressed as the mitogenic:metabolic ratio. Some of the insulin analogs with a high affinity for the IR also have an abnormally high mitogenic:metabolic ratio. One of these high-affinity insulin analogs, AspB10-insulin, which also has a long half-life, has been reported to have a carcinogenic effect on the mammary gland of female rats. At the end of a 24 month treatment period, 44% of mice developed benign breast diseases and 23% developed breast cancer (11). We have recently reported that AspB10-insulin is several-fold more potent than insulin in stimulating growth in both transformed and non-transformed breast cells. In addition, AspB10-insulin may cause phenotypic changes in non-transformed breast cells (12). This abnormally high mitogenic activity has been explained by the formation of receptor–ligand complexes with increased half-life and the consequent prolonged IR and Shc phosphorylation (13). The prolonged time of IR activation may, therefore, cause an imbalance between its metabolic and mitogenic activities in favor of the latter.

IR/IGF-1-R hybrid receptors: a potential target of insulin analogs

Both the insulin receptor (IR) and the IGF-1 receptor (IGF-1-R) are expressed in most human tissues. In addition to homotypic IRs and IGF-1-Rs, formed by identical $\alpha\beta$ receptors that are disulphide-linked into $\alpha 2\beta 2$ tetramers, heterotypic IR/IGF-1-R hybrid receptors have been shown in a variety of human tissues and cultured cells. Hybrid IR/IGF-1-R receptors are believed to be formed in all cells expressing both IR and IGF-1-R (14). IR/IGF-1-R hybrids are heterotetrameric complexes that are formed because a proportion of IR $\alpha\beta$ half-receptors randomly assembles with IGF-1-R $\alpha\beta$ half-receptors, given the high degree of homology between the two receptors. In most cells, hybrid receptor formation, therefore, will depend on the relative abundance of available IR and IGF-1-R half-receptors. Although the biologic role of IR/IGF-1-R hybrids is not yet clear, functional studies with purified hybrid receptors indicate that, as far as ligand binding is concerned, these receptors behave as IGF-1-R rather than IR, since they bind IGF-1 with an affinity similar to that of typical IGF-1-R, while they bind insulin with a much lower affinity (15). Studies focusing on the cell content and relative roles of IRs, IGF-1-Rs and IR/IGF-1-R hybrids have been difficult, given the high structural and functional homology between these receptors. In particular, no direct assay was available for the direct measurement of IR/IGF-1-R hybrids, and these receptors were measured as the proportion of IGF-1 binding sites that were recognized by anti-IR antibodies.

Recently, we developed novel ELISAs that allow to directly measure the content of these three receptors and also their phosphorylation in intact cells exposed to different ligands. By these assays we confirmed that IR/IGF-1-R hybrids bind to and are activated by IGF-1 with an affinity similar to that of typical IGF-1-Rs, and that are activated by insulin with a much lower affinity (16).

The presence of IR/IGF-1-R hybrid receptors may affect cell responsivity to native or pharmaceutical ligands. For instance, preliminary results obtained with AspB10 insulin indicate that this analog partially displaces IGF-1 binding. This displacement occurs at both IGF-1-R and/or IR/IGF-1-R hybrid level (12). Part of the mitogenic activity of the analog may be attributed to this property.

Moreover, cancer cells frequently overexpress IR/IGF-1-R hybrids as a consequence of both IR and IGF-1-R overexpression (16). IR/IGF-1-R activation by locally produced IGFs or by elevated circulating insulin (due to insulin administration) or by insulin analogs may, therefore, stimulate cancer cell growth (16). These data suggest that insulin analogs introduced into clinical use should be tested for their affinity, not only to IGF-1-R but also to IR/IGF-1-R hybrids.

Insulin stimulation of atypical IGF-1-Rs

IGF-1-Rs have been described to be present in cells in different forms, that have small structure and function differences. In MCF-7 breast cancer cells, we observed atypical IGF-1 Rs that were able to bind insulin and IGF-1 with similar affinity (17). These atypical IGF-1 receptors are also present in approximately 8% of breast cancer specimens. Insulin, therefore, especially in hyperinsulinemic patients (insulin-treated, obese) may stimulate and promote growth of some malignant cells via atypical IGF-1-Rs.

THE INSULIN RECEPTOR AS A GROWTH TRANSDUCER

IR intracellular signaling pathways and tissue distribution: similarities and differences with IGF-1-R

Although insulin is primarily considered a metabolic hormone, it is also able to stimulate mitogenesis via its own receptor. This may appear a redundant effect, overlapping the typical IGF-1 effect mediated by a ligand and a receptor that share many similarities with the insulin/IR system. A series of studies have addressed the issue of identifying similarities and differences between the IR and the IGF-1-R mode of action and signaling.

Mastick *et al.* (18) compared some of the signal transduction pathways stimulated by insulin and IGF-1-R in NIH-3T3 cell lines overexpressing similar numbers of either IR or IGF-1 R (approximately 10^6 receptors/cell). They found that the two receptors stimulate similar mitogenic pathways, including Shc phosphorylation, mitogen activated protein (MAP) kinase activation and DNA synthesis. However, quantitative differences were also found (i.e. IRS-1 and a 70 kDa protein were more sensitive to insulin than to IGF-1) (18) and intracellular molecules may be recruited in different amounts or with different timing due to small structure differences of the two receptors.

For instance, Sasoaka *et al.* (19), studying Rat 1 fibroblasts expressing low levels of either IRs or IGF-1-Rs (1.3×10^5 receptors/cell), found that the mitogenic effect was slightly greater for IGF-1 than for insulin, and that this was associated with a more efficient coupling of the IGF-1-R to the MAP kinase activation, possibly due to a delayed Sos phosphorylation. All these differences, however, are small and can hardly explain the different mitogenic potency of IGF-1 in comparison to insulin.

It is likely that most differences between insulin and IGF-1 are due to the different tissue distribution of IR and IGF-1 R, to the episodical secretion of insulin, to the local autocrine/paracrine production of IGF and to the modulation of IGF effects by the IGF-binding proteins. In fact, although the IR is expressed in virtually all tissues, high IR concentrations (more than 200 000 receptors/cell) are present only in terminally differentiated, non-cycling cells such as hepatocytes and adipocytes. Much lower IR levels and, conversely, higher IGF-1-R levels, are expressed by cells able to proliferate (e.g. fibroblasts). This preferential expression of IR in highly differentiated cells and of IGF-1-R in cycling cells may prevent cell proliferation to be activated by circulating insulin and allows a fine modulation of cell proliferation control by the locally produced IGF-1, IGF-2, IGF-binding proteins and type II (mannose-6-phosphate) IGF-2 receptor. In addition to the signal (ligand and receptor) availability, subtle differences in the signaling pathways may also contribute to the prevalent growth activity of IGF-1 and metabolic activity of insulin.

**Insulin receptor isoform A: a fetal insulin and IGF-2 receptor
mainly involved in growth regulation**

In addition to evidence showing that insulin acts as a growth factor via the IR, recent studies have provided evidence suggesting that the isoform A is also a high-affinity receptor for IGF-2, changing previous concepts regarding growth regulation by insulin and its receptor.

The human IR exists in two isoforms. Alternative splicing of a small exon (exon 11) of the insulin receptor gene results in two transcripts, in which 36 nucleotides encoding 12 amino acids at the carboxyl-terminus of the receptor α-subunit are either excluded (Ex11$^-$ or IR-A) or included (Ex11$^+$ or IR-B) (20). The relative expression of the two isoforms varies in a tissue-specific manner. IR-A is predominantly expressed in the central nervous system and hematopoietic cells, while IR-B is predominantly expressed in adipose tissue, liver and muscle, all target tissues for the metabolic effects of insulin. Small functional differences have been described for the two IR isoforms in relation to insulin binding and insulin-mediated β subunit autophosphorylation, with IR-A having a slightly higher binding affinity and IR-B having a more efficient signaling activity, as evaluated by tyrosine kinase and insulin substrate-1 (IRS-1) phosphorylation responses (20).

Until recently it was believed that most, if not all, biological effects of IGF-2 in cells were mediated through the IGF-1 R, as most studies had indicated that IGF-2 binds to the IR with a relatively low affinity (less than 5% that of insulin). However, the presence of 'atypical' IRs with unusually high affinity for IGF-2 had been reported in IM-9 lymphoblasts, immature erythrocytes and fetal tissues (such as human placenta and brain, and chick embryo fibroblasts). Other studies, carried out in transgenic mice, had provided evidence that the growth effect of IGF-2 during fetal development was mediated in part by the IR (21,22). By analyzing mouse dwarfing phenotypes resulting from targeted mutagenesis of the IGF-1 and IGF-2 genes and the cognate IGF-1-R gene, it was demonstrated that this signaling system is determinant for the embryo growth. It was also shown that while IGF-1 interacts exclusively with the IGF-1-R, IGF-2 recognizes an additional receptor, most likely the IR. In fact, the growth retardation in embryos lacking both IGF-1-R and IGF-2 was more severe than in single IGF-1-R mutants, but similar to that obtained in double mutants lacking both IGF-1-R and IR (21,22).

We found that the A but not the B isoform of the IR binds IGF-2 with high affinity, indicating that IR-A is a high affinity receptor for IGF-2 signaling (23). To avoid the interference of IGF-1-R, we employed R cells transfected with either IR-A or IR-B cDNAs. In this system, IGF-2 binds to the IR-A with an affinity that is approximately 30–40% that of insulin. IGF-1 binds with low affinity to both IR isoforms. We also found that IR-A, but not IR-B, was autophosphorylated in response to IGF-2, with a high affinity. By using R cells transfected with the IGF-1-R cDNA we observed that the affinity of IGF-2 for IR-A was very similar to its affinity for IGF-1-R (23).

In cells transfected with the IR-A, exposure to IGF-2 elicited a more marked mitogenic effect than exposure to insulin (Figure 14.1). This difference was associated with a difference in the activation kinetics of receptor and post-receptor intracellular signaling molecules following either insulin or IGF-2 (23).

By analyzing the relative abundance of IR isoforms, we found a predominance of the IR-A in fetal cells and tissues (fibroblasts, muscle, liver and kidney) in respect to adult cells and tissues. Accordingly, in fetal fibroblasts IGF-2 bound with high affinity to the IR-A and had a potent effect in stimulating IR-A autophosphorylation (23). Finally, a predominant IR-A expression was found in three most common human tumors, including breast, lung and colon cancer (23,24). In contrast, IR-B was the predominant isoform in the corresponding normal tissues (Table 14.2). In tumors that predominantly express IR-A, IGF-2 was a potent activator of the IR and, via this receptor, promoted growth. As most of these tumors produce IGF-2, an autocrine/ paracrine loop involving IR-A and IGF-2 represents a novel mechanism that may be relevant for tumor progression.

The molecular mechanisms involved in the development/differentiation regulation of the alternative splicing process of the IR gene are not clear. It has recently been reported that specific regions in intron 10 and exon 11 of the IR gene are involved in this process. In studies carried out in HepG2 human hepatoma cells, which differentiate and predominantly express IR-B after stimulation with glucocorticoids, both splicing enhancer sequences and inhibitory regions have been identified in intron 10 and also sequences involved in splice site selection in exon 11 of the IR gene. Modified alternative splicing for a variety of proteins has been reported in proliferating cells and in malignant cells. In these models, the change in the splicing pattern of pre-mRNAs occurs simultaneously with a change

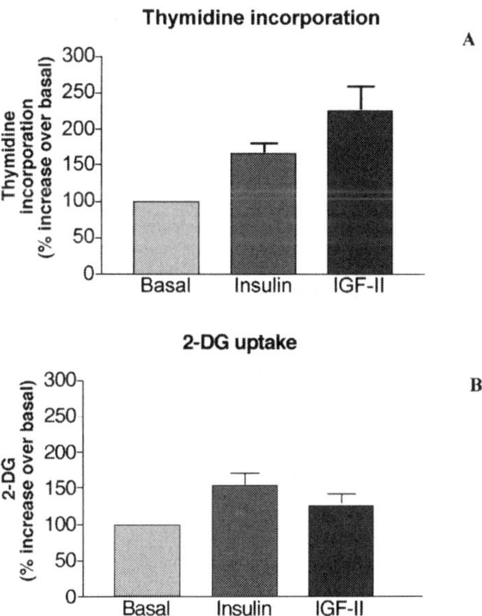

Figure 14.1. Mitogenic (thymidine incorporation, A) and metabolic (2-DG uptake, B) effects of IR-A activated by either insulin or IGF-2. R cells were stably transfected with the IR-A cDNA and subsequently exposed to either insulin or IGF-2 at a concentration of 10 nM

Table 14.1. Relative abundance of IR-A in surgical specimens from either normal breast or breast cancer

	% IR-A transcript content
Normal breast tissue specimens	
N1	47
N2	50
N3	42
N4	27
N5	38
N6	43
N7	46
Mean ± SD	41.9 ± 7.6
Breast cancer tissue specimens	
CA1	52
CA2	90
CA3	95
CA4	81
CA5	65
CA6	60
CA7	74
CA8	77
Mean ± SD	74.2 ± 14.7

in the expression level of some splicing factors of the SR family phosphoproteins that bind pre-mRNA very early during spliceosome assembly and determine the 5′-splice site choice during splicing reaction.

Insulin-resistance and hyperinsulinemia-induced cell mitogenesis

Insulin resistance is a condition of impaired insulin effect, which is usually measured as inadequate glucose uptake and metabolism at the muscle level. Insulin resistance is associated with a variety of disorders, including non-insulin-dependent diabetes mellitus (type 2 diabetes), obesity, functional ovarian hyperandrogenism, essential hypertension, dyslipidemia, and coronary artery disease (25). In these conditions the pancreas is able to secrete more insulin than normal to compensate for the insulin resistance; these patients have, therefore, compensatory hyperinsulinemia (25). Due to the mitogenic effect of insulin, hyperinsulinemia can induce proliferation of certain cell types as ovarian techal cells (causing hyperandrogenism), keratinocytes (causing acanthosis nigricans) and, possibly, tumor cells that overexpress the IR. Several studies have addressed the possibility that conditions of hyper-insulinemia like obesity may be associated with increased risk of developing a variety of cancers (26). Weight gain after the age of 18 has been reported to be associated with significant increase in breast cancer development as well as with insulin resistance and increased risk of type 2 diabetes (27).

CONCLUSION

The mitogenic effects of insulin and its receptor have probably been underestimated because in differentiated tissues the metabolic effects are largely predominant. However, there is a variety of clinical conditions (PCOS, hypertension, atherosclerosis, some malignancies) that are characterized by dysregulated cell proliferation linked to hyperinsulinemia and abdominal adiposity. In addition, the use of insulin analogs, some with an increased mitogenic:metabolic ratio is becoming more common. Attention should be paid to these situations with respect to the possibility that an increased mitogenic action of insulin might produce adverse effects.

REFERENCES

1. Ebina Y, Ellis L, Jarnaglin K, Edery M, Graf L, Clauser E, OU JH, Masiorz F, Kan YW, Goldfine ID *et al*: The human insulin receptor cDNA: the structural basis for hormone activated transmembrane signalling. *Cell* 40:747–758, 1985.
2. Ullrich A, Gray A, Tam AW, Yang-Feng T, Tsubokawa M, Collins C: Insulin-like growth factor I receptor primary structure: comparison with insulin receptor suggests structural determinants that define functional specificity. *EMBO J* 5:2503–2512, 1986.
3 Milazzo G, Giorgino F, Damante, Sung C, Stampfer MR, Vigneri R, Goldfine ID, Belfiore A: Insulin receptor expression and function in human breast cancer cell lines. *Cancer Res* 52:3924–3930, 1992.
4. Mamounas M, Gervin D, Englesberg E: The insulin receptor as a transmitter of a mitogenic signal in Chinese hamster ovary CHO-K1 cells. *Proc Natl Acad Sci USA* 86:9294–9298, 1989.
5. Pillemer G, Lugasi-Evgi H, Scharovsky G, Naor D: Insulin dependence of murine lymphoid T-cell leukemia. *Int J Cancer* 50:80, 1992.
6. Giorgino F, Belfiore A, Milazzo G Costantino A, Maddux B, Whittaker J, Goldfine ID, Vigneri R: Overexpression of insulin receptors in fibroblast and ovary cells induces a ligand-mediated transformed phenotype. *Mol Endocrinol* 5:452–459, 1991.
7. Morrione A, Valentinis B, Xu SQ, Yumet G, Louvi A, Efstratiadis A, Baserga R: Insulin-like growth factor II stimulates cell proliferation through the insulin receptor. *Proc Natl Acad Sci USA* 94(8):3777–3782, 1997.
8. Shafie SM, Gibson SL, Hilf R: Effect of insulin and estrogen on hormone binding in R3230AC mammary adenocarcinoma. *Cancer Res* 37:4641, 1977.
9. Cohen ND, Hilf R: Influence of insulin on growth and metabolism of 7,12 dimethylbenzanthracene-induced mammary tumors. *Cancer Res* 34:3245, 1974.
10. Heuson JC, Legros N: Study of growth-promoting effect of insulin in relation to carbohydrate metabolism in organ culture of rat mammary carcinoma. *Eur J Cancer* 4:1–4, 1968.

11. Drejer K: The bioactivity of insulin analogues from *in vitro* receptor binding to *in vivo* glucose uptake. *Diabet Metab Rev* 8:259–286, 1992.
12. Milazzo G, Sciacca L, Papa V Goldfine ID, Vigneri R: ASPB10 Insulin induction of increased mitogenic responses and phenotypic changes in human breast epithelial cells: evidence for enhanced interactions with the insulin-like growth factor-I receptor. *Mol Carcinogen* 18:19–25, 1997.
13. Hansen BF, Danielsen GM, Drejer K, Sorensen AR, Wiberg FC, Klein HH, Lundemose AG: Sustained signalling from the insulin receptor after stimulation with insulin analogues exhibiting increased mitogenic potency. *Biochem J* 315:271–279, 1996.
14. Soos M, Whittaker J, Lammers R, Ullrich A, Siddle K: Receptor for insulin and insulin-like growth factor-I can form hybrid dimers. *Biochem J* 270:383–390, 1990.
15. Soos MA, Field CE, Siddle K: Purified hybrid insulin/insulin-like growth factor-I receptors bind insulin-like growth factor-I, but not insulin, with high affinity. *Biochem J* 290:419–426, 1993.
16. Pandini G, Vigneri R, Costantino A, Frasca F, Ippolito A, Fujita-Yamaguchi Y, Siddle K, Goldfine ID, Belfiore A: Insulin and IGF-1 receptor overexpression in breast cancer leads to insulin/IGF-1 hybrid receptor overexpression: evidence for a second mechanism of IGF-1 signaling. *Clin Cancer Res* 5:1935–1944, 1999.
17. Milazzo G, Yip CC, Maddux BA, Vigneri R, Goldfine ID: High-affinity insulin binding to an atypical insulin-like growth factor-I receptor in human breast cancer cells. *J Clin Invest* 89:899, 1992.
18. Mastick CC, Kato H, Roberts CT Jr, LeRoith D, Saltiel AR: Insulin and insulin like growth factor-I receptors similarly stimulate deoxyribonucleic acid synthesis despite differences in cellular protein tyrosine phosporylation. *Endocrinology* 135:214–222, 1994.
19. Sasaoka T, Ishiki M, Sawa T, TIshihara H, Takata Y, Imamura T, Usui I, Olefsky JM, Kobayashi M: Comparison of the insulin and insulin-like growth factor I mitogenic intracellular signaling pathways. *Endocrinology* 137:4427–4434, 1996.
20. Mosthaf L, Grako K, Dull TJ, Coussens L, Ullrich A, McClain DA: Functionally distinct insulin receptors generated by tissue-specific alternative splicing. *EMBO J* 9:2409–2413, 1990.
21. Accili D, Drago J, Lee EJ, Johnson MD, Cool MH, Salvatore P, Asico LD, Jose PA, Taylor SI, Westphal H: Early neonatal death in mice homozygous for a null allele of the insulin receptor gene. *Nature Genet* 12:106–109, 1996.
22. Louvi A, Accili D, Efstratiadis A: Growth promoting interaction of IGF-2 with the insulin receptor during mouse embryonic development. *Dev Biol* 189:33–48, 1997.
23. Frasca F, Pandini G, Scalia Pl, Sciacca L, Mineo R, Costantino A, I.D. Goldfine ID, Belfiore A, Vigneri R: The insulin receptor isoform-A: a newly recognized IGF-2 receptor in fetal and cancer cells. *Mol Cell Biol* 19:3278–88, 1999.
24. Sciacca L, Costantino A, Pandini G, Mineo R, Frasca F, Scalia P, Sbraccia P, Goldfine ID, Vigneri R, Belfiore A: Insulin receptor activation by IGF-2 in breast cancers: evidence for a new autocrine/paracrine mechanism. *Oncogene* 18:2471–2479, 1999.
25. Reaven GM: Role of insulin resistance in human diseases. *Diabetes* 37:1595–1607, 1988.
26. Albanes D, Taylor PR: International differences in body height and weight and their relationship to cancer incidence. *Nutr Cancer* 14:69–77, 1990.
27. Barnes-Josiah D, Potter JD, Sellers TA, Himes JH: Early body size and subsequent weight gain as predictors of breast cancer incidence (Iowa, USA). *Cancer Causes Cont* 6:112, 1995.

15

Lipid Metabolism in Type 2 Diabetes

GAETANO CREPALDI and ENZO MANZATO
University of Padua, Padua, Italy

Patients with diabetes mellitus have an increased total mortality as compared to the general population. This higher mortality rate is due to cardiovascular diseases (1). Alterations of the lipid metabolism may be responsible for a large part of the increased atherogenesis observed in diabetic patients.

PREVALENCE OF DYSLIPIDEMIA

The prevalence of hypercholesterolemia in type 2 diabetic patients is similar to that of the non-diabetic population but the prevalence of hypertriglyceridemia is usually reported to be two to three times higher in diabetic patients as compared to normal subjects (2). The prevalence of lipoprotein abnormalities in type 2 diabetic patients is less well documented. The Framingham study suggests that LDL cholesterol concentrations are similar in type 2 diabetic patients as compared to non-diabetic subjects. However, there is a general agreement that HDL cholesterol levels are reduced in type 2 diabetic patients. The frequency of low HDL cholesterol levels (below 30–40 mg/dl) is double in type 2 diabetic patients compared with non-diabetic subjects (3).

It was reported several years ago that diabetic patients are quite often affected by a familial form of hypertriglyceridemia (4). These patients present severe hypertriglyceridemia as well as diabetes, and the treatment of diabetes does not result in a normalization of triglyceride concentrations. Studies of the VLDL metabolism in these patients showed that the synthesis of VLDL

Diabetes in the New Millennium. Edited by U. Di Mario, F. Leonetti, G. Pugliese, P. Sbraccia and A. Signore.
© 2000 John Wiley & Sons, Ltd.

triglycerides was reduced but not normalized by the treatment of the hyperglycemia, while the catabolism of VLDL triglyceride was not significantly affected by metabolic control. These results indicate that a primary or familial form of hypertriglyceridemia is responsible for this type of diabetic dyslipidemia. Severe hypertriglyceridemia with chylomicronemia could be present in diabetic patients during a period of poor metabolic control and insulin deficiency. This type of hypertriglyceridemia is usually corrected by the insulin treatment.

Other observational studies have confirmed that obtaining a good glycemic control in type 2 diabetic patients is not always sufficient to improve the dyslipidemia in these patients. Moreover, non-diabetic subjects from families with type 2 diabetic probands have a prevalence of dyslipidemias similar to that observed in type 2 diabetic patients. Altogether these observations support the hypothesis that familial hypertriglyceridemia and type 2 diabetes are frequently associated. Familial hypercholesterolemia, instead, does not seem to be significantly associated with type 2 diabetes (3).

DYSLIPIDEMIA AND METABOLIC CONTROL

Several studies were performed in order to elucidate the metabolic alterations responsible for lipid abnormalities in diabetic patients and to examine the effects of the antidiabetic treatment on plasma lipoproteins. While in type 1 diabetic patients triglyceride concentrations are related to the degree of the glycemic control, the lipoprotein distribution in type 2 diabetic patients is usually not significantly affected by the degree of the metabolic control, once these patients have reached an acceptable glycemic level. However, plasma triglycerides are usually improved by any antidiabetic treatment, while HDL cholesterol appears to be raised only by insulin treatment (3).

We have examined the cholesterol and triglyceride concentrations in the VLDL, LDL and HDL (isolated by ultracentrifugation) and the apoprotein levels in the whole plasma in a group of well treated type 2 diabetic patients, excluding patients with primary hyperlipoproteinemias. In this study we have also examined and compared in these patients the effects on lipoproteins of different treatments, i.e. diet, sulphonylurea, sulphonylurea plus biguanide, insulin (5).

Compared with controls, total plasma cholesterol concentrations were significantly higher in diabetic patients than in normal subjects, while no significant differences were observed among diabetic groups. Total plasma triglyceride concentrations were higher (but not significantly different) in diabetic patients as compared with controls, and there were not significant differences in plasma triglyceride levels among different groups of diabetic patients. In VLDL the concentrations of triglyceride and cholesterol showed no significant differences between diabetic patients and controls. However, both LDL and HDL triglyceride concentrations were significantly higher in diabetic patients than in controls. No significant differences were observed among different treatment groups.

The apoproteins B and CIII levels were significantly higher in the diabetic group than in controls, while apo-AI, -AII, -CII and -E concentrations were not different. The cholesterol to triglyceride ratio in LDL was significantly lower in diabetic patients in comparison with controls.

Visceral obesity is the type of obesity that is responsible for the metabolic alterations in type 2 diabetic patients as well as in non-diabetic subjects. In fact in our study, obesity, which is frequently observed in type 2 diabetic patients, may explain the variability of HDL cholesterol concentrations. Another possible explanation for the reduced HDL cholesterol could be the increased VLDL triglyceride levels and the HDL cholesterol for VLDL triglyceride exchange, which normally takes place in the plasma by the activity of the lipid transfer proteins. If this is the case, one would expect an increase in HDL triglycerides, along with a HDL cholesterol reduction, as well as no variations in the plasma levels of apo-AI, which is the major apoprotein of HDL. Normal AI levels, reduced HDL cholesterol and increased HDL triglycerides in type 2 diabetes, were indeed reported also by other authors.

In type 2 diabetic patients without primary hyperlipoproteinemias and in good metabolic control (as in our patients), as reported earlier, the degree of the metabolic control does not seem to be relevant to determine the lipoprotein levels. Body weight seems more important than the metabolic control in determining the VLDL plasma concentrations, as already observed also by others. Moreover, from the linear regression analysis of our data, we suggest that in our patients the VLDL triglyceride concentrations are important in determining both the HDL triglycerides and cholesterol concentrations.

Body weight is constantly associated with increased insulin secretion, which in turn strongly influences the hepatic VLDL production. In our diabetic patients the body weight is positively correlated with plasma C peptide basal levels, as already observed also by others.

In conclusion, from a clinical point of view, in well-treated and non-hyperlipoproteinemic type 2 diabetic patients, the body weight seems more important than the glycemic control or the type of treatment in determining the lipoprotein levels. Diabetic patients have a significant increase of total plasma cholesterol (mainly due to LDL), of LDL and HDL triglycerides, and of apo-B and -CIII. Whether these abnormalities have any implication in the increased vascular risk of these patients remains to be established by longitudinal studies, but it is possible.

The type of treatment of type 2 diabetes (whether diet, oral agents or insulin) may also have an important effect on lipoprotein levels. However, this does not seem to be the case when patients are in fair to good metabolic control, as were our patients.

INSULIN RESISTANCE AND DYSLIPIDEMIA

Recently, both cross-sectional and prospective studies have demonstrated the importance of the insulin resistance syndrome or plurimetabolic syndrome as a vascular risk factor (6). Moreover, microalbuminuria has been shown to be linked to insulin resistance in essential hypertension and to hypertension in type 2 diabetic patients.

However, the underlying mechanism accounting for the development of cardiovascular complications in type 2 diabetic patients with hypertension and microalbuminuria remained elusive. This mechanism might be provided by the occurrence of abnormal lipoprotein patterns. Abnormalities in lipoprotein physical properties were recently associated with increased prevalence of cardiovascular disease and with plasma hyperinsulinemia, an index of insulin resistance *in vivo* (7,8).

We investigated whether abnormalities in plasma lipoprotein levels and in the lipoprotein physical properties (in particular the LDL diameter) are shown by type 2 diabetic patients with and without hypertension or microalbuminuria. The relationships among lipoprotein abnormalities and insulin sensitivity were also examined (9). In this study, total plasma cholesterol concentrations were significantly higher in patients without hypertension and microalbuminuria (H^-M^-) and in those with both hypertension and microalbuminuria (H^+M^+) in comparison with non-diabetic controls. Total plasma triglycerides were higher in the H^+M^+ patients than in the H^-M^- and non-diabetic subjects. The other plasma lipid levels are reported in Table 15.1. The mean LDL particle diameter was significantly smaller in H^+M^- and H^+M^+ patients in comparison with H^-M^- and non-diabetic controls. During insulin infusion hepatic glucose output was higher in all type 2 diabetic patients than in controls. Insulin-induced whole body glucose disposal rate was significantly lower in H^+M^+ and H^+M^- patients than in H^-M^- and controls. No differences were found between H^-M^- patients and controls.

This study showed that hypertension, microalbuminuria and obesity are associated with several abnormalities in lipoprotein concentrations and physical properties in a subgroup of type 2 diabetic patients. Moreover, these diabetic patients have an impaired insulin induced carbohydrate uptake by extrahepatic tissues. In contrast, type 2 diabetic patients without hypertension and microalbuminuria have only higher LDL cholesterol (in comparison with controls) and normal insulin sensitivity in extrahepatic tissues (9).

Since hepatic glucose output is less inhibited in both hypertensive and/or microalbuminuric and normotensive diabetic patients than in controls, this study demonstrated that insulin action is impaired in all diabetic patients at the hepatic level. On the other hand, as indicated by whole-body glucose

Table 15.1. Clinical and biochemical features of control subjects and type 2 diabetic patients (mean ± SE)

	Controls	NIDDM patients		
		H^-M^-	H^+M^-	H^+M^+
Number of subjects	20	15	32	22
Age (years)	56 ± 3	56 ± 2	59 ± 2	56 ± 2
Body mass index (kg/m^2)	28.7 ± 1.1	25.5 ± 0.8	30.3 ± 0.7[1]	29.6 ± 1.5[1]
Plasma glucose (mmol/l)	5.2 ± 0.1	9.2 ± 0.9[2]	9.9 ± 0.7[2]	8.8 ± 0.1[2]
Plasma insulin (μU/ml)	15 ± 1	19 ± 2	14 ± 4	11 ± 2
Cholesterol (mmol/l)				
plasma	4.97 ± 0.98	6.05 ± 0.83[2]	5.48 ± 1.22	5.84 ± 0.98[2]
VLDL	0.26 ± 0.21	0.34 ± 0.26	0.44 ± 0.28	0.57 ± 0.54[2]
LDL	3.39 ± 0.96	4.37 ± 0.67[2]	3.93 ± 1.03	4.09 ± 0.91
HDL	1.16 ± 0.18	1.19 ± 0.36	1.01 ± 0.21	1.06 ± 0.23
Triglyceride (mmol/l)				
plasma	1.18 ± 0.67	1.30 ± 0.59	1.63 ± 0.60	2.17 ± 1.32[1,2]
VLDL	0.58 ± 0.43	0.70 ± 0.53	0.99 ± 0.54	1.29 ± 1.10[2]
LDL + HDL	0.49 ± 0.19	0.54 ± 0.14	0.59 ± 0.16	0.82 ± 0.54[2,3]
LDL diameter (nm)	27.2 ± 0.8	26.7 ± 0.8	26.5 ± 0.8[2]	26.0 ± 0.8[2]
Cholesterol-HDL (mmol/l)				
large	0.54 ± 0.41	0.54 ± 0.27	0.37 ± 0.14[1,2]	0.36 ± 0.16[1,2]
small	0.64 ± 0.12	0.66 ± 0.19	0.65 ± 0.14	0.72 ± 0.18
Apoproteins (mg/l)				
AI	1460 ± 230	1540 ± 300	1370 ± 210	1440 ± 240
AII	300 ± 70	320 ± 60	320 ± 70	330 ± 90
B	1030 ± 310	1500 ± 320[2]	1370 ± 330[2]	1510 ± 370[2]
CII	35 ± 17	39 ± 13	47 ± 14	62 ± 26[2,3]
CIII	69 ± 22	84 ± 21	99 ± 34	131 ± 69[2,3]
E	51 ± 14	49 ± 22	47 ± 14	49 ± 18

H^-M^-, normotensive normoalbuminuric; H^+M, hypertensive normoalbuminuric; H^+M^+, hypertensive microalbuminuric.
$p < 0.05$: [1]vs. H^-M^-; [2]vs. C; [3]vs. H^-M^- and H^+M^-.

utilization, extrahepatic carbohydrate metabolism is altered only in diabetic patients with hypertension and microalbuminuria, but not in those without abnormalities in blood pressure and in albumin excretion rate.

In summary, abnormalities in lipoprotein pattern and selective extra-hepatic insulin sensitivity in type 2 diabetic patients are associated with microalbuminuria and/or hypertension. It remains to be established whether extrahepatic insulin resistance is simply associated with these clinical features, or whether it plays a pathogenetic role in the development of altered lipid metabolism. An association of lipid abnormalities, micro-albuminuria and predisposition to cardiovascular disease has been observed in type 1 diabetic patients. A familial clustering of such an association was also described.

PATHOGENESIS OF DYSLIPIDEMIA

Several studies have been carried out to evaluate the metabolic abnormalities responsible for dyslipidemia in type 2 diabetic patients (3). These studies show that VLDL production in type 2 diabetic patients is usually increased. VLDL catabolism is reduced in hyperlipidemic type 2 diabetic patients. VLDL are catabolized through a non-LDL pathway (at least in part via scavenger receptors and/or hepatic receptors) in patients with moderately severe diabetes and through both LDL and non-LDL pathways in those with mild diabetes. Normolipidemic mild diabetic patients have an increased VLDL catabolism through the LDL pathway. During energy restriction in hypertriglyceridemic type 2 diabetic patients, overproduction of VLDL is significantly reduced, while catabolism remains constant. Similar results were obtained utilizing insulin therapy.

In patients with mild type 2 diabetes, both LDL production and LDL catabolism are increased in comparison to those of non-diabetic subjects. In this case, the LDL concentration remains within the normal range. LDL catabolism is impaired in patients with moderately severe diabetes, thus resulting in increased LDL levels.

The low HDL levels in type 2 diabetic patients are due to an increase in HDL catabolism which exceeds the enhanced HDL synthesis.

Lipolytic enzymes play a crucial role in triglyceride metabolism, both in plasma and in adipose tissue. The activities of these enzymes in well-treated type 2 diabetic patients seem to be within the normal range. Intensive insulin therapy results in a significant decrease in VLDL triglycerides and in an increase in HDL. It is also associated with a significant increase in adipose tissue lipoprotein lipase activity, while plasma lipoprotein lipase activity, is unchanged and plasma hepatic lipase activity is reduced.

OTHER LIPOPROTEIN ABNORMALITIES

As already mentioned earlier, several factors may be involved in determining diabetic dyslipidemia. Apo-E isoforms are associated to different LDL cholesterol levels, the apo-E2 isoform being associated to the lowest, the apo-E4 to the highest, and the apo-E3 to the intermediate level. A similar trend in the plasma cholesterol concentrations has also been observed in type 2 diabetic patients. Contrasting results have been reported concerning the association of apo-E isoforms with plasma triglyceride levels. As already observed in non-diabetic subjects, type 2 diabetic patients with apo-E4 isoforms may be resistant to the hypolipidemic therapy, as compared to subjects with apo-E2 isoforms. This may have clinical importance in order to modulate the hypolipidemic treatment (3).

Glycosylation of plasma lipoproteins may also be involved in the genesis of diabetic dyslipidemia and in an increased atherogenicity of plasma lipoproteins.

It appears that the binding and degradation of glycosylated LDL is mediated mainly by the scavenger (atherogenic) receptors, and that the glycosylated LDL of type 2 diabetic patients is more sensitive to oxidation (10).

Lipoprotein(a) [Lp(a)] is an index of vascular risk in non-diabetic subjects. However, there is still little evidence that Lp(a) is a cardiovascular risk factor in type 2 diabetic patients (11).

Plasma Lp(a) levels are genetically determined by the type of apo-A isoforms. Low molecular weight isoforms are associated to high plasma Lp(a) levels and vice versa. The frequency distribution of Lp(a) isoforms in diabetic patients is the same as in the non-diabetic population. Since serum Lp(a) levels are largely (more than 90%) determined by Lp(a) isoforms genetically, it seems that in diabetic patients Lp(a) levels should not differ from those in non-diabetic subjects because of a genetic component.

Some authors have reported that type 1 diabetic patients with micro-albuminuria have increased Lp(a) levels. Increased Lp(a) levels have been observed in type 2 diabetic patients in poor metabolic control. A significant decrease in Lp(a) levels was seen in type 2 diabetic patients in association with an improvement in metabolic control. Other authors observed no relation between Lp(a) levels and the degree of metabolic control. It remains to be established whether Lp(a) levels are affected by the degree of metabolic control in type 2 diabetic patients, since conflicting data are present in the literature.

A limited number of studies are available about the relation between Lp(a) levels and the albumin excretion rate in type 2 diabetic patients. In microalbuminuric type 2 diabetic patients, the Lp(a) levels have been reported normal or increased.

We have examined a group of type 2 diabetic patients to establish whether Lp(a) levels are related to the presence of microalbuminuria or to the degree of metabolic control (12). Our study showed that in type 2 diabetic patients Lp(a) levels were not significantly affected by the presence of micro-albuminuria and were not related to the degree of metabolic control.

DYSLIPIDEMIA AND VASCULAR DISEASE

In type 2 diabetic patients, hyperglycaemia *per se* is a risk factor for macro-vascular disease. Moreover, dyslipidemia, hypertension, cigarette smoking and microalbuminuria all seem to be associated with vascular complications in these patients, as it has already been established in the non-diabetic population (13).

As already reported, diabetic patients often present abnormalities, not only in the quantity (concentration) but also in the quality (chemical composition and/or physical properties) of the lipoproteins which, among other factors, might be responsible for the increased incidence of vascular complications (Table 15.2). Recently, an increased oxidative susceptibility of triglyceride

Table 15.2. Risk categories based on lipid levels in diabetic patients (mg/dl)

Risk	LDL cholesterol	Triglycerides	HDL cholesterol
High	$\geqslant 130$	$\geqslant 400$	< 35
Medium	100–129	200–399	35–45
Low	< 100	< 200	> 45

Reproduced from (18), by permission of the American Diabetes Association.

enriched and small and dense LDL has been demonstrated (14). The LDL oxidation may contribute to the atherosclerotic vascular damage.

It has been suggested that insulin resistance may be a mechanism linking type 2 diabetes to hypertension and to cardiovascular mortality. We investigated the clinical features of patients with type 2 diabetes who develop cardiovascular disease, in comparison with those patients in whom such complication does not occur (15).

Normotensive and normoalbuminuric type 2 diabetic patients were studied during a 6 year follow-up period. These subjects were divided into two groups with insulin-induced whole body glucose utilization below (cohort A) and above (cohort B) the mean value minus one standard deviation in normal controls.

During the follow-up cohort A diabetics more frequently developed hypertension (30% vs. 14%, $p < 0.01$), microalbuminuria (15% vs. 7%, $p < 0.01$) and signs of cardiovascular diseases than did cohort B diabetics. Cohort A patients were also characterized by the so-called 'atherogenic lipoprotein phenotype' (presence of small and dense low density lipoproteins), which is known to be linked to cardiac ischemic disease in non-diabetic populations (7).

Insulin resistance in extrahepatic tissues and the atherogenic lipoprotein phenotype seem to precede the onset of hypertension, microalbuminuria and cardiac ischemic disease in our type 2 diabetic patients.

Our study also shows that a lower rate of insulin induced whole body glucose utilization precedes the development of hypertension and microalbuminuria in type 2 diabetic patients. Moreover, in type 2 diabetic patients the risk of atherosclerotic vascular complications is not present in the whole population, but is limited to those patients who have, at the same time, high blood pressure, increased extrahepatic insulin sensitivity and abnormalities of the lipoprotein pattern. Therefore, it seems unlikely that diabetes *per se* is the only determinant of vascular damage in diabetic patients, and it is possible that other pathogenetic factors are involved in the vascular complications of these patients. The LDL alterations may be responsible for the vascular damage in a subset of type 2 diabetic patients. The identification of the genetic alterations responsible for such an association of clinical abnormalities would allow a better understanding of the pathophysiology of the insulin resistance syndrome and a more effective prevention of vascular clinical events.

Today, we have the demonstration that, by treating diabetic dyslipidemia, we are able to reduce (in some cases by half) the incidence of major cardiovascular events in diabetic patients. Two primary prevention studies, both the Helsinki Heart Study and the Air Force Coronary Atherosclerosis Prevention Study/Texas Coronary Atherosclerosis Prevention Study, enrolled a small number of diabetic patients. In these diabetic patients, hypolipidemic therapy (with gemfibrozil and lovastatin, respectively) reduced the incidence of cardiovascular events.

Three secondary prevention studies with statins, the Scandinavian Simvastatin Survival Study (4S), the Cholesterol And Recurrent Events (CARE) trial, and the Long-term Intervention with Pravastatin in Ischaemic Disease (LIPID) study, showed that cholesterol reduction with simvastatin or pravastatin are able to improve prognosis of diabetic patients with coronary heart disease. A total cholesterol reduction below 200 mg/dl in the 4S diabetic patients was associated within few years with a significant reduction of clinical events (16). Also, in the VA-HIT study, the group of diabetic patients with coronary heart disease treated with gemfibrozil showed a reduction ($p = 0.05$) of recurrent cardiovascular events (17).

The results of these intervention studies with lipid lowering agents are important in order to establish effective therapeutic strategies to reduce the high incidence of coronary events in diabetic patients (18). Hypolipidemic therapy in diabetic patients appears to be more important than an intensive metabolic control or a tight blood pressure control in order to reduce coronary events. In fact in the UK Prospective Diabetes Study (UKPDS), neither metabolic and blood pressure control were associated with a significant reduction in the incidence of coronary events.

CONCLUSIONS

Diabetic dyslipidemia is the result of several factors in each single patient. An important genetic component (e.g. insulin resistance, familial hypertriglyceridemia, apo-E isoforms, etc.) may be prevalent in some patients, while in other patients acquired determinants (e.g. dietary habits, physical activity, metabolic control, etc.) may be more relevant in order to modify the lipoprotein concentrations. Hypolipidemic therapy in diabetic patients was effective in reducing the risk of vascular complications. For this reason, diabetic dyslipidemia must be considered one of the modifiable vascular risk factors, and to prevent the high incidence of cardiovascular complications in these patients it must be adequately treated.

REFERENCES

1. Haffner SM, Lehto S, Ronnemaa T, Pyorala K, Laakso M: Mortality from coronary heart disease in subjects with type 2 diabetes and in nondiabetic subjects with and without prior myocardial infarction. *N Engl J Med* 339:229–234, 1998.

2. Taskinen MR: Hyperlipidaemia in diabetes. *Baillière's Clin Endocr Metab* 4:743–775, 1990.
3. Manzato E, Crepaldi G: Dyslipoproteinemia in manifest diabetes. *J Intern Med* 236 (Suppl 736):27–31, 1994.
4. Brunzell JD, Hazzard WR, Motulsky AG, Bierman EL: Evidence for diabetes mellitus and genetic forms of hypertriglyceridemia as independent entities. *Metabolism* 24:1115–1121, 1975.
5. Manzato E, Zambon A, Lapolla A, Zambon S, Braghetto L, Crepaldi G: Lipoprotein abnormalities in well-treated type II diabetic patients. *Diabet Care* 16:469–475, 1993.
6. Haffner SM, Miettinen H: Insulin resistance implications for type II diabetes mellitus and coronary heart disease. *Am J Med* 103:152–162, 1997.
7. Austin MA, Breslow JA, Hennekens CH, Buring JE, Willett WC, Kraus RM: Low density lipoprotein sub-class pattern and risk of myocardial infarction. *J Am Med Assoc* 260:1917–1921, 1988.
8. Reaven GM, Chen YDI, Jeppesen J, Maheux P, Krauss RM: Insulin resistance and hyperinsulinemia in individuals with small, dense, low density lipoprotein particles. *J Clin Invest* 92:141–146, 1993.
9. Zambon S, Manzato E, Solini A, Sambataro M, Brocco M, Sartore G, Crepaldi G, Nosadini R: Lipoprotein abnormalities in non-insulin-dependent diabetic patients with impaired extrahepatic insulin sensitivity, hypertension, and micro-albuminuria. *Arterioscler Thromb* 14:911–916, 1994.
10. Bowie A, Owens D, Collins P, Johnson A, Tomkin GH: Glycosylated low density lipoprotein is more sensitive to oxidation: implications for the diabetic patient? *Atherosclerosis* 102:63–67, 1993.
11. Haffner SM: Lipoprotein(a) and diabetes: an update. *Diabet Care* 16:835–840, 1993.
12. Zambon S, Baldo-Enzi G, Baiocchi M.R., Nosadini R, Manzato E, Crepaldi G: Lipoprotein(a) levels in type 2 diabetic patients are not influenced by metabolic control or by microalbuminuria. *Diabet Care* 17:1548–1549, 1994.
13. Stamler J, Vaccaro O, Neaton JD *et al*: Diabetes, other risk factors, and 12-yr cardiovascular mortality for men screened in the Multiple Risk Factor Intervention Trial. *Diabet Care* 16:434–444, 1993.
14. Tribble DL, Holl LG, Wood PD, Krauss RM: Variations in oxidative susceptibility among six low density lipoprotein subfractions of differing density and particle size. *Atherosclerosis* 93:189–199, 1992.
15. Nosadini R, Manzato E, Solini A, Fioretto P, Brocco E, Zambon S, Morocutti A, Sambataro M, Velussi M, Cipollina MR, Crepaldi G: Peripheral, rather than hepatic, insulin resistance and atherogenic lipoprotein phenotype predict cardiovascular complications in NIDDM. *Eur J Clin Invest* 24:258–266, 1994.
16. Haffner SM, Alexander CM, Cook JR, Boccuzzi SJ, Musliner TA, Pedersen TR, Kjekshus J, Pyorala K for the Scandinavian Simvastatin Survival Study Group: Reduced coronary events in simvastatin-treated patients with coronary heart disease and diabetes or impaired fasting glucose levels. Subgroup analysis in the Scandinavian Simvastatin Survival Study. *Arch Intern Med* 159:2661–2667, 1999.
17. Bloomfield Rubins H, Robins SJ, Collins D, Fye CL, Anderson JW, Elam MB, Faas FH, Linares E, Schaefer EJ, Schectman G, Wilt TJ, Wittes J, for the Veterans Affairs High-density Lipoprotein Cholesterol Intervention Trial Study Group: Gemfibrozil for the secondary prevention of coronary heart disease in men with low levels of high-density lipoprotein cholesterol. *N Engl J Med* 341:410–418, 1999.
18. American Diabetes Association: Management of dyslipidemia in adults with diabetes. *Diabet Care* 21:179–182, 1998.

16

Evidence-based Therapy of Type 2 Diabetes

MICHAEL BERGER[1] and INGRID MÜHLHAUSER[1,2]
[1]Department of Metabolic Diseases and Nutrition (WHO Collaborating Centre for Diabetes), Heinrich-Heine University, Düsseldorf, Germany; [2]Unit for Health Sciences and Education, University of Hamburg, Germany

With the frightening worldwide rise of its incidence and prevalence rates, type 2 diabetes is becoming a major public health problem; given the demographic and pathophysiological heterogeneity of the disease, a multitude of therapeutic strategies is being advocated as consensus recommendations and guidelines. In addition, the pharmaceutical industry is launching more and more sophisticated and expensive products to combat the endemic growth of type 2 diabetes and its complications. In order to review the different therapeutic strategies, we suggest focusing upon the patient-orientated outcome goals of type 2 diabetes treatment, applying the principles of evidence-based medicine as suggested by Sackett *et al* (1).

Primary therapeutic objectives are to maintain a quality of life as little affected by the disease as possible, the prevention of its acute complications, its hyperglycaemia-induced symptoms and therapeutic collateral effects and the prevention of excess cardiovascular morbidity and mortality, as well as microangiopathic organ damage associated with type 2 diabetes. With excess mortality due to macroangiopathy being the principal clinical problem of type 2 diabetes, it is surprising that only two studies have ever attempted to demonstrate an effect of treatments to lower glycaemia upon the incidence of cardiovascular morbidity and mortality (2,3). All but three randomized controlled trials were conducted to document the effects of attempts to normalize blood glucose on incidence and progression of microangiopathy in

Diabetes in the New Millennium. Edited by U. Di Mario, F. Leonetti, G. Pugliese, P. Sbraccia and A. Signore.
© 2000 John Wiley & Sons, Ltd.

type 2 diabetes (2–4). Sackett *et al* (1) have called for the implementation of evidence-based medicine principles as the integration of best research evidence with clinical expertise and patient values. In this article, we shall comment on the impact of scientific evidence and patient preferences upon the definition of a rational treatment of type 2 diabetes mellitus.

SCIENTIFIC EVIDENCE FOR ANTI-HYPERGLYCAEMIC THERAPY IN TYPE 2 DIABETES MELLITUS

In this context, relevant scientific evidence has to be derived from patient-centred clinical research into the efficacy and safety of therapeutic and preventive regimens. Thus, we shall focus upon data from randomized controlled trials directed at clinically relevant endpoints of type 2 diabetes, i.e. cardiovascular morbidity and mortality and hyperglycaemia-associated organ damage, rather than upon surrogate markers, such as indices of glycaemia or other circulating metabolites. With regard to the incidence of macroangiopathy (cardiovascular morbidity and mortality), neither of the RCTs (2,3) directed at this endpoint were able to detect any significant improvement as a result of blood glucose lowering — with the exception of a positive effect of metformin monotherapy in overweight type 2 diabetic patients upon diabetes-related aggregated vascular complications and death, as well as upon total mortality (5). When hyperglycaemia was lowered by insulin treatment, a significant reduction of microangiopathic organ damage was demonstrated in two randomized controlled trials (2,4). When sulphonylurea drugs were used as antihyperglycaemic agents, contrasting results emerged: with tolbutamide treatment, a significant increase in cardiovascular mortality was observed (6). The pathophysiological plausibility of this phenomenon became only apparent some 30 years later (7); at that time, respective indirect observations indicative of cardiotoxic collateral effects of sulphonylureas on ischaemic hearts were also published (8). With the use of glibenclamide in the UKPDS, no adverse effect on cardiovascular outcomes was observed; however, patients with clinically apparent coronary artery disease were excluded per study protocol (2). At most, those 2% of patients included in the study who have had a myocardial infraction prior to 12 months before being recruited may have to be considered coronary artery patients.

Looking at the aggregate outcomes any diabetes-related endpoint or microangiopathy, the UKPDS revealed a significant benefit resulting from a lowering of HbA_{Ic} levels from a median of 7.9% (conventional treatment) to a median of 7.0% (intensive treatment) — with the 10-year preventive effect of insulin treatment being indistinguishable from the benefit associated with glibenclamide treatment (2). In contrast to the beneficial effects of glibenclamide in this study, chlopropamide — a first-generation sulphonylurea compound—resulted in an increased incidence of arterial hypertension, whereas a significant reduction of microangiopathy was not demonstrated (2). From this diversity concerning the efficacy and safety profile of various sulphonylurea drugs it emerges that—as in other areas of pharmacotherapy (9)—one is not allowed to assume a positive 'class effect' for sulphonylureas based upon the beneficial effects of glibenclamide shown in the UKPDS. In contrast, for any other sulphonylurea drug recommended for use in type 2 diabetes, efficacy and safety still need to be documented. Even for glibenclamide, the therapeutic use in type 2 diabetic patients with coronary artery disease lacks the proof of safety.

Only for glibenclamide (with the above-referenced contraindication in patients with coronary artery disease) and metformin monotherapy in obese type 2 diabetic patients (with the contraindications of biguanide therapy), efficacy and safety have been proven with respect to clinically relevant endpoints. All other oral antidiabetic agents lack the adequate documentation of patient-orientated outcome benefits and can thus not be considered for routine patient care under the principles of evidence-based medicine (10).

When aiming to reduce the excessive cardiovascular morbidity and mortality in type 2 diabetes, it appears adequately justifiable to treat arterial hypertension, hypercholesterolaemia, to stop smoking and to take aspirin (10).

THE INTEGRATION OF PATIENT VALUES BY EVIDENCE-BASED PATIENT INFORMATION AND DECISION MAKING

Sackett *et al* (1) call for the integration of patient values, preferences, concerns and expectations into clinical decisions in order to serve the patient as a basic element in their concept of evidence-based medicine. Inasmuch as possible, the patients' preferences must be based upon informed decision-making processes, as recently described in detail by the UK's General Medical Council (11). This document calls for specific and detailed information on the patient with regard to therapeutic options, their quantitative risks and their uncertainties and concerning the potential conflicts of interests involved in the process; it is specifically stated that a possibility/probability that the patient may decide not to opt for a recommended procedure/treatment must not be a reason for withholding any information. We have recently tried to adapt such recommendations for type 2 diabetic patients about to undergo antidiabetic therapy (12). Such an attempt requires a method to present the quantitative data generated by the three randomized controlled trials (2,3,4) relevant in this area of clinical medicine to the patient in an unbiased and balanced manner.

Table 16.1. Reduction of vascular complications and organ damage by intensive vs. conventional blood glucose control in the UK Prospective Diabetes Study [data from (2,11)]

	Blood glucose control	
	Intensive (median HbA_{Ic} over 10 years 7.0%) $n = 2729$	Conventional (median HbA_{Ic} over 10 years 7.9%) $n = 1138$
Any diabetes related endpoint		
Events per 1000 patient-years	41	46
Absolute risk reduction	5.1	
(% in 10 years)		
NNT	20	
	(95% confidence intervals 10–500)	
p-Value	0.029	
Relative risk reduction	12%	
Microvascular complications		
Events per 1000 patient-years	8.6	11.4
Absolute risk reduction	2.8	
(% in 10 years)		
NNT	36	
	(95% confidence intervals not provided by the authors)	
p-Value	0.0099	
Relative risk reduction	25%	

In quantitative terms, the much-heralded benefit on microvascular disease achieved by intensive blood glucose treatment in the UKPDS was rather modest (2). The exceptional efforts on the part of the patients and the health care system to lower medium HbA_{Ic} levels by 0.9% throughout a decade resulted in a 25% reduction of microvascular endpoints; the absolute risk reduction, however, amounted to a mere 2.8%, i.e. a number needed to treat in order to prevent the occurrence of the aggregate endpoint microvascular complications in one patient was NNT = 36 (13). Similarly sobering findings evolve from the analysis of the aggregate endpoint 'any diabetes-related endpoint' (Table 16.1).

It is this evidence-based analysis of the UKPDS data which is urgently needed to explain the complex sets of data to the patients. At the end of the day, it is up to the patient to decide whether it is worth her/his efforts during a period of 10 years to keep HbA_{Ic} levels at 7.0%, rather than at 7.9%, if the NNT indicative of the probability of a benefit for their own case is in the magnitude of 20 (for any diabetes-related endpoint, with a 95% confidence interval of 10–500). In other words: out of 100 newly diagnosed type 2 diabetic patients, with intensive therapy 95 have no benefit over the next 10 years (when compared with conventional therapy) since they would not have a diabetes-related endpoint (ADREP) with conventional therapy (54 patients) or they will have such an endpoint despite intensive therapy (41 patients).

Even though it is generally felt to be justified to extrapolate from these data to the even greater benefit that may be achievable when initially much higher HbA_{Ic} levels are lowered by appropriate therapy, it is noteworthy that hard data, based upon randomized controlled trials, are only available for relatively young, early manifest type 2 diabetic patients in relatively good (controls, median HbA_{Ic} 7.9%) compared with very good (intensive control, median HbA_{Ic} 7.0%) glycaemic control as followed for a period of 10 years.

On the other hand, it must be assumed that at HbA_{Ic} levels of above 9.0–9.5% an improvement of glycaemic control is justified by the resulting improvement of the patient's well-being and a reduction of a variety of hyperglycaemia-induced sequelae and symptoms.

CONCLUSIONS

Following the principles of evidence-based medicine, it will now be up to patients to decide on their own HbA_{Ic} target level, depending on the risks they are prepared to take and the efforts they are prepared to make. In order to achieve these therapeutic goals, a step-wise approach, including non-drug therapy (14) and insulin treatment with glibenclamide and metformin monotherapy as options for subgroups of patients, is justified by adequate evidence from randomized controlled trials. Furthermore, the efficacy of a multifactorial intervention in slowing the progression of microangiopathic organ damage in type 2 diabetes merits consideration (15).

Enabling the patients to enter into such a decision-making process will require innovative methodological approaches in the area of patient education and communication, which do not yet seem to be available. The systematic integration of patients' preferences on therapeutic goals and strategies based upon informed decision-making processes with the scientific evidence from patient-centred clinical research forms the basis of a treatment of type 2 diabetes mellitus according to the principles of evidence-based medicine.

REFERENCES

1. Sackett DL, Strauss SE, Richardson WS, Rosenberg W, Haynes RB: *Evidence-based medicine. How to practise and teach EBM*, 2nd edn. Edinburgh: Churchill Livingstone, 2000.

2. The University Group Diabetes program: Effects of hypoglycemic agents on vascular complications in patients with adult-onset diabetes. VIII. *Diabetes* 31 (Suppl 5):1–81, 1982.
3. UK Prospective Diabetes Study (UKPDS) Group: Intensive blood-glucose control with sulphonylureas or insulin compared with conventional treatment and risk of complications in patients with type 2 diabetes (UKPDS 33). *Lancet* 352:837–853, 1998.
4. Ohkubo Y, Kishikawa H, Araki E, Miyata T, Isami S, Motoyoshi S, Kojima Y, Furuyoshi N, Shichiri M: Intensive insulin therapy prevents the progression of diabetic microvascular complications in Japanese patients with non-insulin-dependent diabetes mellitus: a randomized prospective 6-year study. *Diabet Res Clin Pract* 28:103–117, 1995.
5. Effect of intensive blood glucose control with metformin on complications in overweight patients with type 2 diabetes (UKPDS 34). *Lancet* 352:854–865, 1998.
6. The University Group Diabetes Program: A study on the effects of hypoglycemic agents on vascular complications in patients with adult-onset diabetes. I. *Diabetes* 19 (Suppl 2): 474–830, 1970.
7. Leibovitz G, Cerasi E: Sulfonylurea treatment of NIDDM patients with cardiovascular disease: a mixed blessing? *Diabetologia* 39:503–514, 1996.
8. Berger M, Mühlhauser I, Sawicki PT: Possible risk of sulfonylureas in the treatment of non-insulin-dependent diabetes mellitus with coronary heart disease (letter). *Diabetologia* 40:1492–1493, 1997; *Diabetologia* 41:744, 1998.
9. Furberg C, Herrington DM, Psaty BM: Are drugs within a class interchangeable? *Lancet* 354:1202–1204, 1999.
10. Berger M, Mühlhauser I: Diabetes care and patient-oriented outcomes. *J Am Med Assoc* 281:1676–1678, 1999.
11. General Medical Council: Protecting patients, guiding doctors. Seeking patients' consent: the ethical considerations. London: General Medical Council, 1999.
12. Mühlhauser I, Berger M: Evidence-based patient information in diabetes. *Diabet Med*, 2000 (in press).
13. Mühlhauser I: UKPDS — Darstellung nach Evidence-based Medicine Kriterien. *Stoffwechsel und Ernährung* 7:267–273, 1998.
14. Kronsbein P, Jörgens I, Mühlhauser I, Scholz V, Venhaus A, Berger M: Evaluation of a structured treatment and teaching programme on non-insulin dependent diabetes. *Lancet* 2:1407–1411, 1988.
15. Gaede P, Vedel P, Parving HH, Pedersen O: Intensified multifactorial intervention in patients with type 2 diabetes mellitus and microalbuminuria: the Steno type 2 randomised study. *Lancet* 353:617–622, 1999.

17

Management of Type 2 Diabetes: Lessons from UKPDS and Other Trials

DAVID LESLIE

Department of Diabetes and Metabolism, St Bartholomew's Hospital, London UK

Diabetes is a potentially devastating disease with a high morbidity and mortality. There is an excess risk of both microvascular and macrovascular complications with diabetes. Recent studies have emphasized and illustrated how we might be able to limit these diabetic complications. UKPDS found that improved control of blood glucose or blood pressure reduced the risk of: major diabetic eye disease, by one quarter; serious deterioration of vision, by nearly one-half; early kidney damage, by one-third; strokes, by one-third, and death from diabetes-related causes, by one-third. Other studies have demonstrated the importance of blood pressure control and reduced cholesterol as well as the use of aspirin in limiting progression of macrovascular disease. Diabetes is no longer viewed as a disease of sugar alone. A more holistic approach is required if our patients are to benefit from the information we have acquired through these recent studies.

BACKGROUND

Diabetes is a world-wide disease. The rate of increase of diabetes is such that there is effectively a global epidemic of the disease. In 1985 the World Health Organization (WHO) estimated that 30 million people had diabetes; today the estimate is around 100 million and projections are that this prevalence will double to 200 million in the next 15 years.

Diabetes in the New Millennium. Edited by U. Di Mario, F. Leonetti, G. Pugliese, P. Sbraccia and A. Signore.
© 2000 John Wiley & Sons, Ltd.

The mortality rates for patients with type 2 diabetes in different countries are up to four times those of the non-diabetic populations and the increased mortality has been attributed mainly to accelerated macrovascular disease, in particular cardiovascular disease (1). Diabetes remains the commonest single cause of limb amputations, as well as the commonest cause of blindness and renal failure in middle-aged adults in developed countries. Epidemiological data indicate that the degree and duration of hyperglycaemia is associated with the microvascular complications of diabetes, including retinopathy, nephropathy and neuropathy (1,3). Recently, it has become apparent that hyperglycaemia may also be a risk factor for macrovascular disease, in addition to hypertension, dyslipidaemia, smoking and thrombotic factors (4–16).

BLOOD GLUCOSE

The introduction of HbA_{1c} as an index of blood glucose control enabled studies of the relationship between HbA_{1c} and microvascular disease from diagnosis (2,3). These studies, including the Diabetes Control and Complications Trial (DCCT) in type 1 diabetic patients, encouraged clinicians, probably correctly as it happens, to believe that optimal blood glucose control was desirable in patients with type 2 diabetes.

The UKPDS was a 20 year study involving 23 centres in the UK. More than 5000 patients with type 2 diabetes were recruited to the study, which cost in excess of £23 million. The study was initiated and coordinated by the late Robert Turner and Rory Holman at the Diabetes Research Laboratories in Oxford. The aim was to determine the impact of intensive blood glucose on 21 predetermined clinical end-points, using, in the case of blood glucose control, sulphonylureas or insulin therapy or, in the overweight patient, treatment with metformin. In addition, the study investigated the impact of intensive blood pressure control on macro- and microvascular complications of diabetes and compared captopril treatment with atenolol.

UKPDS asked whether intensive treatment using different drug therapy (insulin, sulphonylureas or metformin) was better than a 'dietary' policy. Or would it be worse? After all there was real concern about sulphonylureas raised by the UGDP, as well as the argument that insulin therapy could be atherogenic. The primary outcomes concerned unequivocal end-points such as death, severe cardiovascular events, loss of vision and renal failure, assessed together as all diabetes-related events, diabetes-related mortality and all-cause mortality (4–7).

UKPDS glucose control

Some 3867 patients newly diagnosed with type 2 diabetes were randomly assigned to two treatment groups: one group, the intensive treatment group

Table 17.1. Results of UKPDS Glucose Control Study (risk reduction)

12%	For any diabetes-related endpoint	$p = 0.029$
25%	For microvascular endpoints	$p = 0.0099$
16%	for myocardial infarction	$p = 0.052$
24%	for cataract extraction	$p = 0.046$
21%	for retinopathy at 12 years	$p = 0.0015$
33%	for albuminuria at 12 years	$p = 0.000054$

(aim, fasting plasma glucose <6 mmol/l), took either one of three oral sulphonylurea drugs (chlorpropamide, glibenclamide or glipizide) or insulin; the second group (aim, fasting plasma glucose <15 mmol/l without symptoms), initially only received dietary treatment, i.e. a diet high in carbohydrate and fibre and low in saturated fats (4). In the study design, the failure of diet or drugs to maintain targets glucose levels led to the introduction of drugs or the use of different drugs, respectively. Thus, patients in the diet-alone arm might end up on a number of drugs or taking insulin. As a result there was substantial overlap in therapy between the groups for comparison. The definition of diabetes was a plasma blood glucose higher than 6.0 mmol/l, which is lower than the current definition of higher than 7.0 mmol/l, so that a fraction of the patients may have had impaired glucose tolerance and not frank diabetes. The discrepancies in the definition of diabetes might have limited the power of the study, but should not have influenced the positive results.

It was found that patients on intensive therapy had better blood glucose control than patients on conventional treatment (4). The mean HbA_{1c} over 10 years was 7.0% in the intensive group and 7.9% in the conventional group, a difference of 0.9%, which was highly significant although with some overlap between the two groups. There was no difference in the HbA_{1c} using different drugs. Importantly, while the difference in HbA_{1c} persisted throughout the study period, the HbA_{1c} did increase gradually in both groups during the study after an initial fall in the first year after diagnosis. The results were analysed as endpoints and as aggregate endpoints over 15 years (4). The significant differences are shown in Table 17.1. Note that the risk reduction for myocardial infarction falls just short of statistical significance. Of diabetes-related endpoints, 564 of 963 were macrovascular in the intensive group, as were 259 of 438 in the smaller conventional group. In other words, in both groups macrovascular endpoints were observed more often than microvascular events. Nevertheless, intensive therapy had the biggest impact on micro-vascular events. There was no advantage in terms of outcome between sulphonylureas and insulin. Side-effects occurred, predominantly hypogly-caemia and weight gain. Hypoglycaemia was more common in the intensive group than in conventional group and more common with insulin than sulphonylureas.

UKPDS Glucose Control Study — metformin

1704 patients newly diagnosed with type 2 diabetes who were overweight (>120% ideal body weight) were randomly assigned to three treatment groups: one group, an intensive treatment group (aim, fasting plasma glucose <6 mmol/l), took either one of three oral sulphonylurea drugs (chlorpropamide, glibenclamide or glipizide) or insulin; the second group (aim, fasting plasma glucose <15 mmol/l without symptoms), initially only received dietary treatment involving a diet high in carbohydrate and fibre and low in saturated fats; while a third group received metformin (aim, fasting plasma glucose <6 mmol/l) (5).

It was found that patients on intensive therapy including metformin had better blood glucose control than patients on conventional treatment (5). The HbA_{1c} was, on average over 10 years, 7.4% in the metformin group and similar in the intensive group, but 8.0% in the conventional group — on average, a difference of 0.6%, which was highly significant, although with some overlap in the HbA_{1c} between the groups. There was no difference in the HbA_{1c} between agents used in the intensive group. Patients allocated metformin, compared with the conventional group, showed a risk reduction of 32% for any diabetes-related endpoint, and 36% for all-cause mortality (5). These risk reductions on metformin were significantly greater than with the sulphonylureas or insulin. The early introduction of metformin with sulphonylureas was associated with an increase in diabetes-related deaths as compared with continued sulphonylurea therapy by itself. However, combination therapy with sulphonylureas and metformin was not, overall, associated with an increased risk of diabetes-related death. Side-effects on metformin in UKPDS included hypoglycaemia, which surprisingly was more common (34% of patients over the study period) than in the diet group (4.2%).

UKPDS summary

These studies showed that intensive blood glucose control with either sulphonylureas, metformin or insulin substantially decreased the risk of microvascular complications. In overweight type 2 diabetic patients, metformin may be the drug of choice. No therapy had an adverse effect on cardiovascular disease.

Comparison of UKPDS with DCCT

It is worth comparing the results of DCCT with UKPDS. DCCT was also designed to compare the impact of intensive blood glucose control on microvascular, but not macrovascular, complications in type 1 and not type 2 diabetic patients (2). Comparable HbA_{1c} assays were used in both studies, so that comparisons could be made. In DCCT, the initial mean HbA_{1c} was 8.9% (compared with about 6.2% in UKPDS) (2,4). In DCCT the achieved mean HbA_{1c} in the intensive group was about 7%, as compared with about 9% in the conventional group—a difference of 2% (compared with 0.9% in UKPDS). There was no inexorable rise in HbA_{1c} throughout DCCT, as occurred in UKPDS. The results of DCCT demonstrated that intensive care aimed at optimal glycaemic control could reduce the risk of developing microvascular complications. For example, the risk of developing retinopathy was reduced by 76% and the risk of progression of retinopathy by 50% in the intensive group. Similar levels of reduction were observed with the development of microalbuminuria, proteinuria and neuropathy. By implication, all patients with type 1 diabetes, irrespective of their degree of complications, could benefit from improved glycaemic control. The risk reductions appeared to be proportional in both studies to the HbA_{1c} differences; thus, progression of retinopathy was diminished by 63% in DCCT and 21% in UKPDS, and for albuminuria by 54% and 34% respectively (2,4). Notably, the HbA_1 levels in UKPDS were overall lower than in DCCT, suggesting that improved blood glucose control can still be beneficial at levels not far short of the normal range. On the other hand, not all patients with optimal glycaemic therapy will be protected from complications; for example, in the DCCT by 8 years 25% of patients in the intensive care group progressed to microalbuminuria, as did about 18% in UKPDS (2,4). This observation raises the possibility that factors other than blood glucose are important in the pathogenesis of diabetic complications. In neither DCCT nor UKPDS did intensive blood glucose control have an impact on macrovascular events (2,4). In UKPDS the 16% reduction of myocardial infarction fell just short of statistical significance ($p = 0.052$), while in DCCT the risk of macrovascular disease, not an aim of the study, was reduced by 41%, but the numbers were small and the effect not significant. In contrast, the UKPDS blood pressure control study found a striking 44% reduction in stroke, which was highly significant.

Implications of UKPDS and DCCT

Taken in conjunction with DCCT and other studies, notably from Scandinavia and Japan, the results confirm the glucose hypothesis (2–5). For every 1% fall in HbA_{1c} there is a reduction in microvascular risk by about 25%, irrespective of type of diabetes.

Use of hypoglycaemic drugs

The means of obtaining an improvement in blood glucose using current therapies is apparently irrelevant, although there may be some value in using metformin initially in overweight type 2 diabetic patients (5). The metformin study in the UKPDS was something of an afterthought, as metformin was originally one of the drugs to be used in the intensive group and not for independent assessment. Whilst a seemingly minor point, this concern is a real one, given the substantial number of statistical comparisons that have been made in the studies, allowing ample opportunity for occasional random significant results. Nevertheless, it is difficult to avoid the conclusion that metformin should be the initial drug of choice in the obese type 2 diabetic patient, and its beneficial effect on glucose was comparable in obese and non-obese patients. There remains the observation that sulphonylurea-treated patients given metformin at an early stage had a marked increase in both diabetes-related (96% increase) and all-cause (60% increase) deaths (5). Is this observation the inevitable consequence of multiple statistical comparisons, as a further analysis of the data suggests, or are there real risks in using combined sulphonylurea and metformin therapy? A subsequent study from Sweden confirmed a higher mortality in patients on sulphonylureas and metformin. It is possible that the increased mortality in this group simply reflects a more aggressive type of diabetes requiring combination therapy.

In broad terms, combination therapy has proved successful, at least in terms of reducing HbA_{1c}. Several double-blind studies have been performed using metformin and insulin in both type 1 and type 2 diabetic patients. The evidence consistently suggests that in type 2 diabetes there is an insulin-sparing effect in adding metformin, and that the combination provides a safe strategy to achieve better blood glucose control, with a limited risk of hypoglycaemia and weight gain. Combining insulin with a glitazone can also be beneficial, reducing the HbA_{1c} in one study of insulin-treated patients by a mean of 1.2% with an associated reduction in insulin requirement.

Blood glucose targets

The targets for blood glucose control are surely much clearer now. There are no thresholds within the diabetic range of blood glucose for risk of microvascular complications. Target HbA_{1c} should be as normal as is practical, given that normal levels may be unrealistic, due to either the inadequacies of our treatment, ourselves or our patients. Early diagnosis will be important.

BLOOD PRESSURE

The critical questions in terms of blood pressure management are who should be treated, what should they be treated with, and what target blood pressure should we aim to achieve? In considering these questions, the important variables are the type of diabetes (type 1 or type 2) and the presence of coexisting microvascular or macrovascular disease. The assumption that treatment of hypertension is worthwhile is based on the value of such treatment in non-diabetic subjects studied in large randomized controlled studies. Since hypertension associated with diabetes carries a high risk, those patients with type 1 or type 2 diabetes are immediately identified as at risk and are candidates for anti-hypertensive therapy when the blood pressure is more than 130 (possibly 140) systolic or 85 diastolic.

UKPDS Blood Pressure Control Study

A randomized controlled trial of 1148 patients with type 2 diabetes compared tight control of blood pressure, aiming at a blood pressure of < 150/85 mmHg, with less tight control, aiming at a blood pressure of < 180/105 mmHg (6). Patients on intensive therapy had lower blood pressure (mean 144/82 mmHg) than patients assigned less tight control (154/87 mmHg) (6). There was no difference in the blood pressure using either captopril or atenolol (11). After 9 years, 29% of the tight control group required three or more drugs.

The significant differences are shown in Table 17.2. Patients allocated tight control, compared with the conventional group, showed a risk reduction of 24% for any diabetes-related endpoint and 44% in strokes, but no significant effect on all-causes mortality (6). The risk reductions on captopril were similar to atenolol; in particular, progression to albuminuria was similar (7). Side-effects were no different with captopril and atenolol, apart from weight gain, which was greater with atenolol.

Summary

It was concluded that tight blood pressure control in patients with hypertension and type 2 diabetes achieves a clinically important reduction in the risk of deaths related to diabetes, complications related to diabetes, progression of diabetic retinopathy and deterioration in visual acuity (6). Blood pressure lowering with captopril or atenolol was similarly effective (7)—although beware, because the study did not have sufficient power to exclude such a difference. In this respect type 2 diabetic patients may differ from type 1 patients. Combinations of drugs were often required to achieve the target blood pressure. The controversy about the value of calcium channel blocking drugs was not considered. The goal for blood pressure can probably be set at less than 140/85 mmHg but there was no threshold effect as with glucose (10–15).

Blood pressure trials

Apart from UKPDS, there have been four other major studies testing angiotensin-converting enzyme inhibitors (ACEIs). In these, the results favoured the use of an ACEI in comparison with nisoldipine (in ABCD) and

Table 17.2.   Results of UKPDS Blood Pressure Control Study (risk reduction)

24%	for any diabetes-related endpoint	$p = 0.0046$
32%	for diabetes-related deaths	$p = 0.019$
44%	for stroke	$p = 0.013$
37%	for microvascular disease	$p = 0.0092$
56%	for heart failure	$p = 0.0043$
34%	for retinopathy progression	$p = 0.0038$
47%	for deterioration of vision	$p = 0.0036$

amlodopine (in FACET) but not in a Finnish study using nitrendipine (11). In ABCD treatment with nisoldipine ($n = 235$) vs. enalapril ($n = 235$) over a 5 year follow-up showed a higher risk of fatal and non-fatal myocardial infarction in the former (11). On the other hand, there were no differences in the primary end-points, namely total or cardiovacular mortality. The FACET study of amlodipine ($n = 188$) vs. fosinopril ($n = 188$) over 3.5 years showed an increased risk of cardiovascular events in the former, but the analysis was *post hoc*, following the results of ABCD, and therefore of limited value. In none of these studies was there a placebo group, so the results did not exclude a beneficial effect of calcium channel blockers, indeed, in the Finnish study these agents were particularly beneficial in older patients.

The HOPE study of diabetic patients over the age of 55 years with one other cardiovascular risk factor (hypertension, elevated total cholesterol, low HDL cholesterol, cigarette smoking, or microalbuminuria) benefit from therapy with an ACEI, in this case ramipril (14). There was a 25% reduction in the combined risk of myocardial infarction, stroke and cardiovascular death in patients receiving ramipril (10 mg/day) as compared with a placebo after 4.5 years. The benefit was achieved with only a 3 mmHg difference in systolic blood pressure between the group so that only 40% at best, it is argued, of the benefit could be attributed to the blood pressure effect. This 40% effect is based on meta-analysis of different populations from those studied in HOPE, so there is still discussion on the blood pressure independent benefits of ACEIs.

Which antihypertensive drug?

One risk of these antihypertensive drugs is that they may have a detrimental metabolic effect, particularly β-blockers and thiazides. In a study of 12 550 adults without diabetes, it was noted that those on thiazides had no excess risk of diabetes and neither had patients on ACEIs or calcium channel blockers (13). However, patients on β-blockers had a 28% higher risk of diabetes than those taking no medication. The effect was not due to weight gain. Interestingly, patients with hypertension were almost 2.5 times more likely to develop diabetes than those without hypertension. The use of smaller doses of thiazides and chlortalidone in recent studies may account for the lack of adverse action of diuretics in more recent studies, as compared with older studies that did identify a diabetogenic action of these drugs. The use of α-blockers has suffered a set-back following the premature halt to ALLSTAT, a trial in which α-blockers were unexpectedly linked to an increased risk of cardiac failure. In selecting the ideal agent for treatment of hypertension, the Sixth Report of the Joint National Committee on the treatment of hypertension recommended ACEIs as initial agents for lowering blood pressure in patients with type 2 diabetes. Nevertheless, α-blockers and diuretics have beneficial effects. Calcium channel blockers are, in my opinion and subject to further information, still of value.

In diabetic and non-diabetic patients with proteinuria there is substantial evidence that ACEIs have a renoprotective effect, independent of the effect on hypertension. In these patients with proteinuria the initial treatment of choice is an ACEI, irrespective of whether the patient does or does not have coincident hypertension. In patients intolerant of ACEIs there is enough evidence to support a beneficial effect of antihypertensive agents to use other agents.

What blood pressure target?

Isolated systolic hypertension is highly prevalent in the elderly population and more than 70% of adults over 64 years of age are considered to be hypertensive (systolic BP >or = 140 mmHg and/or diastolic > or = 90 mmHg). Systolic pressure is a better predictor of cardiovascular events than diastolic pressure and a wide pulse pressure is a better predictor than either alone. Both the SHEP and SYST-Eur trials, studying elderly patients irrespective of their diabetes status, showed clear cardiovascular benefit in treating isolated systolic hypertension (10). In a subgroup of 492 diabetic patients, there was a dramatic reduction in cardiovascular mortality (down 76%), such that the excess risk of diabetes was almost completely abolished by treatment which included nitrendipine, enalapril and or a thiazide. Current recommendations suggest lowering systolic pressure by no more than 20 mmHg initially to limit postural hypotension.

It is worthwhile treating a systolic blood pressure of 160 or more and a diastolic pressure of 90 or more. Less clear is what constitutes blood pressure control. It could be said that hypertension is best defined as that level of blood pressure above which treatment does more good than harm. Studying the target of therapy, the hypertension optimal therapy trial (HOT) studied 18 790 patients randomized to three target blood pressures (12). After 3.8 years follow-up, the BP levels achieved were 139.7/ 81.1; 141/83.2; 143.7/85.2 mmHg. The nadir of cardiovascular mortality was at 82.6 mmHg diastolic and of cardiovascular mortality at 86.5 mmHg. In the substantial subgroup of diabetic patients ($n = 1501$), major cardiovascular events were reduced by 51% in those that achieved a diastolic blood pressure of 81.1 mmHg. In UKPDS there was no evidence for a threshold of microvascular complications risk above 130 mmHg systolic. A question arising from these studies is whether we should treat all people with blood pressure over, say, 140/85. Those studies to date have not considered this point and in the absence of an evidence base, the recommended targets are speculative.

CHOLESTEROL

The evidence from UKPDS is that improving glycaemic control has a major impact on microvascular disease but, if anything, a small effect on macrovascular disease. Thus, management of risk from macrovascular disease requires measures other than glycaemic control. Recent studies have identified the clear and substantial benefit in reducing mortality by reducing blood cholesterol levels. Analysis of earlier studies, particularly primary prevention studies which did not use statins, led to concern that lowering cholesterol might increase death from non-cardiovascular causes. Meta-analysis and case studies indicated that this concern was needless and that the excess of non-cardiac deaths, including suicides and accidents, occurred by chance. Secondary prevention studies using dietary modification resulted in a substantial reduction in mortality at 2 years, and even demonstrated angiographically improved cardiovascular disease on diet alone. The most striking and convincing results came from the Scandinavian Simvastatin Survival Study (4S) which studied 4444 patients with cardiovascular disease whose serum cholesterol was between 5.5–8.0 mmol/l (8). A subgroup analysis of the 4S identified 202 diabetic subjects, 99 of whom were randomized to a placebo and 105 to simvastatin. Most of the diabetic subjects had type 2 diabetes, as only 12% of them were on insulin. As a group compared with the non-diabetic subjects, they tended to be older, have higher blood pressure, body mass index and triglycerides, and a lower HDL-cholesterol. Nevertheless, these diabetic subjects may not be representative of type 2 diabetes patients in general, as those with triglyceride levels greater than 2.5 mmol/l were excluded. The treated diabetic patients showed a similar fall in cholesterol to the non-diabetics, with a fall in cardiovascular events, both major and all-events, by 55% (8). There was also a 37% reduction in total mortality, although this did not reach statistical significance. It was concluded that simvastatin is also beneficial in type 2 diabetes patients with cholesterol levels of 5.5–8.0 mmol/l and with evidence of macrovascular disease. It was estimated that 6 years of treatment with simvastatin in 100 patients with established cardiovascular disease with cholesterol levels of 5.5–8.0 mmol/l could prevent cardiovascular events in 9/29 non-diabetic subjects and 29/49 subjects with diabetes. By implication, then, the potential benefits of lowering blood cholesterol with simvastatin in diabetic patients could be even greater than in non-diabetic subjects.

The extent of vascular disease in patients with type 2 diabetes is such that they may, it would appear, be reasonably treated in a similar way to those with established cardiovascular disease (9). This was the conclusion of a 7-year incidence study of myocardial infarction in 1059 type 2 diabetic and 1373 non-diabetic subjects. Incidence rates in the diabetic subjects with and without myocardial infarction at baseline were 45% and 20.2%, respectively, ($p<0.001$), and in non-diabetic subjects 18.8% and 3.5%, respectively ($p<0.001$) (9). Thus, even diabetic subjects without previous clinical heart disease had a similar risk of myocardial infarction to the non-diabetic subjects with previous myocardial infarction.

SMOKING

There remains perhaps the most potent risk factor for cardiovascular disease, cigarette smoking. It is estimated that stopping smoking could reduce the risk of progression to cardiovascular disease by up to 70% in the non-diabetic population and we have no reason to believe that the benefit will be less in diabetic patients (15).

ASPIRIN AND VITAMIN E

Activated aggregating platelets are important in the development of acute coronary events and aspirin can prevent platelets aggregating. Aspirin has been assessed in the primary and secondary prevention of macrovascular disease (15–20).

Primary prevention

Aspirin has been used for the primary prevention of cardiovascular disease, that is it has been given to subjects with no evidence of vascular disease to see if it would prevent the development of such disease. In broad terms the results of these studies have been inconclusive, showing no unequivocally beneficial effect of aspirin, although this negative result might have been a consequence of this very low absolute risk of cardiovascular disease.

In the British Doctors' Trial, 500 mg of aspirin daily had no significant effect after 6 years on cardiovascular events, myocardial infarction or stroke (20); however, in the US Physicians' Health Study, aspirin did reduce myocardial infarction by 44%, albeit with a slight increase in haemorrhagic stroke (19).

Myocardial infarction occurred in 231/10 763 (2.0%) of the cohort on placebo therapy, but in only 128/10 750 (1.2%) on aspirin therapy (19). Of the 22 071 male physicians studied, 533 had diabetes. In these, the risk reductions for myocardial infarction were similar to those for the entire cohort, consistent with a beneficial effect of aspirin on diabetic as well as non-diabetic men. There was no difference in risk reduction in diabetic and non-diabetic men, indicating that there was no additional benefit of aspirin in diabetic patients, although the study was not powered to make this comparison (19). In the HOT study there was a significant reduction of 2.5 myocardial infarctions per 1000 patient years of aspirin treatment in patients with diabetes given aspirin as primary prevention (12).

Oxidative modification of low-density lipoprotein (LDL) is an important step in the development of atherosclerosis, and antioxidants such as vitamin E have been shown to slow atherosclerosis (15). In a recent study, vitamin E had no apparent effect on cardiovascular disease (16).

Summary

In summary, primary prevention trials using aspirin have been limited and focused on groups with a very low risk of the disease. The lack of a clear advantage for aspirin might be due to the limited power of the studies. In broad terms, there was some evidence for an effect of aspirin, in diabetic as in non-diabetic patients, but the results did not provide sufficiently clear evidence to use aspirin as a primary prevention therapy in my opinion.

Secondary prevention cardiac events

The potential benefit of aspirin increases along with the risk of cardiovascular disease in the cohort under study. Thus, in a subgroup analysis of the US Physicians' Health Study, 333 men with chronic stable angina had a reduced risk of progression to myocardial infarction (19). There is little information regarding the impact of aspirin on the risk of progression to myocardial infarction in patients with diabetes. A subgroup analysis of the antiplatelet trial collaboration involving more than 4500 patients with diabetes suggested a benefit of antiplatelet therapy, which was similar in diabetic and non-diabetic patients (17). The Early Treatment Diabetic Retinopathy Study (ETDRS) also reported a beneficial effect of aspirin (in secondary end-points) (18); there was no effect on overall mortality but an 18% reduction in important cardiovascular events (just statistically significant) and a significant reduction in myocardial infarction. These differences resulting from aspirin treatment were not so striking at 7 year review (20).

Cerebrovascular events

There are no studies of patients with diabetes using aspirin to prevent cerebrovascular disease although in non-diabetics, risk of recurrent transient ischaemic attack or stroke is reduced and suggests a 25% reduction in non-fatal stroke.

Microvascular disease

There is only one study of aspirin in the prevention of microvascular disease in diabetes, which showed no beneficial effect (18). The ETDRS used 3711 patients with a mixture of type 1 and type 2 diabetes, nearly half of whom had cardiovascular disease; patients were given aspirin 650 mg over a 5 year period. There were 289 myocardial infarctions (a secondary end-point) in the aspirin group (16%) and 336 in the placebo group (18%, $p = 0.038$), but no difference in mortality. Importantly, there was no increased risk of microvascular complications in patients taking aspirin.

Dosage of aspirin

The platelet release reaction is exquisitely sensitive to inhibition by aspirin. In this regard, it has been shown that a dose as low as 75 mg of enteric-coated aspirin is just as effective as higher doses of either plain or enteric-coated aspirin in inhibiting thromboxane synthesis.

Summary and recommendations

The American Diabetes Association advise aspirin therapy as a secondary prevention strategy in diabetic men and women who have evidence of large vessel disease. This includes diabetic men and women with a history of myocardial infarction, vascular bypass procedure, stroke or transient ischaemic attack, peripheral vascular disease, claudication, and/or angina. In addition, they advise aspirin therapy as a primary prevention strategy in high-risk men and women with diabetes, in particular in those with a combination of cardiovascular risk factors.

FUTURE MANAGEMENT STRATEGY

The goals of management of diabetes are, at first glance, easily established. We know that the excess mortality associated with diabetes is due to macrovascular disease, whilst the morbidity due to diabetes results from both macrovascular and microvascular disease. Since the aim of therapy is to normalize excess mortality and morbidity, it follows that therapy should be aimed at risk factors for both macrovascular and microvascular disease. Risk factors for macrovascular disease are known to include hypertension, hypercholesterolaemia, obesity, smoking and hyperglycaemia, and those for microvascular disease include hyperglycaemia and hypertension. Since many type 2 diabetic patients have a combination of these risk factors, it is likely that patients will require a combination of drugs to manage their diabetes.

The management of type 2 diabetes may, therefore, be complex and the physician will have to consider the interplay between the psychosocial background, various risk factors and several therapeutic agents before deciding on a regimen appropriate for any given individual. In practical terms, the therapy of type 2 diabetes involves a trade-off between what is desirable and what is practically possible. UKPDS hints at a new era in the management of type 2 diabetes. New drugs promise a substantial expansion of the current, rather limited, therapeutic options. Finally, an increasing appreciation of the importance of patient education suggests that these scientific advances can be transformed into real benefit for the patient.

REFERENCES

1. Stamler J, Vaccaro O, Neaton JD, Wentworth D: Diabetes, other risk factors, and 12 yr cardiovascular mortality for men screened in the Multiple Risk factor Intervention Trial. *Diabet Care* 16:434–444, 1993.
2. Diabetes Control and Complications Trial Research Group: The effect of intensive treatment of diabetes on the development and progression of long term complications in insulin-dependant diabetes mellitus. *N Engl J Med* 329:977–986, 1993.
3. Klein R: Hyperglycaemia and microvascular and macrovascular disease in diabetes. *Diabet Care* 18:258–271, 1995.
4. UK Prospective Diabetes Study Group: Intensive blood glucose control with sulphonylureas or insulin compared with conventional treatment and risk of complications in patients with type 2 diabetes (UKPDS 33). *Lancet* 352:837–853, 1998.
5. UK Prospective Diabetes Study Group: Effect of Intensive blood glucose control with metformin on complications in overweight patients with type 2 diabetes. (UKPDS: 34). *Lancet* 352:854–865, 1998.
6. UK Prospective Diabetes Study Group. Tight blood pressure control and risk of macrovascular and microvascular complications in type 2 diabetes (UKPDS 38. *BMJ* 317:703–713, 1998.
7. UK Prospective Diabetes Study Group: Efficacy of atenolol and captopril in reducing risk of macrovascular and microvascular complications in type 2 diabetes: UKPDS 39. *Br Med J* 317:713–720, 1998.
8. Pyorala K, Pedersen TR, Kjekshus J. Faergeman O, Olsson AG, Thorgeirsson G and the Scandinavian Simvastatin Survival Study (4S) Group: Cholesterol lowering with Simvastatin improves prognosis of diabetic patients with coronary heart disease. *Diabet Care* 20:(61)14–20, 1997.

9. Haffner SM, Lehto S, Ronnemaa T, Pyorala K, Laakso M: Mortality from coronary heart disease in subjects with type 2 diabetes and in non-diabetic subjects with and without prior myocardial infarction. *N Engl J Med* 339: 229–234, 1998.

10. Staessen JA, Fagard R, Thijs L *et al*: Randomised double blind comparison of placebo and active treatment for older patients with isolated systolic hypertension. (SYS-EUR trial). *Lancet* 350: 757–764, 1997.

11. Estacio RO, Jeffers BW, Miatt WR *et al*: The effect of nisoldipine as compared with enalapril on cardiovascular outcomes in patients with non-insulin-dependent diabetes and hypertension (ABCD trial). *N Engl J Med* 338: 645–652, 1998.

12. Hansson L, Zachetti A, Carruthers SG *et al*: Effects of intensive blood pressure lowering and low-dose aspirin in patients with hypertension: principal results of the hypertension optimal treatment (HOT) randomised trial. *Lancet* 351:1755–1762, 1998.

13. Gress TW, Nieto FJ, Sharar E *et al*: Hypertension and antihypertensive therapy as risk factors for type 2 diabetes mellitus. *N Engl J Med* 342: 905–912, 2000.

14. The Heart Outcomes Prevention Evaluation (HOPE) Study Investigators: Effect of ramipril on cardiovasular and microvascular outcomes in people with diabetes mellitus: results of the HOPE study and MICRO-HOPE substudy. *Lancet* 355: 253–259, 2000.

15. Braunwald E Shattock lecture — cardiovascular medicine at the turn of the millennium: triumphs, concerns, and opportunities. *N Engl J Med* 337:1360–1369, 1997.

16. The Heart Outcomes Prevention Evaluation (HOPE) Study Investigators: Vitamin E supplementation and cardiovascular events in high-risk patients. *Lancet* 342:154–160, 2000.

17. Antiplatelet Trialists' Collaboration: Collaborative overview of randomised trials of antiplatelet therapy I: prevention of death, myocardial infarction, and stroke by prolonged antiplatelet therapy in various categories of patients. *Br Med J* 308:71–72, 81–106, 1994.

18. ETDRS Investigators: Aspirin effects on mortality and morbidity in patients with diabetes mellitus: *J Am Med Assoc* 268:1292–1300, 1992.

19. Steering Committee of the Physicians' Health Study Research Group: Final report on the aspirin component of the ongoing Physicians' Health Study. *N Engl J Med* 321:129–135, 1989.

20. Patrono C: Aspirin as an antiplatelet drug. *N Engl J Med* 330:1287–1294, 1994

18

From Metabolic Disorder to Diabetic Complications

ANTONIO TIENGO[1], ANGELO AVOGARO[1],
ROBERTO TREVISAN[2] AND STEFANO DEL PRATO[1]

[1]Department of Clinical and Experimental Medicine, University of Padova, Italy
[2]Diabetes Section, Ospedali Riuniti di Bergamo, Italy

Diabetes is the most common metabolic disease and its frequency will increase with the characteristic of an epidemic. The major concern with respect to the disease remains the burden of chronic micro- and macroangiopathic complications. There is an overwhelming bulk of epidemiological and intervention data linking these complications to the metabolic alteration of diabetes mellitus and in particular to chronic hyperglycemia. None the less, the intimate mechanism(s) responsible for the structural modification leading to diabetic complication is only partially understood.

Both insulin deficiency (i.e. type 1 diabetes) and insulin resistance (i.e. type 2 diabetes) are characterized by an inappropriate increase of plasma glucose concentration, which is often associated with accelerated plasma free fatty acids (FFA) metabolism. Both glucose and FFA are major energetic substrates and energy homeostasis is highly regulated and conserved in living organisms.

It has been suggested that a moderate degree of hyperglycemia could provide the required drive to satisfy energy requirement in the face of defective insulin-mediated glucose utilization (1). Therefore, an initial increase in plasma glucose might be seen as an adaptive process, with negative effects developing whenever the process becomes a constant one. In this presentation we will revise the available information supporting this view, together with some of the possible mechanisms through which the chronic metabolic disturbance may predispose to long-term diabetic complications.

Diabetes in the New Millennium. Edited by U. Di Mario, F. Leonetti, G. Pugliese, P. Sbraccia and A. Signore.
© 2000 John Wiley & Sons, Ltd.

METABOLIC DISTURBANCES IN DIABETES MELLITUS

While in type 1 diabetes metabolic disturbance is the direct consequence of the lack of endogenous insulin secretion, a more complex pathogenetic process leads to hyperglycemia in type 2 diabetes, with insulin resistance playing a major role (2). When assessed by the euglycemic (~ 5 mmol/l) hyperinsulinemic (~ 250 pmol/l) clamp technique, a condition of insulin resistance was demonstrated both in type 1 (3) and type 2 diabetic patients (4). While in the former, the degree of insulin sensitivity appears to be a function of the glycemic control (3), in the latter insulin resistance is a more intrinsic defect. We have previously shown that the defect of insulin action involves several steps of intracellular glucose metabolism (4). In our hands, insulin sensitivity of type 2 diabetic patients with moderately severe fasting hyperglycemia (~ 10 mmol/l) was reduced by 54% compared with non-diabetic individuals. By means of a multiple tracer approach, we also measured glucose disposition through intracellular glucose metabolic pathways, showing that glycogen deposition was reduced by 75%, glycolytic flux by 36% and glucose oxidation by 57% (4). Conversely, non-oxidative glycolysis was significantly increased. An overall picture of the disposition of plasma glucose that is taken up by cells under conditions of euglycemia and physiologic hyperinsulinemia indicates that, from the quantitative standpoint, the impairment in glycogen synthesis is approximately two-fold greater than the impairment in total body glycolysis. On a percentage basis, glycogen synthesis and glycolysis accounted for 44% and 56%, respectively, of total body glucose uptake in control subjects, whereas this ratio was shifted to 26% and 74% in type 2 diabetic patients (4). Not only glucose metabolism but also insulin-mediated FFA metabolism is altered in the diabetic condition. At physiologic plasma insulin concentration, both concentration and turnover of plasma FFA rate remain significantly higher as compared with non-diabetic individuals (5).

The defect in insulin-mediated glucose uptake observed in type 2 diabetic patients under conditions of euglycemic (~ 5 mmol/l) hyperinsulinemia (~ 250 pmol/l), was completely normalized upon a 10 mmol/l elevation of plasma glucose concentration (~ 15 mmol/l), although this was not sufficient to correct intracellular glucose metabolism. In particular, glucose oxidation was still reduced as compared with normal individuals with a persistent excess of non-oxidative glycolysis (4). A similar capacity of hyperglycemia to ensure 'normal' glucose uptake in response to insulin stimulation has been observed in type 1 diabetic patients as well (3). These results are not surprising if one considers that tissue glucose uptake occurs via a facilitated transport system with prevailing plasma glucose and insulin concentrations as the main regulatory factors. Plasma glucose concentation influences its own utilization by a mass action effect which is independent of insulin, but the integrity of this process in the diabetic condition requires specific exploration. Definition of glucose-mediated glucose uptake is of importance, since it has been suggested that in normal man, as much as half of the decline in plasma glucose concentration following glucose administration is due to the mass effect of hyperglycemia (6), and that in pancreatectomized diabetic dogs, hyperglycemia provides a compensatory mechanism to maintain normal rates of glucose uptake in the presence of insulin deficiency (7). Therefore, we have examined the mass action effect of hyperglycemia by fixing the plasma insulin at the basal level in normal and diabetic individuals (8).

Our results demonstrate that the ability of hyperglycemia to promote whole-body glucose uptake is impaired in both type 1 and type 2 diabetic patients, a defect which is accounted for by a reduction in both glycogen deposition and glucose oxidation. Moreover, the reduction of plasma FFA in response to stepwise increase in plasma glucose concentration was blunted in diabetic patients, as compared with control individuals (8).

To summarize, the diabetic condition is associated with both insulin and glucose resistance, accounting for inappropriate elevation in plasma glucose and FFA concentration.

MAINTENANCE OF HYPERGLYCEMIA AS A PHYSIOLOGIC MECHANISM

Whether these defects are intrinsic to the diabetic condition or could be induced was then explored in normal individuals. We reasoned that a condition of insulin resistance is equivalent to a reduced generation of the biological hormone signal. Therefore, this condition can be recreated by reducing the insulin concentration of the cell it is exposed to. In order to accomplish that, a hyperglycemic ($+10$ mmol/l) clamp was carried out in normal individuals, while plasma insulin concentration was either maintained at fasting level or inhibited by somatostatin infusion. Under these conditions there was no difference in whole-body glucose uptake ($20\,\mu$mol/kg/min), but with endogenous insulin suppression a major impairment in the oxidative glycolytic flux became apparent, with a concomitant increase in both the non-oxidative glycolytic rate and the activity of the Cori cycle. The latter was also positively correlated with the rate of endogenous glucose production. It is of interest to note that the pattern of intracellular glucose disposition observed in normal individuals with basal hypoinsulinemia (i.e. reduced insulin signal at the cell level), was virtually identical to that described for type 2 diabetic patients studied at equivalent plasma glucose concentration and spontaneous plasma insulin levels (i.e. insulin resistance). We conclude that under conditions of hypoinsulinemia and/or insulin resistance, some degree of hyperglycemia is needed to ensure 'normal' glucose diposal, although is not sufficient to ensure its normal disposition among the different intracellular metabolic pathways.

Nonetheless, the disturbed glucose disposition favoring anaerobic glycolysis and the activation of the Cori cycle may contribute to glucose production and hyperglycemia.

This tentative conclusion is supported by results obtained in forearm studies carried out in hyperglycemic type 2 diabetic patients, as compared with euglycemic normal individuals (9). The difference in plasma glucose (10 vs. 4.7 mmol/l), exerted enough mass effect to ensure comparable glucose uptake by the forearm muscle in both diabetic and non-diabetic individuals. However, when the lactate–pyruvate interconversion rate was assessed, this was five-fold higher in diabetic individuals, suggesting a hampered pyruvate entry into Krebs cycle. The difference between the conversion from pyruvate to lactate and back provides an estimate of lactate production available for feeding the Cori cycle, and it was calculated to be twice as much in diabetic patients (6 vs. 3 μmol/l/min).

On the basis of these findings, we suggest that the maintenance of hyperglycemia may represent a physiological attempt to maintain an adequate glucose flux at the level of peripheral tissues under conditions of transient insulin resistance. An impairment of insulin action is indeed a feature of all stress conditions, such as infection, trauma, surgery, etc., all of which require an adequate energy supply. Under this condition the maintenance of adequate substrates (glucose, FFA) is crucial in order to meet the energy demand. However, for such a mechanism to be recognized as a physiologic one, an intrinsic regulatory activity must be demonstrated. In both *in vitro*, in cultured myotubes, and *ex vivo*, muscle acute hyperglycemia induces a significant increase in GLUT4 translocation (10), an effect which seems to be mediated by an increased activation of protein kinase C. However, this effect is limited over time, since prolonged hyperglycemia does induce insulin-resistance, as demonstrated in diabetes mellitus (8), suggesting that a potentially favorable effect may become a negative one if insulin sensitivity is not restored and hyperglycemia becomes constant. This effect is likely to be the result of the activation of the hexosamine pathway (12). In the normal condition, 2–3% of total glucose flux entering the cell is diverted from fructose-6-phosphate to glucosamine-6-phosphate via the glutamine-fructose-6-phosphate aminotransferase (GFAT), leading to the formation of end-products of the hexosamine pathways and glucosamine-*O*-linked protein. The activation of this pathway is regulated by the availability of fructose-6-phosphate and therefore, by glucose utilization. With the increase in glucose transport and phosphorylation, more fructose-6-phosphate is funneled into the hexosamine pathways, with end-products exerting a negative feedback on GLUT4 translocation (11). It has been recently shown that similar effects can be obtained as the result of increased fructose-6-phosphate pool due to inhibition of the glycolytic flux induced by FFA (12). The final result is the downregulation of glucose transport and insulin resistance. However, more recent results have suggested that the activation of this peculiar enzymatic pathway is associated with regulation of PK-C activity (13) and expression of TGFs and fibronectin, all potential mechanisms related to the development of the diabetic complication.

THE METABOLIC DISTURBANCE AND MECHANISM OF DIABETIC COMPLICATIONS

Abundant evidence shows that patients with type 1 diabetes or type 2 diabetes are at high risk for cardiovascular disorders: coronary heart disease, stroke, peripheral arterial disease, cardiomyopathy and congestive heart failure. Cardiovascular complications are now the leading cause of diabetes-related morbidity and mortality. Diabetes has long been recognized to be an independent risk factor for CVD. The adverse influence of diabetes extends to all components of the cardiovascular system: the microvasculature, the larger arteries and the heart, as well as the kidneys. There is a substantial evidence that vasodilation mediated by endothelium-derived nitric oxide is impaired in animal models of diabetes and in patients with both insulin-dependent and non-insulin-dependent diabetes mellitus. Nitric oxide possesses a variety of antiatherogenic properties, including inhibition of leukocyte adhesion, platelet aggregation and vascular smooth muscle proliferation. Thus, the pathogenesis of diabetic vascular disease may involve an abnormality in the bioavailability of endothelium-derived nitric oxide, contributing to the development and pathological consequences of atherosclerosis through a loss of these protective properties. Acute hyperglycemia attenuates endothelium-dependent vasodilatation in normal man, as assessed in response to metacholine stimulation (14). In type 2 diabetic individuals, chronic hyperglycemia is associated with impaired endothelium-dependent vasodilatation and insulin resistance (15), a condition which is likely to be worsened by the coexistence of the typical alteration of the metabolic syndrome. If accurate selection of type 2 diabetic patients is carried out in order to minimize the impact of factors known to affect *per se* vascular reactivity, endothelium-dependent and endothelium-independent vascular relaxation appears to be more conserved (16). Conversely, the coexistence of arterial hypertension is associated with a more dramatic defect in the nitroergic response induced by transient ischemia of the forearm.

Beside hyperglycemia, substrates other than glucose may play a negative role on endothelial function. Conditions of insulin resistance are characterized by inappropriate elevation of plasma FFA. The increase in the circulating levels of these substrates may affect insulin action by impairing the intrinsic ability of insulin to promote glucose utilization (expressed by the arteriovenous glucose difference), either by competition with glucose at the level of the oxidative pathway or by affecting glucose transport and phosphorylation.

Experimental data exist to show that oleic acid inhibits constitutive nitric oxide synthase (NOS) in cultured bovine pulmonary artery endothelial cells. These findings lend support to the hypothesis that increased FFA availability might affect insulin-mediated vasodilatation. When we exogenously infused lipid emulsion to increase their plasma FFA concentration to a value close to 2 mM, the percentage increase in forearm blood flow (FBF) in response to intra-arterial acetylcholine infusion was blunted. Moreover, there was no specific chain-length effect of FFA molecule, and these negative effects of increased plasma FFA levels on acetylcholine-mediated vasodilatation were evident, not only on a percentage basis but also in terms of absolute changes from baseline (17).

The negative impact of hyperglycemia is not limited to endothelial function in terms of nitric oxide release. Several studies have demonstrated that hyperglycemia could cause its adverse effects by activating diacylglycerol (DAG)-sensitive protein kinase C (PKC). PKC activity is increased in the retina, aorta, heart and renal glomeruli of diabetic rats, as well as in cultured vascular cells or tissues exposed to elevated levels of glucose. Literature findings have shown that PKC activation in monocytes may affect the steps involved in monocyte capture/tethering, rolling and transmigration. Thus, elevated plasma glucose concentration would favour early events of atherosclerotic lesion by stimulating PKC activity. In order to assess this hypothesis *in vivo*, we have determined the effect of hyperglycemia on PKC activity and on the distribution of Ca^{++} and phospholipid sensitive PKC isoforms in monocytes from type 2 diabetic patients. Moreover, in order to define whether these parameters were affected by hyperglycemia *per se* independent of diabetes, monocytes were harvested after normalization of plasma glucose concentration by means of insulin infusion. We found that: (a) membrane PKC activity is increased in monocytes from type 2 diabetic patients; (b) monocytes express the glucose-sensitive $PKC_{\beta 2}$ isoform, which is increased in diabetic patients; (c) in these individuals, the normalization of circulating plasma glucose by insulin infusion results in a slight reduction of $PKC_{\beta 2}$ isoform along with a significant reduction of PKC activity; (d) in normal subjects, an acute rise of plasma glucose increases PKC activity and membrane $\beta 2$ isoform (18). Therefore, these data indicate that PKC activation in type 2 diabetic patients is largely accounted for by hyperglycemia, and that the glucose-induced alterations in monocyte PKC activity may be relevant for the development of diabetic complications and of atherosclerosis. This view is further supported by the demonstration that PKC activity in fibroblasts from type 1 diabetic patients is markedly stimulated by high glucose and phorbol esters, as compared with cells derived from non-diabetic subjects. A more accurate analysis revealed that high glucose levels represented a specific challenge for the PKC-α isoform.

Previous reports have indicated that PKC activity may be modulated not only by DAG synthesis, but also via the activation of the hexosamine pathways (13). Therefore, as briefly discussed above, the hexosamine pathway is a legitimate candidate to link the effect of chronic hyperglycemia to the development of diabetic complications.

Preliminary studies from our laboratory indicate a direct relationship between GFAT expression in response to glucose and fibronectin secretion in fibroblasts from type 1 diabetic patients.

CONCLUSION

Diabetes mellitus is a condition characterized by peculiar abnormalities in the energy metabolism, with hyperglycemia as its hallmark. However, hyperglycemia may represent an attempt to compensate for impaired glucose utilization, a process which may be physiologically operative. However, the compensation effect must be short-lived in nature because the persistence of hyperglycemia may worsen insulin resistance and activate intracellular signals capable of triggering the transcription and synthesis of several factors involved in the pathogenesis and progression of micro- and macroangiopathy. Hyperglycemia is not the only substrate change in the diabetic individual as any alteration in glucose utilization seems to be associated with abnormalities in lipid (FFA) metabolism. The increase of circulating FFA is likely to worsen insulin resistance, but also to accelerate the negative impact of hyperglycemia on the risk of complications itself. The mechanism(s) translating the negative impact of metabolic disturbances onto the cellular damage are likely to represent a complex maze. The initial clues on how to escape from the maze are now being discovered.

REFERENCES

1. Best JD, Kahn SE, Ader M, Watanabe RM, Ni TC, Bergman RN: Role of glucose effectiveness in the determination of glucose tolerance. *Diabet Care* 19: 1018–1030, 1996.
2. De Fronzo RA, Bonadonna RC, Ferrannini E: Pathogenesis of NIDDM. In *International Textbook of Diabetes Mellitus*. Alberti KGMM, Keen H, De Fronzo RA, Zimmet P Eds, Wiley, Chichester, 1992, pp. 197–220.
3. Del Prato S, Nosadini R, Tiengo A *et al*: Insulin-mediated glucose disposal in type 1 diabetes: evidence for insulin resistance. *J Clin Endocrinol Metab* 57: 904–910, 1983.
4. Del Prato S, Bonadonna RC, Bonora E *et al*: Characterization of cellular defects of insulin action in type 2 (non-insulin-dependent) diabetes mellitus. *J Clin Invest* 91: 484–494, 1993.

5. Groop LC, Bonadonna RC, Del Prato S *et al*: Glucose and free-fatty acid metabolism in non-insulin-dependent diabetes: evidence for multiple insulin resistance. *J Clin Invest* 84: 205–213, 1989.

6. Ader M, Pacini G, Ysug YI, Bergman RN: Importance of glucose per se to intravenous glucose tolerance. Comparison of the minimal model prediction with direct measurements. *Diabetes* 34: 1092–1103, 1985.

7. Soskin S, Levine R: A relationship between the blood sugar and the rate of sugar utilization affecting theories of diabetes. *Am J Physiol* 120: 761–770, 1937.

8. Del Prato S, Matsuda M, Simonson DC *et al*: Studies on the mass action effect of glucose in NIDDM and IDDM: evidence for glucose resistance. *Diabetologia* 40: 687–697, 1997.

9. Avogaro A, Miola M, Valerio A *et al*: Intracellular lactate–pyruvate-interconversion rates are increased in muscle tissue of non-insulin dependent diabetic individuals. *J Clin Invest* 98: 108–115, 1996.

10. Galante P, Mosthaf L, Kellerer M *et al*: Acute hyperglycemia provides an insulin-independent inducer for GLUT4 translocation in C2C12 myotubes and rat skeletal muscle. *Diabetes* 44: 646–651, 1995.

11. McClain DA, Crook ED: Hexosamines and insulin resistance. *Diabetes* 45:1003–1009, 1996.

12. Hawkins M, Barzilai N, Liu R, Hu M, Chen W, Rossetti L: Role of the glucosamine pathway in fat-induced insulin resistance. *J Clin Invest* 99: 2173–2182, 1997.

13. Filippis A, Clark S, Proietto J: Increased flux through the hexosamine biosynthesis pathway inhibits glucose transport acutely by activation of protein kinase C. *Biochem J* 324: 981–985, 1997.

14. Williams SB, Goldfine AB, Timimi FK *et al*: Acute hyperglycemia attenuates endothelium-dependent vasodilation in humans *in vivo*. *Circulation* 97: 1675–1701, 1998.

15. Makimattila S , Virkamaki A, Groop P-H *et al*: Chronic hyperglycemia impairs endothelial function and insulin sensitivity via different mechanisms in insulin-dependent diabetes mellitus. *Circulation* 94: 1276–1282, 1996.

16. Avoaro A, Piarulli F, Valerio A *et al*: Forearm nitric oxide balance, vascular relaxation, and glucose metabolism in non-insulin dependent diabetic patients. *Diabetes* 41: 1040–1046, 1997.

17. Vigili De Kreutzenberg S, Crepaldi C, Marchetto S *et al*: Plasma free-fatty acids and endothelium-dependent vasodilation: effects of chain-length and cyclo-oxigenase inhibition. *J Clin Endocrinol Metab* 85: 793–798, 2000.

18. Cxeolotto G, Gallo A, Miola M *et al*: Protein kinase C is acutely regulated by plasma glucose concentration in human monocytes *in vivo*. *Diabetes* 48: 1316–1322, 1999.

19

Hyperglycemic Pseudohypoxia and Hypoxia in the Pathogenesis of Diabetic Complications

JOSEPH R. WILLIAMSON and YASUO IDO
Diabetes and Metabolism Unit, Boston University Medical Center Hospital,
Boston, MA, USA

The concept of 'hyperglycemic pseudohypoxia', i.e. cytosolic reductive stress caused by elevated glucose levels, and the hypothesis that this redox change could play an important role in the pathogenesis of diabetic complications was postulated in 1993 (1). Since that time a number of studies have been reported, some supporting the hypothesis, some not. In this same time frame, we have gained a better understanding of the potential impact of this redox change on energy metabolism and signaling pathways, as well as the caveats of experimental models and the limitations of pharmacological tools currently available for evaluating the hypothesis. Overall, subsequent testing of this hypothesis has provided support for an important role of cytosolic reductive stress in the pathogenesis of retinopathy, nephropathy, peripheral neuropathy and diabetic vascular dysfunction in general. On the other hand: (a) different (as yet unidentified) mechanisms may be more important than reductive stress in the development of autonomic neuropathy; and (b) osmotic stress appears to be of primary importance in cataractogenesis. In addition, the role of this 'pseudohypoxic' redox change in diabetic vascular dysfunction has led to new insights into redox signaling of increased blood flow evoked by physiological neural and muscle activity.

We will first review the background of the concept of 'pseudohypoxia' and discuss recent evidence linking this cytosolic redox change to other metabolic imbalances implicated in the pathogenesis of diabetic complications. We will

Diabetes in the New Millennium. Edited by U. Di Mario, F. Leonetti, G. Pugliese, P. Sbraccia and A. Signore.
© 2000 John Wiley & Sons, Ltd.

then consider a number of caveats in the interpretation of data reported by several investigators, which appear to be discordant with a role for this redox change in the pathogenesis of diabetic complications. For a current, more in-depth review of these issues, see (2).

BACKGROUND

Initial studies of possible mechanisms by which increased metabolism of glucose (in the cytoplasm) through the sorbitol pathway (Figure 19.1) causes complications of diabetes pointed to an important role for osmotic stress (resulting from accumulation of sorbitol) in cataractogenesis. In other tissues such as retina and nerve, however, sorbitol levels appeared to be insufficient to cause substantial osmotic stress. Considerable attention was focused on the possibility that competition between aldose reductase, glutathione reductase and nitric oxide synthase for the cofactor NADPH might impair the activity of glutathione reductase to maintain adequate levels of reduced glutathione to prevent oxidative stress. To this day, there is little if any credible evidence that NADPH levels are limiting for the activities of these enzymes. Our attention was drawn to the potential importance of the second step of the sorbitol pathway, since an increased rate of reduction of NAD^+ to NADH, coupled to oxidation of sorbitol to fructose, might increase the ratio of $free_{(f)}$ $cytosolic_{(c)}$ $NADH_{fc}/NAD_{fc}^+$ and associated metabolic imbalances, thereby mimicking the effects of the same redox change induced by hypoxia (Figure 19.2).

This hypothesis was tested by adding sorbitol at normal glucose levels to granulation tissue growing in skin chambers in non-diabetic rats (3,4). Blood flow was increased just as by addition of glucose and as observed in retina, peripheral nerve and kidney in rats with diabetes of short duration, in non-diabetic rats with acute hyperglycemia of only 5 hours duration, and by acute hypoxia. Furthermore, increased blood flow induced by sorbitol was prevented by an inhibitor of sorbitol dehydrogenase (SDI) but not by inhibitors of aldose

Sorbitol Pathway

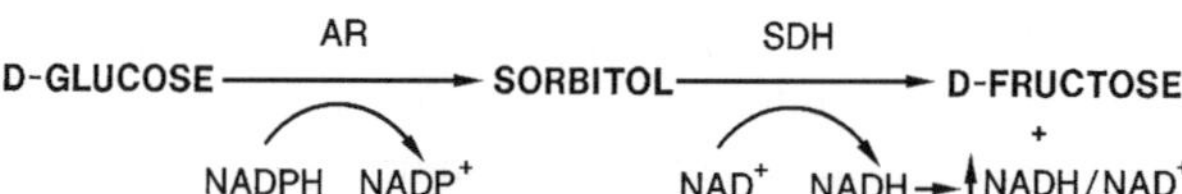

Figure 19.1. The sorbitol pathway. In the first step of this pathway, glucose is reduced to sorbitol coupled to oxidation of NADPH to $NADP^+$ by aldose reductase (AR). In the second step of the pathway sorbitol is oxidized to fructose coupled to reduction of NAD^+ to NADH by sorbitol dehydrogenase (SDH). Since the rate of this reaction is faster than NADH can be reoxidized to NAD^+, the ratio of reduced NADH to oxidized NAD^+ increases resulting in 'cytosolic reductive stress'

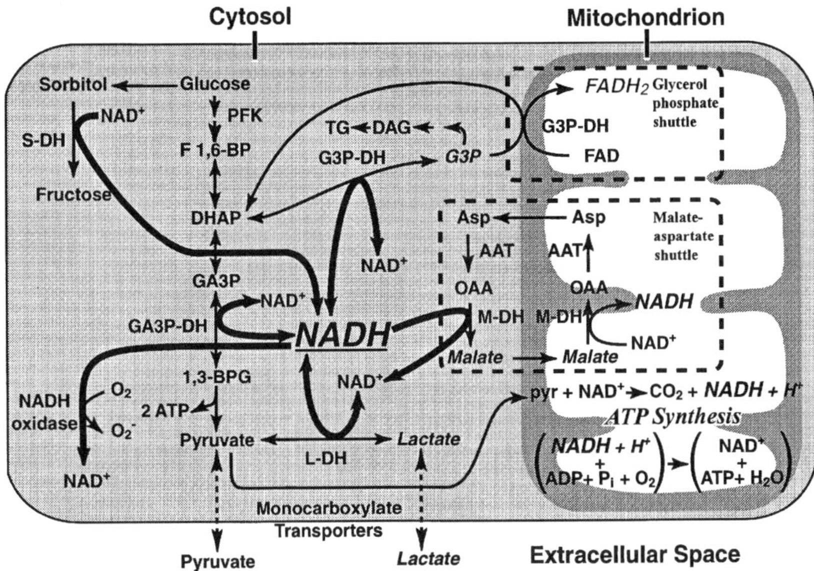

Figure 19.2. Linkage of redox cycling of free cytosolic$_{(fc)}$ $NAD_{fc}^+ \rightleftharpoons NADH_{fc}$ to electron transport, energy metabolism, and redox metabolite-coupled signaling pathways. Oxidation of substrates (e.g. sorbitol and glyceraldehyde 3-phosphate (GA3P) produced from glucose by glycolysis) by dehydrogenase (DH) enzymes is coupled to transfer of electrons to NAD_{fc}^+ which is reduced to $NADH_{fc}$. Electrons carried by $NADH_{fc}$ can be reoxidized by several different pathways under normoxic conditions. These include the malate–aspartate shuttle (via malate-DH, M-DH), the glycerol phosphate shuttle (via cytosolic glycerol 3-phosphate-DH (G3P-DH), lactate dehydrogenase (L-DH), and $NADH_{oxidase}$. As the cumulative rate of reduction of NAD^+_{fc} to $NADH_{fc}$ (e.g. by glycolysis and the sorbitol pathway) increases, the capacity of the electron shuttles to reoxidize $NADH_{fc}$ is exceeded and increasing amounts of $NADH_{fc}$ are reoxidized by signaling pathways that generate superoxide by $NADH_{oxidase}$ and *de novo* synthesis of diacylglycerol (DAG) and activation of protein kinase C. Acceptance of electrons from GA3P by NAD is limited by availability of NAD_{fc}^+ and the activity of GA3P-DH is impaired by the increased ratio of $NADH_{fc}/NAD_{fc}^+$, with the result that levels of GA3P, DHAP- and fructose 1,6-bisphosphate (F1,6-BP) are elevated. Increased levels of these triose phosphates (which are in equilibrium) provide higher levels of substrate to drive glycolysis. The elevated triose phosphate levels also, however, are substrate for formation of methylglyoxal, a highly reactive glycating agent

reductase (ARI), and by coadministration of pyruvate which is reduced to lactate coupled to oxidation NAD_{fc}^+ to $NADH_{fc}$ by lactate dehydrogenase (DH). Subsequent studies demonstrated that SDI as well as ARI prevented vascular and neural dysfunction manifested by impaired motor nerve conduction velocity (MNCV) in diabetic rats. In addition, an increase in $NADH_{fc}/NAD_{fc}^+$ in peripheral nerve of diabetic rats was prevented by ARI and SDI (1,2) without normalizing increases in free mitochondrial$_{(fm)}$ $NADH_{fm}/NAD_{fc}^+$ (5).

These observations indicate that elevated glucose levels increase the rate of transfer of electrons from sorbitol to NAD_{fc}^+ faster than $NADH_{fc}$ can be reoxidized. The resulting increased ratio of reduced $NADH_{fc}$ to oxidized NAD_{fc}^+ ($NADH_{fc}/NAD_{fc}^+$) constitutes 'cytosolic reductive stress', which can develop independent of an increase in $NADH_{mc}/NAD_{mc}^+$. Cytosolic reductive stress also develops in association with hypoxia as a consequence of an increase in $NADH_{mc}/NAD_{mc}^+$ which impairs transfer of electrons from $NADH_{fc}$ into mitochondria (by the glycerol phosphate and malate–aspartate electron shuttles) for oxidation by the electron transport chain.

The physiological importance of the redox state of $NADH_{fc}/NAD_{fc}^+$ is that this pyridine nucleotide couple is the major carrier of electrons from substrates for energy metabolism, i.e. for ATP synthesis. NAD_{fc}^+ is the initial acceptor of electrons (coupled to reduction to $NADH_{fc}$) from glucose-derived metabolites, i.e. glyceraldehyde 3-phosphate (GA3P) during glycolysis in the reaction catalyzed by GA3P-DH. Further metabolism of products of this reaction is coupled to ATP synthesis by substrate phosphorylation (SP) and production of pyruvate for ATP synthesis by mitochondrial oxidative phosphorylation (OP). ATP synthesis from glucose in the cytosol by SP and in mitochondria by OP depends on continuous redox cycling of $NAD_{fc}^+ \rightleftharpoons NADH_{fc}$. Under aerobic conditions $NADH_{fc}$ is reoxidized to NAD_{fc}^+ largely by lactate-DH and by the glycerol phosphate and malate–aspartate electron shuttles.

LINKS BETWEEN CYTOSOLIC REDUCTIVE STRESS, ENERGY METABOLISM, AND METABOLIC PATHWAYS IMPLICATED IN THE PATHOGENESIS OF DIABETIC COMPLICATIONS

Changes in the ratio of reduced to oxidized NAD ($NADH_{fc}/NAD_{fc}^+$), regardless of the cause, e.g. hypoxia or elevated glucose levels, impact on levels of reduced and oxidized substrates of numerous cytosolic dehydrogenase enzymes that utilize NAD as the cofactor for electron transfer reactions. As the ratio of $NADH_{fc}/NAD_{fc}^+$ increases to exceed the capacity of electron shuttles, more $NADH_{fc}$ is reoxidized by pathways that generate signaling molecules. Thus, an increase in $NADH_{fc}/NAD_{fc}^+$ favors reduction of dihydroxyacetone phosphate (DHAP) to glycerol 3-phosphate (G3P). This is the first step both for: (a) one pathway for *de novo* synthesis of diacylglycerol to activate protein kinase C; and (b) the glycerol phosphate shuttle. Recent studies have demonstrated that ARI block synthesis of diacylglycerol and activation of protein kinase C in glomeruli (6,7).

An increase in $NADH_{fc}/NAD_{fc}^+$ also increases the level of triose phosphates (GA3P, DHAP-dihydroxyacetone phosphate, and fructose 1,6-bisphosphate in equilibrium) which are substrates for GA3P-DH and precursors of methylglyoxal (a toxic highly reactive glycating agent). Statil, an inhibitor of aldose reductase, prevents accumulation of methylglyoxal in lens, whole blood and renal medulla (but not renal cortex) of diabetic rats (8).

To the extent that an increase in $NADH_{fc}/NAD_{fc}^{+}$ is associated with an increase in $NADH_{fc}$ (which is highly likely in view of the very low ratio of $NADH_{fc}/NAD_{fc}^{+}$ under physiological conditions), more $NADH_{fc}$ is available for $NADH_{oxidase}$ for reduction of oxygen to superoxide coupled to oxidation of $NADH_{fc}$ to NAD_{fc}^{+} (9). Thus, an increase in $NADH_{fc}/NAD_{fc}^{+}$ increases availability of substrates for synthesis of superoxide, diacylglycerol to activate protein kinase C, and methylglyoxal.

Several lines of evidence support a signaling cascade whereby an increase in superoxide increases intracellular calcium, which activates constitutive nitric oxide synthase to increase blood flow, as observed in non-diabetic rats with acute hyperglycemia and in rats with diabetes of short duration. Recent observations in the skin chamber granulation tissue model and in cultured cells support an important role for an increase in $NADH_{fc}/NAD_{fc}^{+}$ (induced by elevated levels of glucose or sorbitol) in mediating increased production of VEGF, which is prevented by SDI. In addition, increased blood flows induced by elevated levels of glucose or sorbitol are prevented by VEGF, antibodies (3,4).

CAVEATS IN ASSESSING THE ROLE OF HYPERGLYCEMIC PSEUDOHYPOXIA IN METABOLIC, VASCULAR, AND NEURAL DYSFUNCTION INDUCED BY DIABETES

Several investigators who have examined the role of sorbitol pathway-mediated cytosolic reductive stress in the pathogenesis of diabetic complications have challenged the concept of 'hyperglycemic pseudohypoxia' as well as its putative role in diabetic complications. In reviewing these studies, however, it is evident that there are important caveats in interpreting the observations in all of these studies, which negate the credibility and validity of the authors' conclusions. The basic problem with many of these studies is that the investigators have not recognized that $NADH_{fc}/NAD_{fc}^{+}$ can be modulated, under the conditions of their experiments, independent of the sorbitol pathway. In view of the importance of these and other related issues, they are discussed below in some detail.

In vivo studies

A potent selective inhibitor of sorbitol-DH with pharmacokinetic properties like those of aldose reductase inhibitors would be an invaluable tool for evaluating the role of cytosolic reductive stress in mediating sorbitol pathway-induced complications of diabetes. Unfortunately, the only inhibitor available to date has a very short plasma half-life (less than 1 hour vs. 6–10 hours for three different aldose reductase inhibitors—zopolrestat, sorbinil and WAY-121509). In addition, while neither ARI or SDI affect tissue glucose levels (substrate for aldose reductase), elevated sorbitol levels in diabetic rats are normalized by ARI, whereas they are further increased by SDI. In our studies, and in the report by Cameron *et al* (10), SDI increase sciatic nerve sorbitol levels ~10-fold in non-diabetic rats to equal levels in diabetic rats and increase sorbitol levels another ~four-fold in diabetic rats. Thus, this sorbitol-DH inhibitor is a double-edged sword. If SDI levels fall to concentrations that do not completely inhibit sorbitol-DH, the 10-fold higher sorbitol levels in non-diabetic rats can be rapidly oxidized to fructose (even transiently), just as in diabetic rats. And in diabetic rats the four-fold higher levels of sorbitol induced by inhibitory levels of SDI may transiently drive reduction of NAD_c^+ to NADH at an even higher rate than in untreated diabetics when SDI levels fall. The cytosolic redox change resulting from these brief periods of increased flux of sorbitol to fructose is comparable to transient hypoxia. In this regard, it is noteworthy that even brief periods of moderate hypoxia once or twice daily for only 1 or 2 hours significantly increase proliferation of cultured endothelial cells and reduce structural vascular resistance of chick retinal vessels almost as effectively as continuous hypoxia (11).

These considerations explain the paradoxical observations in our initial studies with SDI, in which the inhibitor attenuated vascular dysfunction and impaired motor nerve conduction velocity (MNCV) in diabetic rats, but caused slight impairment of MNCV in control rats (12). When the dose of the inhibitor was increased in subsequent studies, no adverse effects were observed in control rats and the inhibitor prevented impaired MNCV (and associated increased $NADH_{fc}/NAD_{fc}^+$) and vascular dysfunction in diabetic rats as well as ARI.

Our experiments described above were designed to assess the efficacy of SDI to prevent vascular and neural dysfunction induced by diabetes, and the SDI was administered from the onset of diabetes. Cameron *et al* (10) recently compared the efficacy of an ARI vs. an SDI in reversing sciatic nerve vascular and electrophysiological dysfunction in diabetic rats. Both inhibitors were administered for 2 weeks following 6 weeks of untreated diabetes. Although the anticipated effects of both inhibitors were observed on sorbitol and fructose levels in nerve and other tissues, SDI failed to reverse neural dysfunction which was normalized by ARI. Significantly decreased 'endoneurial nutritive blood flow' in surgically exposed nerves in control rats given the SDI suggests that tissue SDI levels had fallen before nerve functional assessments were performed. The authors concluded that '. . . ARIs have beneficial actions on nerve perfusion and conduction in experimental diabetes, whereas SDIs lack these effects'.

The caveat to this study by Cameron *et al* is that, since sorbitol levels are normalized by ARI but are markedly increased by SDI, it is reasonable to predict that reversal of diabetes-induced dysfunction might take longer with an SDI than with an ARI. We tested this prediction in a protocol which duplicated that of Cameron *et al*. Two weeks after initiating treatment, improvement of nerve conduction was distinctly better with the ARI than with the SDI. After 4 weeks of treatment nerve conduction was normalized by the SDI as well as the ARI (13).

The recent observations of Obrosova *et al* (14), that the SDI was ineffective (an ARI was not examined) in preventing oxidation and metabolic imbalances in peripheral nerve of diabetic rats, may be explained by the low dose of the SDI administered (in view of the very short half-life, noted above).

Perhaps the most surprising paradoxical observation yet reported is that while treatment with the SDI prevents impaired MNCV in peripheral nerve in diabetic rats, the frequency of neuroaxonal dystrophic changes in autonomic nerves is markedly increased in the same animals (15) (the MNCV data were not included in the publication of the effects of the SDI on neuroaxonal dystrophic changes). On the other hand, this finding is consistent with evidence that autonomic and peripheral neuropathy differ in their pathogenesis.

Likewise, while SDI as well as ARI ameliorate vascular and electro-physiological dysfunction in diabetic rats, the SDI appears to slightly accelerate the rate of cataractogenesis in our studies and in those of Kador *et al* (16). Since osmotic stress and depletion of lens antioxidant osmolytes are generally believed to be much more important in cataractogenesis than in other complications of diabetes, the finding that SDI increased the rate of cataract formation in diabetic rats is not surprising. The additional observation of Kador *et al*, that SDI had no impact on cataractogenesis in galactose-fed rats, also is not surprising, since galactitol is a poor substrate for sorbitol-DH; thus the SDI would not be expected to impact significantly on polyol accumulation or on potential redox changes associated with oxidation of galactitol to tagatose by polyol-DH. On the other hand, we have recently demonstrated that lactate/pyruvate-$NADH_{fc}/NAD_{fc}^+$ ratios are increased in human erythrocytes exposed to elevated galactose levels and that this redox change is coupled to oxidation of galactose to galactonate by galactose-DH, which is inhibited by tolrestat (an ARI) (17). Thus tolrestat is not as specific an inhibitor of aldose reductase as generally believed.

In vitro studies with cultured cells and incubated tissues

Perhaps the most important caveat/limitation in the use of cultured cells and incubated tissues for assessing sorbitol pathway-induced cytosolic reductive stress and sequelae is the potential for development of marked increases in $NADH_{fc}/NAD_{fc}^+$ independent of glucose levels and/or increased sorbitol pathway metabolism. This is because lactate released from cells accumulates in the medium, causing the lactate/pyruvate ratio to increase. Since extracellular and intracellular lactate/pyruvate ratios are in near-equilibrium with each other and with intracellular $NADH_{fc}/NAD_{fc}^+$, an increase in the lactate/pyruvate ratio in the culture medium can mimic the effects of elevated glucose levels and hypoxia to increase $NADH_{fc}/NAD_{fc}^+$ and sequelae, including increased synthesis of diacylglycerol, activation of PKC, superoxide produc-tion, etc. In contrast, excess lactate produced by cells *in vivo* diffuses into plasma and is taken up by the liver and utilized for synthesis of glucose, which diffuses back into blood as substrate for use by the same cells.

Thus, if the culture medium is not changed often enough, extracellular lactate/pyruvate and intracellular free $NADH_{fc}/NAD_{fc}^+$ will increase in proportion to the initial glucose content of the medium and will be unaffected by ARI or SDI. In most published studies no data are provided for initial and/or final lactate and pyruvate levels in the cultured cells or medium; in the few studies in which such data are available, the values are highly unphysiological.

Thus, Thomas *et al* (18) and Gilles *et al.* (19) reported that elevated glucose levels did not increase lactate/pyruvate ($NADH_{fc}/NAD_{fc}^+$) ratios in cultured human retinal pigment epithelial (RPE) cells (18) or bovine retinal capillary endothelial cells (19). In the report by Thomas *et al*, RPE lactate/pyruvate ratios (134 and 114, in 5 mM and 30 mM glucose, respectively) were ~five-fold higher than values reported in most freshly isolated normal tissues and ~10-fold higher than ratios reported by Salceda *et al.* (20) in freshly isolated RPE from control rats and rats with diabetes of up to 3 weeks duration. Thomas *et al* reported that addition of 3 mM pyruvate to the medium had no effect on RPE lactate/pyruvate ratios assessed 6 hours later when pyruvate levels had fallen to 0.84 and 0.89 mM in media, with initial glucose concentrations of 5 and 20 mM glucose. To the extent that extracellular and intracellular levels of pyruvate and lactate were in near-equilibrium, intra- and extracellular lactate concentrations would be 90 to 100 mM, i.e. ~100 times normal plasma levels. At the other extreme, Gilles *et al* (19) reported that lactate/pyruvate ratios in the medium of capillary endothelial cells exposed to 5 and 30 mM glucose at room temperature were infinitesimal, i.e. 9.1×10^{-3} and 7.9×10^{-3}, respectively. The culture medium obtained from the manufacturer was specified to contain 1.2 mM pyruvate, but no lactate (normal plasma lactate and pyruvate levels are 1 and 0.1 mM, respectively); at the end of the incubation medium lactate was determined to be ~6 mM (6 × normal plasma levels), but pyruvate was not measured (personal communication from M. Gillies).

Xia *et al* (21) reported that sorbinil (an ARI) failed to prevent increased *de novo* synthesis of DAG (induced by elevated levels of glucose and galactose) by cultured bovine retinal capillary endothelial cells and rat aortic endothelial and smooth muscle cells; the effects of sorbinil on PKC activity were not reported. Lee *et al* (22) reported that sorbinil prevented increased sorbitol levels and impaired ouabain-sensitive Na^+, K^+-ATPase activity induced by elevated glucose levels in bovine retinal capillary endothelial cells, but did not prevent increased protein kinase C activity; DAG levels were not assessed. Lactate and pyruvate were not measured in either report. The discordant effects of sorbinil on Na^+, K^+-ATPase and PKC activity may be explained by evidence that sorbinil binds to bovine renal Na^+, K^+-ATPase and counteracts inhibition of Na^+, K^+-ATPase activity by fluorescein isothiocyanate, with a K_{50} of 3.9×10^{-6} (23); the concentration of sorbinil in the experiments of Lee *et al* was 10.0×10^{-6}.

In view of numerous reports that sorbinil and other ARI prevent a wide spectrum of retinal, neural, and renal changes *in vivo* in diabetic rats (1,2,24), the failure of sorbinil to prevent increased DAG synthesis and PKC activation by elevated glucose levels in these experiments implies either that: (a) increased DAG synthesis and PKC activation contribute little to the pathogenesis of vascular and neural changes induced by diabetes; or (b) the *in vitro* milieu of their cultured cells is unsuitable for investigating mechanisms that mediate increased DAG synthesis and PKC activation in diabetic animals. The latter view is supported by beneficial effects of protein kinase C inhibitors in diabetic animals (25,26) as well as studies demonstrating that ARI prevent increased DAG synthesis, activation of PKC and phospholipase A_2, and related changes induced by elevated glucose levels in cultured human and rat mesangial cells and rat glomerular explants (6,7,27).

Kuruvilla and Eichberg (28) recently reported that depletion (by elevated glucose levels) of phospholipid arachidonoyl-containing molecular species (ACMS) in a human Schwann cell line was prevented by an ARI (zopolrestat) but not the SDI. Interestingly, addition of sorbitol or mannitol to the media had no effect on ACMS, whereas addition of fructose mimicked the effects of glucose. These, and other observations in their studies, were considered to be consistent with a role for increased ROS and/or '. . . diminished availability of NADPH which may reduce . . . desaturase activities, thereby interfering with arachidonic acid formation, and . . . weakening antioxidant defenses by impairing . . . the NADPH-requiring glutathione cycle'. In any case, their findings are consistent with the important function of NADP as an electron carrier for reductive synthetic reactions vs. the function of NAD as the major carrier of electrons for energy metabolism.

Retinal incubations

Winkler *et al* (29) recently reported that their experiments and calculations did not support the concept of hyperglycemia-induced cytosolic reductive stress in incubated retinas from normal rats. These investigators measured retinal lactate, but not pyruvate, levels; thus retinal lactate/pyruvate-free $NADH_{fc}/NAD_{fc}^{+}$ ratios are unknown. They also asserted that if the 30 mM glucose-induced increase in retinal lactate/pyruvate ratio, reported by Van den Enden *et al* (30), was due to increased flux of glucose through the sorbitol pathway to fructose, then increases in retinal lactate levels should be equimolar to fructose accumulation. This unfounded assertion exemplifies the widespread naiveté among investigators regarding: (a) the redox metabolite indicator method for assessing free $NADH_{fc}/NAD_{fc}^{+}$ (31); (b) the marked quantitative differences between lactate/pyruvate and free $NADH_{fc}/NAD_{fc}^{+}$ ratios established by lactate-DH; and (c) pathways for reoxidation of $NADH_{fc}$ produced by the sorbitol pathway that are independent of lactate-DH, e.g. glycerolipid synthesis, the glycerol phosphate and malate–aspartate shuttles, and $NADH_{oxidase}$.

Nishikawa *et al* (32) recently reported that blocking increased mitochondrial superoxide production by cultured bovine aortic endothelial cells exposed to elevated glucose levels prevented sorbitol accumulation, activation of protein kinase C, formation of advanced glycation end-products, and NF–κB activation. Although the authors suggested that superoxide activated aldose reductase by overcoming inhibition of aldose reductase caused by increased nitric oxide production, this interpretation is inconsistent with evidence that nitric oxide upregulates aldose reductase in cultured cells (33). Most interesting, but not resolved by the experiments in this report, is the source of the electrons that fueled the increased superoxide production. The authors reported that rotenone, an inhibitor of mitochondrial complex I, had no effect on superoxide production, whereas inhibition of complex II was effective. Since electrons carried by mitochondrial$_{(m)}$ $NADH_m$ are donated to complex I (as noted by the authors), these observations indicate that the immediate source of electrons fueling superoxide production was not $NADH_m$ produced by oxidation of pyruvate in the tricarboxylic cycle (the source suggested by the authors) or from the malate–aspartate shuttle (which transports electrons from $NADH_{fc}$ to $NADH_m$). Their findings suggest that the major carrier of electrons that fueled superoxide production was $FADH_2$, which donates its electrons to complex II. The origin of the electrons carried by $FADH_2$ could be the glycerol phosphate shuttle, which transports electrons from $NADH_{fc}$ to mitochondrial FAD_m, reducing it to $FADH_2$. Thus the source of electrons that fueled superoxide could be the sorbitol pathway, since sorbitol accumulation was increased three-fold by elevated glucose levels.

Another observation of interest in these studies was the finding that inhibition of pyruvate transport into mitochondria (by a monocarboxylate transporter inhibitor) for oxidation the tricarboxylic acid cycle prevented superoxide production. Halestrap and Denton (34) reported that this same inhibitor (at a slightly lower concentration) markedly decreased the lactate/pyruvate ($NADH_{fc}/NAD_{fc}^+$) ratio in the perfused heart. Unfortunately, the effects of an aldose reductase inhibitor on superoxide formation were not examined, neither were lactate and pyruvate measurements reported in the publication by Nishikawa *et al* (32).

CONCLUSIONS

In conclusion, a growing body of evidence supports an important role for cytosolic reductive stress (apparently largely the consequence of increased flux of glucose via the sorbitol pathway) in the pathogenesis of many diabetic complications. Reports suggesting that cytosolic reductive stress is of no consequence appear to be based largely on observations in experimental models and/or under experimental conditions that may not be appropriate for testing the hypothesis. On the other hand, it is clear that multiple metabolic imbalances associated with the diabetic milieu, some of which are independent of cytosolic reductive stress, contribute to diabetic complications. The contributions of these metabolic imbalances appear to vary considerably in different tissues.

REFERENCES

1. Williamson JR, Chang K, Frangos M, Hasan KS, Ido Y, Kawamura T, Nyengaard JR, Van den Enden M, Kilo C, Tilton RG: Hyperglycemic pseudohypoxia and diabetic complications. *Diabetes* 42:801–813, 1993.
2. Williamson JR, Ido Y: The vascular cellular consequences of hyperglycemia. In *Diabetic Angiopathy*. Tooke JE (ed.) London: Chapman & Hall, pp. 161–185, 1999.
3. Tilton RG, Kawamura T, Chang KC *et al*: Vascular dysfunction induced by elevated glucose levels in rats is mediated by vascular endothelial growth factor. *J Clin Invest* 99:2192–2202, 1997.
4. Sherwood SJ, Tilton RG: Glucose-induced VEGF production by cultured human aortic smooth muscle cells is linked to increased sorbitol pathway activity. *Diabetes* 49:A277, 2000.
5. Ido Y, Ostrow E, Mylari BL, Oates PJ, Williamson JR: Decreased motor nerve conduction velocity (MNCV) in diabetic rats is linked to cytosolic reductive stress. *Diabetologia* 40 (Suppl 1):A33, 1997.
6. Keogh RJ, Dunlop ME, Larkins RG: Effect of inhibition of aldose reductase on glucose flux, diacylglycerol formation, protein kinase C, and phospholipase A_2 activation. *Metabolism* 46:41–47, 1997.
7. Ishii H, Tadda H, Isogai S: An aldose reductase inhibitor prevents glucose-induced increase in transforming growth factor-β and protein kinase C activity in cultured human mesangial cells. *Diabetologia* 41:362–364, 1998.
8. Phillips SA, Mirrlees D, Thornalley PJ: Modification of the glyoxalase system in streptozotocin-induced diabetic rats: effect of the aldose reductase inhibitor Statil. *Biochem Pharmacol* 46:805–811, 1993.
9. Wolin MS: Reactive oxygen species and vascular signal transduction mechanisms. *Microcirculation* 3:1–17, 1996.
10. Cameron NE, Cotter MA, Basso M, Hohman TC: Comparison of the effects of inhibitors of aldose reductase and sorbitol dehydrogenase on neurovascular function, nerve conduction and tissue polyol pathway metabolites in streptozotocin-diabetic rats. *Diabetologia* 40:271–281, 1997.
11. Adair TH, Gay WJ, Montani JP: Growth regulation of the vascular system: evidence for a metabolic hypothesis. *Am J Physiol* 259:R293–R404, 1990.
12. Tilton RG, Chang K, Nyengaard JR, Van den Enden M, Ido Y, Williamson JR: Inhibition of sorbitol dehydrogenase: effects on vascular and neural dysfunction in streptozocin-induced diabetic rats. *Diabetes* 44:234–242, 1995.
13. Ido Y, Chang K, Oates PJ, Mylari BL, Williamson JR: Inhibitors of sorbitol dehydrogenase (SDI) and aldose reductase (ARI) reverse impaired morator nerve conduction velocity (MNCV) in diabetic rats. *Diabetes* 48(Suppl 1):A150, 1999.
14. Obrosova IG, Fathallah L, Lang HJ, Greene DA: Evaluation of a sorbitol dehydrogenase inhibitor on diabetic peripheral nerve metabolism: a prevention study. *Diabetologia* 42:1187–1194, 1999.
15. Schmidt RE, Dorsey DA, Beaudet LN, Plurad SB, Williamson JR, Ido Y: Effects of sorbitol dehydrogenase inhibition on experimental diabetic autonomic neuropathy. *J Neuropathol Exp Neurol* 57:1175–1189, 1998.
16. Kador PF, Inoue J, Secchi EF *et al*: Effects of sorbitol dehydrogenase inhibition on sugar cataract formation in galactose-fed and diabetic rats. *Exp Eye Res* 67:203–208, 1998.

17. Berry GT, Wehrli S, Reynolds R *et al*: Elevation of erythrocyte redox potential linked to galactonate biosynthesis: elimination by tolrestat. *Metabolism* 47:1423–1428, 1998.

18. Thomas TP, Porcellati F, Kato K, Stevens MJ, Sherman WR, Greene DA: Effects of glucose on sorbitol pathway activation, cellular redox, and metabolism of myo-inositol, phosphoinositide, and diacylglycerol in cultured human retinal pigment epithelial cells. *J Clin Invest* 93:2718–2724, 1994.

19. Gillies MC, Su T, Stayt J, Simpson JM, Naidoo D, Salonikas C: Effect of high glucose on permeability of retinal capillary endothelium in vitro. *Invest Ophthalmol Vis Sci* 38:635–642, 1997.

20. Salceda R, Vilchis C, Coffe V, Hernández-Muñoz R: Changes in the redox state in the retina and brain during the onset of diabetes in rats. *Neurochem Res* 23:893–897, 1998.

21. Xia P, Inoguchi T, Kern TS, Engerman RL, Oates PJ, King GL: Characterization of the mechanism for the chronic activation of diacylglycerol-protein kinase C pathway in diabetes and hypergalactosemia. *Diabetes* 43:1122–1129, 1994.

22. Lee TS, MacGregor LC, Fluharty SJ, King GL: Differential regulation of protein kinase C and (Na,K)-adenosine triphosphatase activities by elevated glucose levels in retinal capillary endothelial cells. *J Clin Invest* 89:90–94, 1989.

23. Garner MH, Spector A: Stimulation of glucosylated lens epithelial Na,K-ATPase by an aldose reductase inhibitor. *Exp Eye Res* 44:339–345, 1987.

24. Cameron NE, Cotter MA: The relationship of vascular changes to metabolic factors in diabetes mellitus and their role in the development of peripheral nerve complications. *Diabet Metab Rev* 10:189–224, 1994.

25. Koya D, King GL: Protein kinase C activation and the development of diabetic complications. *Diabetes* 47:859–866, 1999.

26. Kowluru RA, Jirousek MR, Stramm L, Farid N, Engerman RL, Kern TS: Abnormalities of retinal metabolism in diabetes or experimental galactosemia. V. Relationship between protein kinase C and ATPases. *Diabetes* 47:464–469, 1998.

27. Derylo B, Babazono T, Glogowski E, Kapor-Drezgic J, Homan T, Whiteside C: High glucose-induced mesangial cell altered contractility: role of the polyol pathway. *Diabetologia* 41:507–515, 1998.

28. Kuruvilla, R., Eichberg, J: Depletion of phospholipid arachidonoyl-containing molecular species in a human Schwann cell line grown in elevated glucose and their restoration by an aldose reductase inhibitor. *J Neurochem* 71:775–783, 1998.

29. Winkler BS, Dang L, Malinoski C, Easter SS Jr: An assessment of rat photoreceptor sensitivy to mitochondrial blockade. *Invest Ophthalmol Vis Sci* 38:1569–1577, 1997.

30. Van den Enden MK, Nyengaard JR, Ostrow E, Burgan JH, Williamson JR: Elevated glucose levels increase retinal glycolysis and sorbitol pathway metabolism: implications for diabetic retinopathy. *Invest Ophthalmol Vis Sci* 36:1675–1685, 1995.

31. Williamson DH, Lund P, Krebs HA: The redox state of free nicotinamide-adenine dinucleotide in the cytoplasm and mitochondria of rat liver. *Biochem J* 103:514–527, 1967.

32. Nishikawa T, Edelestein D, Du XL, Yamagishi S, Matsumura T, Kaneda Y, Yorek MA, Beebe D, Oates PJ, Hammes HP, Giardina I, Brownlee M: Normalizing mitochondrial superoxide production blocks three pathways of hyperglycaemic damage. *Nature* 404:787–790, 2000.

33. Seo HG, Nishinaka T, Yabe-Nishimura C: Nitric oxide upregulates aldose reductase expression in rat vascular smooth muscle cells: a potential role for aldose reductase in vascular remodeling. *Mol Pharmacol* 57:709–717, 2000.

34. Halestrap AP, Denton RM: The specificity and metabolic implications of the inhibition of pyruvate transport in isolated mitochondira and intact tissue preparations by alpha-Cyano-4-hydroxycinnamate and related compounds *Biochem J* 148:97–106, 1975.

20

Hyperglycaemia and Endothelial Dysfunction

RICCARDO GIORGINO

Dipartimento dell'Emergenza e dei Trapianti di Organi,
Università degli Studi, Bari, Italy

Diabetes mellitus represents one of the most frequent causes of mortality and morbidity in contemporary society. In the Italian population, the prevalence of diabetes mellitus is estimated to be 3%, and probably rises to 6–10% if we include undiagnosed diabetic individuals, with type 2 diabetes being 20 times more prevalent than type 1 diabetes.

Diabetes mellitus is associated with several microvascular and macro-vascular complications that shorten life expectancy of diabetics by 5–10 years as compared to non-diabetic individuals. Macrovascular complications are responsible for more than 50% of total mortality from diabetes, but microvascular disease also contributes to increased morbidity and mortality. Diabetic macrovascular disease (coronary, CNS and peripheral artery disease) occurs as an early and rapidly evolving atherosclerotic process. Mortality from coronary artery disease is two- to six-fold higher in diabetic subjects compared to non-diabetic individuals. In addition, heart failure with impairment of diastolic function is quite common in diabetic patients and may represent a specific diabetes-related cardiomyopathy. Diabetic subjects are also more prone to cerebral stroke, which is two to three times more frequent than in non-diabetic subjects, and show an increased intima-media thickness of the common carotid artery, which is considered one of the earliest signs of atherosclerosis, even in the absence of clinical signs of cerebral artery disease (1). Peripheral artery disease is five to ten times more frequent in diabetic than in non-diabetic subjects and typically localizes to the arteries below the knee.

Diabetes in the New Millennium. Edited by U. Di Mario, F. Leonetti, G. Pugliese, P. Sbraccia and A. Signore.
© 2000 John Wiley & Sons, Ltd.

Microvascular disease in diabetes includes retinopathy, nephropathy and neuropathy. Diabetic retinopathy is the second cause of visual loss in the general population, after cataracts, and is responsible for 2–8% of blindness in the diabetic population. Renal failure from diabetic nephropathy represents the cause of death in 35–42% of type 1 diabetics and in 6–12% of type 2 diabetics. Proteinuria is found in about 20% of diabetic subjects. According to data obtained from a recent analysis carried out in the province of Turin, Italy, about 6% of type 2 diabetic subjects have clinical proteinuria and 21% have microalbuminuria (2). About one-third of subjects entering dialysis programs are diabetics, and these are mostly type 2 diabetics. In type 1 diabetic subjects, the prevalence and incidence of proteinuria increase with the duration of diabetes, even though two incidence peaks are observed 10 and 30 years, respectively, after the onset of the disease (3), suggesting the existence of a genetic susceptibility to develop renal alterations.

Increasing experimental evidence suggests that endothelial dysfunction plays a major role in the pathogenesis of vascular damage in diabetes mellitus. Under normal conditions, the endothelium accomplishes multiple functions (Table 20.1): (a) it regulates vascular tone through nitric oxide (NO) production, resulting in a vasodilator effect, and endothelin, a vasoconstrictor agent; (b) it inhibits platelet adhesion and aggregation through prostacyclin, NO and coagulation factors; (c) it participates in maintaining the structure and regulating the function of several tissues through the synthesis of extra-cellular matrix (ECM) proteins, growth factors and hormones; (d) it actively regulates the flux of molecules from the vascular lumen to the interstitial space by acting as a selective barrier. 'Endothelial dysfunction' is a condition in which one or more of these properties are found to be altered.

The functions of the endothelium can be studied *in vitro* by using cultured endothelial cells of human (HUVEC) or animal (BREC) origin. In humans *in vivo* these functions can be investigated by analysing the expression and the activity of the NOS enzyme, by measuring the plasma levels of specific proteins produced by the endothelium (endothelin, growth factors, von Willebrand factor (vWF), ECM proteins), and by evaluating *in vivo* the reactivity to pharmacological stimuli and the permeability to circulating molecules.

Table 20.1. Functions of the vascular endothelium

Regulation of vascular tone (nitric oxide and endothelin)
Inhibition of platelet adhesion and aggregation (prostacyclin, NO, coagulation factors)
Modulation of tissutal structure and function (ECM proteins, growth factors, hormones)
Regulation of the flux of molecules from the vascular lumen to the interstitium

It has been suggested that endothelial dysfunction may play a major role in the pathogenesis of both macrovascular and microvascular disease in diabetes mellitus (Table 20.2). Abnormalities of the permeability and vascular tone, quantitative and qualitative characteristics of ECM proteins, and factors regulating the thrombohaemostatic balance are frequently observed in the early phases of diabetic vascular disease, as demonstrated by studies performed in experimental animal models of diabetes and diabetic patients (4). Moreover, changes in NO release are detectable at various levels in diabetic patients. For example, the activity of the circulating NO synthase (c-NOS) is decreased in diabetic subjects (5). In addition, changes in NO and endothelin levels in the kidney contribute to the dysregulation of ECM synthesis seen in diabetes, as evidenced by recent studies on kidneys of diabetic rats. NOS alterations represent an important pathogenetic step in the development of endothelial dysfunction (6), even though little is known about the role of this enzymatic system in selected populations of diabetic subjects and in organ-specific vascular districts.

The cellular and molecular mechanisms leading to endothelial dysfunction in diabetes have not yet been clarified. Metabolic abnormalities, including hyperglycaemia and associated oxidative stress, are thought to play an important role in this process. High glucose concentrations reduce proliferation of cultured endothelial cells and promote the synthesis of altered ECM components, which appear to be abnormal both in quantity (i.e. increased glycoprotein content) and quality (i.e. relative increase in galactose and sialic acid residues). The induction of acute hyperglycaemia in normal subjects results in measurable changes of haemodynamic parameters (systolic and diastolic blood pressure, heart rate), blood viscosity and platelet aggregation, and this probably occurs through an increased production of free radicals (7). Hyperglycaemia is associated with increased oxidative stress in type 1 diabetic subjects (8), and this abnormality is thought to be a major mechanism leading to endothelial dysfunction in these subjects (9). In addition to hyperglycaemia, other environmental factors may contribute to endothelial damage in diabetes.

Table 20.2. Endothelial dysfunction in diabetes mellitus

Abnormal vascular tone
Reduced endothelium-dependent vasodilatation
Reduced barrier function
Increased thickness of the carotid intima-media
Changes in NOS expression and activity
Impaired synthesis of peptides, hormones and ECM proteins
Elevated homocysteine levels
Impaired pro-thrombotic:anti-thrombotic ratio
Higher free radical levels

Recent results obtained *in vivo* in humans suggest that poorly controlled diabetes is characterized by excessive NO production not fully explained by the degree of hyperglycaemia (10), raising the possibility that high ketone concentrations and acidosis may also promote NO synthesis independently of hyperglycaemia. Homocysteine, a compound derived from methionine metabolism, has recently gained considerable interest as a potential mediator of vascular damage. Elevated homocysteine plasma levels could lead to endothelial dysfunction through multiple potential mechanisms, which include formation of reactive molecular species (i.e. free radicals), neutralization of the vasodilator effects of NO and inhibition of t-PA binding to the vascular wall. Importantly, circulating homocysteine concentrations are higher in diabetic subjects compared to controls. Therefore, hyperglycaemia, poor metabolic control and high levels of homocysteine may act together to promote an increased oxidative stress of endothelial cells. The resulting activation of specific intracellular signalling pathways may lead to multiple abnormalities of endothelial function, including abnormal ECM synthesis, reduced barrier function, and impaired synthesis of vasoactive substances, peptides, and other endothelium-specific molecules.

While substantial evidence supports the concept that hyperglycaemia contributes to endothelial dysfunction, exposure to the diabetic milieu does not fully explain the variable incidence and progression of vascular complications in diabetic individuals, nor the coexistence of different microvascular and/or macrovascular complications in the same diabetic subject. The heterogeneous appearance of distinct vascular complications in the diabetic population underlines the importance of genetic factors that may confer a specific susceptibility to endothelial damage. Therefore, the molecular analysis of genes involved in the regulation of endothelial function may provide valuable information relevant to the understanding of how the vascular disease develops in diabetes mellitus. Candidate genes for this analysis include: (a) genes encoding proteins specifically synthesized by endothelial cells, such as endothelial nitric oxide synthase (ec-NOS) and endothelin-1 (Et-1); (b) genes involved in the protection from oxidative stress (receptor for oxidized LDL, ORL-1, NADH/NADPH oxidase, glutathione S-transferase (GST) isoforms); and (c) genes involved in homocysteine metabolism, such as the methylentetrahydrofolate reductase (MTHFR). Also, mutations and/or polymorphisms of genes involved in lipoprotein metabolism are known to be associated with increased cardiovascular risk. These include: (a) the Trp64Arg mutation of the β_3-adrenergic receptor gene, which is associated with central obesity, insulin resistance, early onset of type 2 diabetes, and altered lipid profile (11); (b) the *Hind*III polymorphism of the lipoprotein lipase (LPL) gene, which is associated with visceral fat accumulation, higher plasma levels of triglyceride, and lower HDL cholesterol (12); and (c) a polymorphism of the PAI-1 gene involving 4G/5G insertion/deletion, which is associated with high plasma levels of triglyceride and PAI-1 activity (13). Finally, the genetic susceptibility to endothelial and vascular damage may also involve proteins mediating the intracellular insulin and IGF-1 signalling cascade in the endothelial cell. Preliminary studies have demonstrated that the Gly972Arg mutation of the IRS-1 gene (i.e. the major substrate for both insulin and IGF-1 receptor tyrosine kinases) represents an independent risk factor for coronary artery disease, particularly in insulin-resistant subjects (14). The potential role of this IRS-1 mutation in the mechanisms leading to vascular damage has not been investigated. Since insulin can directly stimulate NO synthesis, structural changes of IRS-1 protein may possibly contribute to abnormalities in lipid profile and NO-mediated endothelial regulation.

The identification of genetic and environmental factors responsible for the development and evolution of the vascular complications in diabetes is instrumental in reducing the social costs due to this disease. The availability of reliable diagnostic tools for a timely recognition of diabetic individuals subject to vascular disease would be extremely useful, allowing early treatment strategies to be set up. Candidate markers of early vascular damage have been investigated in this context. The increased thickness of the carotid intima-media is associated with a higher risk of myocardial infarction and cerebral stroke in the general population, independently of other risk factors. Increased levels of prothrombotic factors (i.e. fibrinogen, PAI-1, vWF, factor VII) and changes of antithrombotic and fibrinolytic factors (i.e. t-PA, protein C, antithrombin III) have been associated with increased prevalence of atherosclerosis (15,16). Increased levels of vWF are also associated with an increased cardiovascular risk in patients with type 2 diabetes (17). Moreover, resistance to activated protein C, another important cardiovascular risk factor (18), is particularly frequent in type 1 diabetics (19) and in obese patients. In regard to nephropathy, increased vWF concentrations are associated with microvascular disease both in type 1 (6) and type 2 (20) diabetes. Increased vWF levels are found in type 2 diabetics with histopathologic signs of renal disease, but not in microalbuminuric subjects with normal glomerular structure (21). Other authors have shown that type 2 diabetic subjects have higher circulating levels of E-selectin and vascular cell adhesion molecule-1 (VCAM-1), which are both released by the damaged endothelium (22). As stated above, increased plasma levels of homocysteine may be a marker of vascular damage, and mild hyperomocysteinaemia seems to represents an independent risk factor for atherosclerosis in diabetic subjects (23).

Since the majority of diabetic patients are obese and the majority of fat people have insulin resistance and hyperinsulinaemia, it is to be expected that obesity and insulin resistance may have an independent deleterious effect on endothelial function. Relevant to this concept, endothelial dysfunction has been suggested to precede type 2 diabetes. Obesity is a well-known independent cardiovascular risk factor and can accelerate the early development of atherosclerosis. Indeed, patients with central obesity show a thickening of the intima-media of the common carotid artery (24). Patients with central obesity also have higher plasma levels of inflammatory proteins, such as ceruloplasmin (25) and C-reactive protein (De Pergola *et al* unpublished data), which are predictive of myocardial infarction. Homocysteine has been also suggested to link obesity and cardiovascular disease. In regard to endothelial function in obesity, plasma levels of vWF and PAI-1, which are mainly produced by endothelial cells, are significantly higher in obese patients as compared to normal weight individuals. The concentrations of these prothrombotic factors are independently correlated with abdominal fat, suggesting that visceral fat accumulation *per se* may induce endothelial dysfunction (26). PAI-1 is also produced by adipocytes and, notably, a direct relationship between PAI-1 plasma levels and body fat mass has been shown in obese women (27). Interestingly, the metabolic syndrome, which includes visceral obesity, is statistically associated with a polymorphism of PAI-1 gene involving 4G/5G insertion/deletion (28). In addition, the waist-to-hip ratio has been shown to represent an independent predictor of lower endothelium-dependent vaso-dilatation (29). Lastly, higher free radical plasma levels have been reported in non-diabetic obese compared to normal subjects, suggesting that obesity may facilitate oxidative stress (30).

Insulin resistance may also contribute to the thickening of the arterial wall in obese patients, independently of the extent of body fatness and the levels of glycaemia (31). A direct correlation between free radicals and plasma insulin levels has also been shown in non-diabetic obese patients independently of body mass index, suggesting that hyperinsulinaemia may induce oxidative stress and endothelial dysfunction in the absence of hyperglycaemia (31). Even though chronic hyperinsulinemia may be responsible for endothelial dysfunc-tion, the reverse possibility has also been suggested, i.e. that endothelial dysfunction may cause insulin resistance. This may occur as a consequence of reduced interaction between insulin and insulin receptors expressed in insulin-sensitive tissues, due to lower flow-dependent vasodilatation in the arteriolae and capillary bed (32).

Finally, it should emphasized that, independently of diabetes and insulin resistance, the family history of type 2 diabetes may amplify the unfavourable effects of the excess of body fat. In support of this concept, non-diabetic siblings of subjects with type 2 diabetes have been shown to be characterized by the thickening of the common carotid artery intima-media complex (33), higher plasma levels of factor VII, fibrinogen, fibrin D-dimers, and vWF (34,35), and lower sensitivity to the antithrombotic effect of activated protein C (De Pergola *et al*, unpublished observations).

Altogether, these studies are consistent with the hypothesis that, although hyperglycaemia exerts a pivotal role in the development and maintenance of endothelial dysfunction, multiple factors (i.e. obesity, insulin resistance, genes associated with family history of type 2 diabetes) present before the onset of hyperglycaemia in the prediabetic individual also contribute to trigger endothelial cell damage. These factors may be particularly important to induce endothelial dysfunction in subgroups of selected individuals at high risk of cardiovascular disease.

REFERENCES

1. Pujia A, Gnasso A, Irace C, Colonna A, Mattioli PL: Common carotid arterial wall thickness in NIDDM subjects. *Diabet Care* 17:1330–1336, 1994.
2. Bruno G, Cavallo Perin P, Bargero G, Borra M, Calvi V *et al*: Prevalence and risk factors for micro- and macroalbuminuria in an Italian population-based cohort of non-insulin-dependent diabetic subjects. *Diabet Care* 19:43–47, 1996.
3. Krolewski AS, Warram JH: Natural history of diabetic nephropathy. *Diabet Rev* 3:447–459, 1995.
4. Roy S, Maiello M, Lorenzi M: Increased expression of basement membrane collagen in human diabetic retinopathy. *J Clin Invest* 93:438–442, 1994.
5. Martina V, Bruno GA, Trucco F, Zumpano E, Tagliabue M *et al*: Platelet cNOS activity is reduced in patients with IDDM and NIDDM. *Thromb Haemost* 79:520–522, 1998.
6. Jensen T, Bjerre-Knudsen J, Feldt-Rasmussen B, Deckert T: Features of endothelial dysfunction in early diabetic nephropathy. *Lancet* 1(8636):461–463, 1989.
7. Giugliano D, Marfella R, Coppola L, Verrazzo G, Acampora R *et al*: Vascular effects of acute hyperglycemia in humans are reversed by L-arginine. Evidence for reduced availability of nitric oxide during hyperglycemia. *Circulation* 95:1783–1790, 1997.
8. Santini SA, Marra G, Giardina B, Cotroneo P, Mordente A *et al*: Defective plasma antioxidant defenses and enhanced susceptibility to lipid peroxidation in uncomplicated IDDM. *Diabetes* 46:1853–1858, 1997.
9. Baynes JW: Role of oxidative stress in development of complications in diabetes. *Diabetes* 40:405–412, 1991.
10. Avogaro A, Calò L, Piarulli F, Miola M, de Kreutzenberg S *et al*: Effect of acute ketosis on the endothelial function of type 1 diabetic patients. The role of nitric oxide. *Diabetes* 48:391–397, 1999.
11. Sakane N, Yoshida T, Umekawa T, Kondo M, Sakai Y *et al*: Beta 3-adrenergic-receptor polymorphism: a genetic marker for visceral fat obesity and the insulin resistance syndrome. *Diabetologia* 40:200–204, 1997.
12. Vohl MC, Lamarche B, Moorjani S, Prud'homme D, Nadeau A *et al*: The lipoprotein lipase HindIII polymorphism modulates plasma triglyceride levels in visceral obesity. *Arterioscler Thromb Vasc Biol* 15:714–720, 1995.
13. Ossei-Gerning N, Mansfield MW, Stickland MH, Wilson IJ, Grant PJ: Plasminogen activator inhibitor-1 promoter 4G/5G genotype and plasma levels in relation to a history of myocardial infarction in patients characterized by coronary angiography. *Arterioscler Thromb Vasc Biol* 17:33–37, 1997.
14. Baroni MG, D'Andrea MP, Montali A, Panitteri G, Campagna F *et al*: A common mutation in the insulin receptor substrate-1 gene is a genetic marker for the insulin resistance syndrome in patients with coronary artery disease. *Arterioscl Thromb Vasc Biol* 19:2975–2980, 1999.

15. Cortellaro M, Cofrancesco E, Boschetti C, Mussoni L, Donati MB *et al*: Increased fibrin turnover and and high PAI-1 activity as predictors of ischemic events in atherosclerotic patients: a case-control study. *Arterioscler Thromb* 13:1412–1417, 1993.

16. Thompson SG, Kienast J, Pyke SD, Haverkate F, van de Loo JC: Hemostatic factors and the risk of myocardial infarction or sudden death in patients with angina pectoris. *N Engl J Med* 332:635–641, 1995.

17. Stehouwer CD, Nauta JJ, Zeldenrust GC, Hackeng WH, Donker AJ *et al*: Urinary albumin excretion, cardiovascular disease, and endothelial dysfunction in non-insulin-dependent diabetes mellitus. *Lancet* 340:319–323, 1992.

18. Hainaut P, Azerad MA, Lehmann E, Schlit AF, Zech F *et al*: Prevalence of activated protein C resistance and analysis of clinical profile in thromboembolic patients. A Belgian prospective study. *J Intern Med* 241:427–433, 1997.

19. Gruden G, Olivetti C, Cavallo-Perin P, Bazzan M, Stella S *et al*: Activated protein C resistance in type 1 diabetes. *Diabet Care* 20:424–425, 1997.

20. Porta M, La Selva M, Molinatti PA: von Willebrand factor and endothelial abnormalities in diabetic microangiopathy. *Diabet Care* 14:167–172, 1991.

21. Fioretto P, Mauer M, Brocco E, Velussi M, Frigato F *et al*: Patterns of renal injury in NIDDM patients with microalbuminuria. *Diabetologia* 39:1569–1576, 1996.

22. Bannan S, Mansfield MW, Grant PJ: Soluble vascular cell adhesion molecule-1 and E-selectin levels in relation to vascular risk factors and to E-selectin genotype in the first degree relatives of NIDDM patients and in NIDDM patients. *Diabetologia* 41:460–466, 1998.

23. Hoogeveen EK, Kostense PJ, Beks PJ, Mackaay AJ, Jakobs C *et al*: Hyperhomocysteinemia is associated with an increased risk of cardiovascular disease, especially in non-insulin-dependent diabetes mellitus: a population-based study. *Arterioscler Thromb Vasc Biol* 18:133–138, 1998.

24. Ciccone M, Maiorano A, De Pergola G, Minenna A, Giorgino R, Rizzon P: Microcirculatory damage of common carotid artery wall in obese and non obese subjects. *Clin Hemorrheol Microcirc* 21:365–374, 2000.

25. Cignarelli M, De Pergola G, Picca G, Sciaraffia M, Pannacciuli N, Tarallo M, Laudadio E, Turrisi V, Giorgino R: Influence of obesity and body fat distribution on ceruloplasmin serum levels. *Int J Obesity* 20:809–813, 1996.

26. De Pergola G, De Mitrio V, Sciaraffia M, Pannacciulli N, Minenna N, Giorgino F, Petronelli M, Laudadio E, Giorgino R: Lower androgenicity is associated with higher plasma levels of pro-thrombotic factors irrespective of age, obesity, body fat distribution and related metabolic parameters in men. *Metabolism* 46:1287–1293, 1997.

27. De Mitrio V, De Pergola G, Vettor R, Marino R, Sciaraffia M, Pagano C, Scaraggi FA, Di Lorenzo L, Giorgino R: Plasma plasminogen activator inhibitor-1 (PAI-1) is associated with plasma leptin, irrespective of body mass index, body fat mass, and plasma insulin and metabolic parameters in premenopausal women. *Metabolism* 48:960–964, 1999.

28. Sartori MT, Vettor R, Saggiorato G, Lombardi AM, De Pergola G, Patrassi GM, Federspil G, Girolami A: Insulin resistance and PAI-1 levels in obesity: influence of the 4G/5G polymorphism of PAI-1. *Int J Obesity* 24 (Suppl 1):137, 2000.

29. Sarabi M, Millgard J, Lind L: Effects of age, gender and metabolic factors on endothelium-dependent vasodilation: a population-based study. *J Intern Med* 246:265–274, 1999.

30. Ciccone M, Pestrichella V, Rossi O, Maiorano A, Modugno M, De Pergola G, Giorgino R, Rizzon P: Oxidative stress is an early marker of endothelial disfunction? *Clin Hemorheol Microcirc* 21:341–342, 2000.
31. De Pergola G, Ciccone M, Pannacciulli N, Modugno M, Sciaraffia M, Minenna A, Rizzon P, Giorgino R: Lower insulin sensitivity as an independent risk factor for carotid wall thickening in normotensive nondiabetic non-smoker normal weight and obese premenopausal women. *Int J Obesity* (in press).
32. Pinkney JH, Stehouwer CDA, Coppack SW, Yudkin JS: Endothelial dysfunction: cause of the insulin resistance syndrome. *Diabetes* 46(Suppl 2):S9–S13, 1997.
33. De Pergola G, Sciaraffia M, Pannacciulli N, Minenna A, Laudadio E, Tarallo M, Giorgino R: Intima media thickness of common carotid artery is increased in siblings of NIDDM patients more than in subjects without family history of diabetes. *Diabetologia* 39(Suppl 1):181, 1996.
34. Mansfield MW, Heywood DM, Grant PJ: Circulating levels of factor VII, fibrinogen, and vonWillebrand factor and features of insulin resistance in first-degree relatives of patients with NIDDM. *Circulation* 94:2171–2176, 1996.
35. Fernandez-Castaner M, Camps I, Fernandez-Real JM, Domenech P, Martinez-Brotons F: Increased prothrombin fragment 1 + 2 and D-dimer in first-degree relatives of type 2 diabetic patients. *Acta Diabetol* 33:118–121, 1996.

21

Cell to Cell Communication Abnormalities in the Diabetic Milieu

FLAVIA PRICCI[1], GAETANO LETO[2], GIULIO ROMEO[2],
SAMANTHA CORDONE[2], ROSALBA CIPRIANI[2],
ANNARITA GABRIELE[2], CLAUDIA BRUFANI[2]
and UMBERTO DI MARIO[2]

[1]Laboratory of Metabolism and Pathological Biochemistry,
Istituto Superiore di Sanità, Rome, Italy;
[2]Division of Endocrinology, Department of Clinical Sciences,
"La Sapienza" University, Rome, Italy

Cell-to-cell communication in vessels occurs via both physical interaction (i.e. tight and gap junctions, and adhesion molecules) and/or the action of soluble mediators. This cross-talk is essential for the maintenance of structure and function of the whole vessel, thus responding to changes in its environment. Therefore, disruption of any of this may be responsible for vascular remodelling associated with microangiopathy/macroangiopathy (1).

Diabetic vascular disease is characterized by a process of dysregulated tissue remodeling leading to an increased deposition of extracellular matrix (ECM), due to an imbalance between its synthesis and degradation, associated with impaired vascular cell growth and turnover and inflow of non-resident vascular cells, particularly monocyte/macrophages and platelets. This phenomenon is accompanied by deranged hemodynamics, with increased blood flow in the early phase and reduced peripheral circulation in the advanced stages, increased permeability with leakage of circulating macromolecules and cells

Diabetes in the New Millennium. Edited by U. Di Mario, F. Leonetti, G. Pugliese, P. Sbraccia and A. Signore.
© 2000 John Wiley & Sons, Ltd.

within the vessel wall, and enhanced procoagulant activity and altered rheological properties, with increased thrombotic tendency.

At present, the diabetic milieu is considered to be capable of inducing an altered expression or peripheral action of autocrine/paracrine factors modulating tissue remodeling as well as hemodynamics, permeability and coagulation. This cascade of events is not specific for diabetic vascular disease, but represents the 'common final pathway' operating in other inflammatory or degenerative vascular diseases. However, it appears to be specifically triggered by hyperglycemia and the biochemical abnormalities associated with excess glucose disposal, including increased flux through the polyol and hexosamine pathways, protein kinase C (PKC) activation, non-enzymatic glycation and oxidative stress resulting from enzymatic and non-enzymatic glucose metabolism. Moreover, in view of the different susceptibility to vascular complications exhibited by diabetic patients independent of metabolic control, the pathogenetic sequence is thought to be modulated by environmental and, particularly, genetic factors, which either predispose to or protect from development of clinical manifestations of target organ disease (Figures 21.1 and 21.2).

STRUCTURAL ALTERATIONS

Extracellular matrix accumulation

Several experimental observations have indicated that various ECM components accumulate during vascular complications of diabetes and both

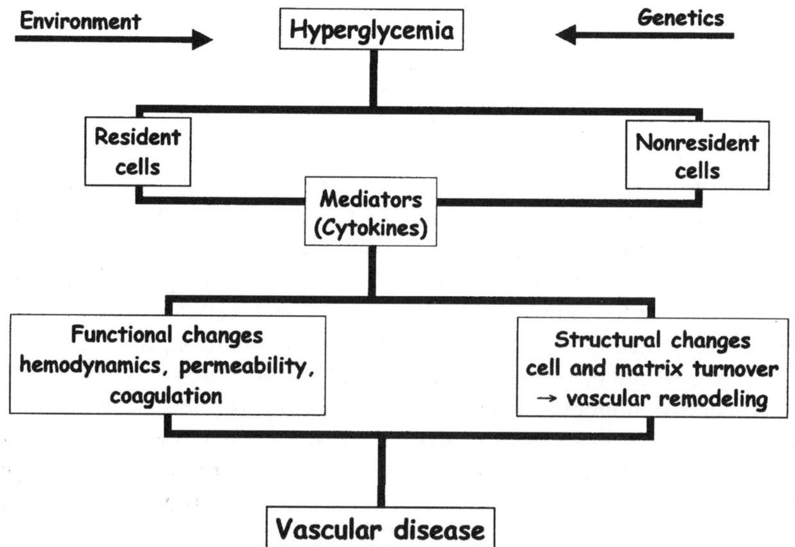

Figure 21.1. Pathogenetic cascade in diabetic vascular disease

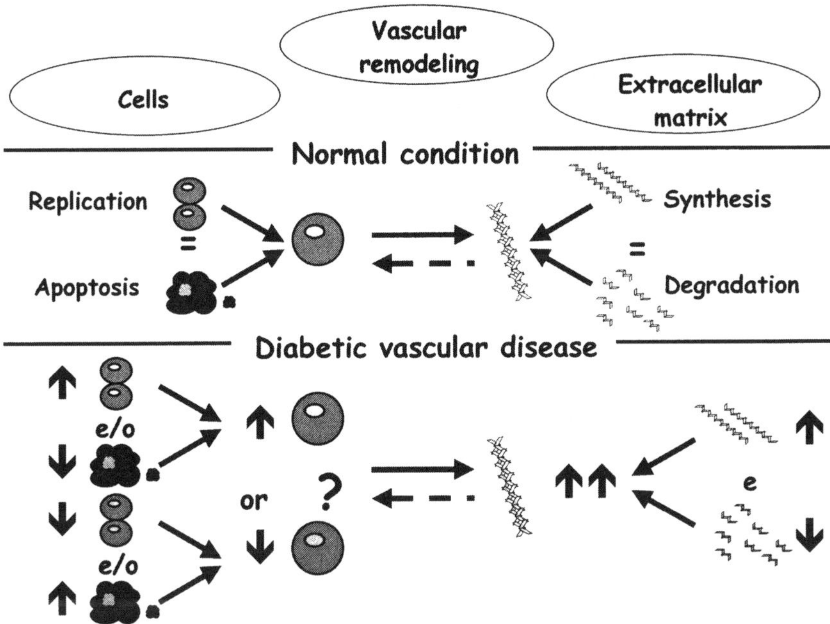

Figure 21.2 Vascular remodeling under normal conditions and in diabetic vascular disease

quantitative and qualitative changes contribute to this increased ECM deposition occurring in diabetes (2,3).

Increased matrix synthesis has been demonstrated in retinal or umbilical vein endothelial cells (4–6), retinal pericytes (7) and glomerular mesangial cells (8,9) cultured in high glucose by measuring either the levels of transcripts for the correspondent genes or the amounts of the various matrix components released in the medium. These changes have been demonstrated to persist after withdrawal of glucose supplementation of culture media of endothelial cells, indicating that these cells maintain, at least temporarily, a memory of the effects of glucose on transcription activity (5). At the retinal level, thickening of the basement membrane is a hallmark of diabetic retinopathy (10). It is related to an increased synthesis or reduced degradation of matrix components. In fact, overexpression of the ECM components fibronectin and collagen IV has been demonstrated in retinas from diabetic humans (11–12).

Within the glomerulus, ECM accumulation involves both the glomerular basement membrane and mesangial matrix, although only the increased deposition of the latter correlates with deterioration of renal function (13). In particular, type IV, V and VI collagen was demonstrated to increase with age and diabetes (14–16) and, in the more advanced stages of glomerular disease, type I collagen was also shown to be present in the diabetic lesions (15). The glomerular content of heparan sulphate proteoglycan was shown to be reduced, either absolutely or relatively to other matrix components (17–19), and also the sulphation of glycosaminoglycans was reported to be decreased (20). The accumulation of glomerular matrix has been referred to both increased production and reduced degradation in mesangial cells exposed to high glucose concentrations and/or in glomeruli isolated from diabetic rats (21–24).

Altered cell turnover

Delayed replication, disturbed cell cycle and accelerated death have been demonstrated in different cell culture systems in diabetic conditions (25,26).

In the retinal vasculature, endothelial cell (EC)–pericyte direct interaction occurs through gaps in the capillary basement membrane; at this level, EC are known to control differentiation and growth of pericytes by means of soluble factors such as PDGF and heterotypic cell contact (27). Diabetes and high glucose increase retinal EC and pericyte cell death by apoptosis, which heralds the formation of acellular capillaries (28). As a speculation, dying cells might affect viability of neighboring cells because of contact loss or activation of death membrane receptors such as Fas or TNF-R. Accelerated cell turnover might lead to altered vascular remodeling of retinal capillaries because of limited replicative potential of such cells.

With regard to macroangiophathy, abnormal vascular cell apoptosis and proliferation of VSMC, associated with increased adhesiveness of inflammatory cells, are all mechanisms that may contribute to plaque formation and progression (1).

In the kidney, studies in diabetic animals failed to detect an increase in cell proliferation at the glomerular level (23,29), despite evidence of transient (30) or persistent (31) increase of PCNA expression. Likewise, studies in cell culture systems showed that high glucose and glucose-modified proteins exert an inhibitory, rather than a stimulatory, effect on the replicative activity of mesangial cells. In diabetes, studies in experimental animals showed unchanged death rate at the glomerular level, with increased apoptosis in the tubuli (32,33), possibly due to epithelial cell injury induced by glycosuria and consequent glycogenesis.

MEDIATORS

Several studies in experimental animal models and cell culture systems have attempted to evaluate the role of various autocrine and paracrine factors in microvascular diabetic complications and indicate that several mediators may be implicated in the pathogenesis of diabetic vascular disease, although no single factor has been so far identified as that playing a causative role in the development of this complication.

These substances include the cytokines regulating the process of tissue remodeling, as well as vascular permeability, hemodynamics and coagulation (34) and also the adhesion molecules mediating cell-to-cell and cell-to-matrix interactions (35). In fact, the adhesion molecules are capable of influencing back the activity of the cells expressing them (the so called 'outside-in signaling', as opposed to the 'inside-out signaling' inherent to the classical adhesive function), due to their close association with cytoskeletal proteins, signaling molecules and growth factor receptors; as a consequence, the adhesion molecules participate in cell cycle control, thus regulating cell proliferation and death (36).

Various experimental evidence indicates that hyperglycemia could interfere with different mediators in *in vivo* and *in vitro* models of diabetic vascular disease, leading to both altered tissue remodeling and hemodynamic modifications.

Among the cytokines suspected of being implicated in the pathogenesis diabetic vasculopathy, transforming growth factor β (TGFβ), together with the renin–angiotensin system (RAS), and insulin-like growth factor (IGF)-1, either alone or as a component of the GH–IGF-1 axis, have received particular attention, due to the numerous observations indicating a key role for these peptides. Other growth factors, such as platelet-derived growth factor (PDGF), basic fibroblast growth factor (bFGF), epidermal growth factor (EGF) and vascular endothelial growth factor (VEGF), vasoactive substances, such as endothelin-1 (ET-1), nitric oxide (NO) and eicosanoids, and factors modulating coagulation and fibrinolysis, such as plasminogen activator inhibitor-1 (PAI-1), have also been implicated in the pathogenesis of the functional and structural changes observed in the diabetic kidney (Figure 21.3).

TGF-β

Recent experimental studies have now demonstrated that TGFβ is a key factor in tissue remodeling and in particular is involved in experimental models of diabetic kidney disease, as well as in human diabetic nephropathy and in fibrotic disorder of other organs.

In vitro, TGFβ has been demonstrated to upregulate various matrix proteins, including collagens, fibronectin, laminin, tenascin and proteoglycans and their integrin receptors in mesangial and other cell types, and to reduce ECM breakdown by decreasing MMP and increasing TIMP synthesis. It was also shown to induce mesangial cell hypertrophy and to exert a bimodal effect on cell cycle with prevailing inhibition at higher doses. These action are part of a complex response to injury targeted to obtain a rapid wound closure, thus preventing blood loss and sepsis (37,38). TGFβ is the major local effector of

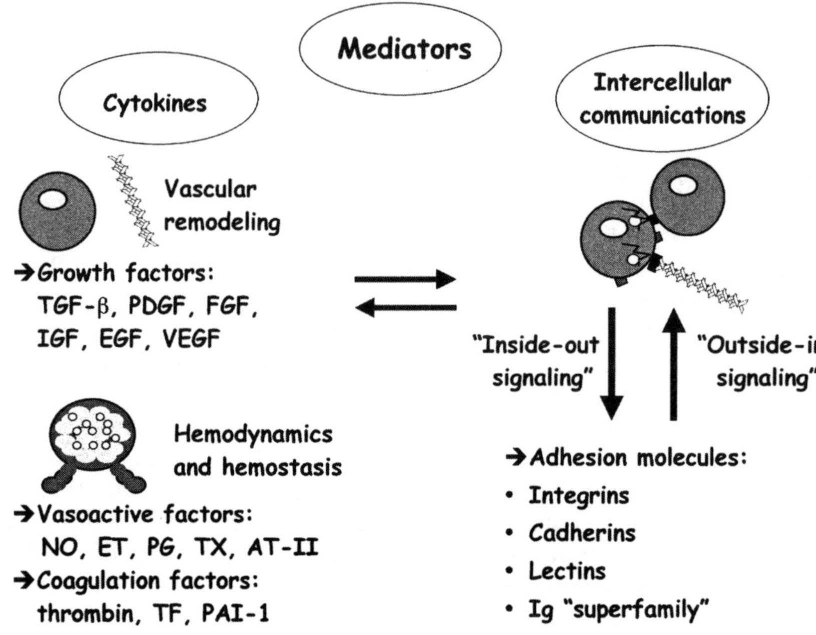

Figure 21.3.   Mediators of vascular remodeling

this response, which includes also (a) chemoattraction of monocyte/ macrophages and fibroblasts, to remove debris and initiate matrix deposition, respectively; (b) autoinduction of TGFβ, to amplify the biologic effect; (c) suppression of the pro-inflammatory action of interleukin-1, tumor necrosis factor α (TNFα) and NO, to favor repair; and (d) activation of PDGF, bFGF and ET-1, to promote cell proliferation and angiogenesis in association with synthesis of new matrix. In addition, TGFβ is capable of terminating the process upon completion of repair. However, in case of repeated or continuing injury, TGFβ activation may persist and promote progressive tissue fibrosis; this mechanism is now considered to be operating in various fibrotic disorders of the kidney and other organs, including diabetic glomerular disease (37,38) due to the fact that hyperglycemia could represent a chronic stimulus for persistent activation of TGFβ. *In vitro* experiments have confirmed this hypothesis, demonstrating that high glucose stimulates type I collagen synthesis in cultured mesangial cells, with a reduced effects in the presence of anti-TGFβ antibodies (39); moreover, in animal models of experimental diabetes, short-term hyperglycemia has been shown to stimulate renal TGFβ mRNA expression and neutralizing anti-TGFβ antibodies inhibited diabetes-induced matrix overexpression (40, 41).

Regarding to the mechanism which underlie these effects, due to the very early upregulation of TGFβ, glucose may directly activate transcription of

TGFβ, as suggested by the recent identification of a glucose-responsive element in the TGFβ promoter (42), and/or may indirectly stimulate this cytokine through PKC activation.

Another aspect is that TGFβ has significant interplay with the RAS, which represent the major systemic effector of the response to injury. By inducing vasoconstriction and stimulating the release of aldosterone, angiotensin II (Ang II) maintains blood pressure and intravascular volume despite blood loss from the site of injury. When RAS is activated, infusion of TGFβ has been shown to induce renal vasoconstriction. In addition, Ang II favors wound repair by stimulating TGFβ production. In recent human studies it has been demonstrated that the Ang II receptor blocker, losartan, significantly lowers circulating TGFβ1 levels (43). This effect has been observed also in cultured glomerular mesangial and endothelial cells, suggesting that the renal fibrogenic potential attributed to Ang II is actually mediated by TGFβ (44).

Moreover, TGFβ might interfere with the regulation of vascular tone, which is reduced in the early stage of diabetic vascular disease despite an upregulation of vasoconstrictors, by decreasing the release of intracellular calcium via the inositol 1,4,5-triphosphate (IP$_3$)-receptor, a key process common to vasoactive and mitogen factors, thus leading to their reduced effect. This process has been demonstrated in mesangial and vascular smooth muscle cells chronically treated with the cytokine, and these data are associated with a reduced protein and mRNA expression of type I IP$_3$R and an upregulation of TGFβ in the diabetic kidney (45).

IGF system

The studies investigating the IGF system in diabetes were based on the notion that IGF-1 is a progression factor for cells and stimulates matrix protein synthesis (46,47).

In diabetic nephropathy and in unilateral nephrectomy, an increased IGF-1 content has been demonstrated, whose origin is not known; this alteration is accompanied to several modifications of IGF receptors and IGF binding proteins (IGFBP) (48–50). It is of interest that transgenic mice for GH or GHRH show glomerulosclerosis similar to diabetic nephropathy and that transgenic mice for the GH variant, which function as an antagonist of GH, do not develop diabetic glomerular lesions (51–54). Moreover, the hemodynamic and hypertrophic alterations typical of diabetic nephropathy confirm the suspicion that the IGF system may be involved in the pathogenesis of diabetic vasculopathy. The role of IGF-1 in diabetic vascular disease is also suggested by several observations both *in vivo* and *in vitro*. In diabetic patients, GH deficiency and associated low IGF-1 levels can prevent or reverse proliferative retinopathy (55), and some authors have described high IGF-1 contents in vitreous and serum of patients with proliferative diabetic retinopathy (56,57).

Moreover, in retinal vessels, a single intravitreous injection of a large dose of hrIGF-1 produces microangiopathy that has a prolonged time of onset and remains stable 2 to 6 months after injection. Some aspects of this angiopathy resemble diabetic retinopathy, suggesting growth factor effects in the morphologic vascular changes of diabetes (58).

Finally, when examining the relevance of changes in the IGF system in the pathogenesis of diabetic complications, it should also be considered the potential role of variations in circulating insulin levels (and peripheral sensitivity) in relation to the type of diabetes and hypoglycemic treatment. For many decades, increased insulin levels, from either endogenous or exogenous sources, have been suspected of exerting an unfavorable effect on diabetic vascular disease (59), due the growth potential of this hormone, possibly mediated via the IGF-1 receptor. Recent findings in mesangial cell cultures have indicated that insulin potentiates the effects of Ang II on TGFβ production (60) and studies in vascular smooth muscle cells have shown that insulin increases PAI-1 production and reduces the fibrinolytic potential independently of glucose (61). In addition, reduced insulin levels may also produce negative effects by participating in the decreased activity of the NO-synthase enzyme, whose activity and vasodilating effect are stimulated by insulin (62). Recent findings on the relationship between IGF-1 and VEGF might account for the possible potentiating effect of increasing IGF-1 levels, due to rapid normalization of hyperglycemia on the worsening of diabetic retinopathy (63).

NO

Nitric oxide is synthesized by endothelial cells from arginine and acts as a potent vasodilator, thus promoting relaxation of neighboring smooth muscle cells. NO also inhibits platelet aggregation and adhesion and reduces smooth muscle and fibroblast mitogenesis. Based on these actions, it has been suggested that altered production of NO may be responsible for impaired vascular tone regulation and remodeling in diabetes.

Data on the synthesis and release of NO by cells and tissues in diabetes are very controversial, suggesting either NO or NOS activity impairment. Hyperglycemia and AGEs have been demonstrated to suppress endothelial constitutive NO-synthase (EcNOS) expression both *in vitro* and *in vivo* (64); AGEs are capable of quenching NO released in their vicinity and could regulate EcNOS through the receptor-mediated induction of PKC. Moreover, impaired NO-dependent glomerular cGMP generation in diabetic rats has been shown to be mediated by high levels of tromboxane A_2 and PKC, thus suggesting that these compounds may act by quenching NO production (65). In diabetic BB rats, the diminished endothelium-mediated relaxation might be due to quenching of NO by increased levels of superoxide anion, with formation of peroxynitrite, or decreased substrate availability (66,67). In fact, during acute hyperglycemia (68), EcNOs levels and activity appear to be increased without NO elevation, probably due to excess consumption of this compound by the increased amounts of superoxide anion (69), thus indicating the importance of the balance between the two free radicals (70).

VEGF

Vascular endothelial growth factor (VEGF) is a highly conserved protein which exists in four isoforms in the human (71); it is a potent angiogenetic factor and an endothelial cell-specific mitogen (72). Moreover, VEGF acts as a survival factor for newly formed retinal vessels (73) and its effects are exerted by binding to two receptors, Flt-1 and Flk-1.

The findings that VEGF is induced by hypoxia (74) and is produced by a number or retinal cells, i.e. EC, pericytes, pigment epithelial cells and Müller cells, have suggested a role for this factor in diabetes-induced vascular permeability and neovascularization in the retina.

Aiello *et al* (75) have found that VEGF levels were significantly increased in the vitreous of patients with active proliferative diabetic retinopathy (PDR), when compared to retinopathy-free diabetic individuals or patients with quiescent PDR. In a mouse model of neovascularization, VEGF inhibition achieved by VEGF-neutralizing chimeric proteins was able to abrogate retinal vessel proliferation (76). Interaction/synergism with other growth factors is possibly needed for VEGF-induced angiogenesis. For example, systemic administration of an IGF-R1 antagonist was shown to prevent retinal neovascularization in the mouse model of ischemia-induced proliferative retinopathy (63). Whereas the role of VEGF in the advanced, neovascular phase of DR is well established, some controversy remains regarding the contribution of VEGF to retinal permeability in early background DR.

Several investigations have pointed out an increase in VEGF expression in rat diabetic retinas at a time when vessel leaking is appreciated (77). By contrast, Gerhardinger *et al* (78) have not detected significant difference in VEGF synthesis or localization in the retina of patients with background DR, when compared to age- and sex-matched non-diabetic individuals.

While it is conceivable to make a case for VEGF inhibition in preventing retinal neovascularization, a number of trials is currently under way in which VEGF agonism is used to stimulate therapeutic angiogenesis (79). This applies to patients with coronary ischemia, severe limb ischemia and other instances.

With regard to diabetes, it is known that NOD mice show reduced hindlimb neovascularization after femoral artery ligation and that adenovirus-mediated VEGF gene transfer by intramuscular injection was able to ameliorate the defect in vascular collateralization (80).

Adhesion molecules

Alterations of numerous adhesion molecules have been described in different vascular areas, such as retinal capillaries. Blood–retinal barrier (BRB) impairment, whose integrity relies, at least in part, on communication between retinal endothelial cells, pericytes or mural cells and glial cells, causes increased vascular permeability, which is observed early in diabetic retinopathy (81) and may lead to macular edema.

Antonetti *et al* (82) have shown a decrease in occludin, a fundamental component of interendothelial tight junctions, in the retina of diabetic rats as well as in cultured retinal EC exposed to VEGF. Decrease in occludin protein was correlated with increased vascular permeability. By contrast, other investigations have suggested an increased expression of occludin, which might impact as well on BRB integrity (83).

Glial cell communication with both ECs and pericytes is a key factor in BRB integrity. In the course of diabetes, glial cell invasion in occluded, non-perfused vessels has been demonstrated (84) before occludin content increase (83).

Regarding the aorta and large vessels, the role of direct cell-to-cell interaction in diabetes-induced atherosclerosis remains unclear. Kuroki *et al* have shown decreased gap junction activity associated with increased levels of phosphory-lated connexin 43 in VSMC exposed to HG (85). Whether VSMC growth inhibition may be altered by connexin 43 change has still to be elucidated.

Moreover, endothelial cells incubated with sera of diabetic patients or HG show an increased adhesiveness to leukocyte under laminar flow, when compared to respective controls. This phenomenon was mediated by adhesion molecules ICAM-1 and VCAM-1 in a NF–κB-dependent manner (86). Since NF–κB activation was observed in VSMC cultured under HG (87) and in EC, VSMC and macrophages of carotid endoarterectomy specimens form non-diabetic patients (88), this pathway might operate in diabetic macroangiopathy as well.

PKC activation

The demonstration that PKC activation is capable of increasing vascular permeability, ECM synthesis, cytokine actions, smooth muscle cell contractility, leukocyte adhesion, cell growth and angiogenesis has prompted the hypothesis that this abnormality may play a central role in the pathogenesis of diabetic vascular complications (89). PKC is a family of serine and threonine kinases which acts as an intracellular signal transduction system for many cytokines and hormones and includes at least 11 isoforms that can be classified according to their structural differences into: conventional PKCs (α, $\beta1$, $\beta2$, γ), sensitive to both Ca^{2+} and diacylglycerol (DAG); new PKC (δ, ε, η, θ, μ), sensitive to DAG; and atypical PKCs (ζ, λ), sensitive to other phospholipids (91). The major fraction of cellular DAG is derived from the hydrolysis of polyphosphoinositides or phosphatidylcholine by phospholipase C or D, respectively. Increases in cellular DAG content have been demonstrated in many target tissues of the diabetic vascular complications, such as retina, aorta, heart and renal glomeruli from diabetic patients and animal models of diabetes (89–91). The mechanism by which PKC is activated by diabetes and hyperglycemia appears to be related to an increased *de novo* synthesis of DAG through the glycolytic pathway. The activation of PKC by hyperglycemia may be tissue-specific, since it was noted in the retina, aorta, heart and glomeruli but may not occur in the brain and peripheral nerves (92). Among the various PKC isoforms in vascular cells, PKCα, β1, β2 and isoforms appear to be preferentially activated in the retina, PKCα, β1, δ and ε isoforms in the glomerular cells and PKCβ, δ in aorta and heart of diabetic rats. Several biochemical and functional alterations have been related to the activation of the DAG–PKC pathway. An important biochemical change induced by DAG–PKC activation is the inhibition of Na$^+$-K$^+$-ATPase, an integral component of the sodium pump, which is involved in the maintenance of cellular integrity and functions such as cell contractility, growth and differentiation. Na$^+$-K$^+$-ATPase inhibition has been demonstrated in the vascular and neural tissues of diabetic patients and experimental diabetic animals (92,93).

Abnormalities in vascular blood flow and contractility have been found in many organs of diabetic patients or animals, including kidney, retina, peripheral arteries and microvessels of peripheral nerves (92). Multiple lines of evidence supported the hypothesis that the decrease in retinal blood flow, possibly due to vasocostriction induced by endothelin-1 (ET-1) (94), is linked to PKC activation. Injection of phorbol ester, a PKC agonist, into the retina decreased retinal blood flow, and the use of PKC inhibitors normalized it.

Abnormalities in hemodynamics (elevated renal glomerular filtration rate and modest increases in renal blood flow) have been clearly documented to precede diabetic nephropathy. Diabetic glomerular hyperfiltration is likely to be the result of an hyperglycemia-induced decrease in arteriolar resistance of the afferent arterioles, resulting in an increase of the glomerular filtration pressure. The glomerular hyperfiltration in diabetes could be due to an overproduction of vasodilatatory prostanoids, such as prostaglandin E$_2$ (PGE$_2$) and prostaglandin I$_2$ (PGI$_2$) through the activation of cytosolic phospholipase A$_2$ (cPLA$_2$) mediated by mitogen activated protein kinase (MAPK), which is dependent on diabetes-induced activation of PKC (95). An increase in the activity of nitric oxide (NO), a potent vasodilator, may also enhance glomerular filtration; NO production might be increased in diabetes through PKC-induced NO synthase (iNOS) over expression. PKC activation can directly increase the permeability of endothelial cells, probably by phosphorilating cytoskeletal proteins of intracellular junctions (92). Phorbol ester-induced increases in endothelial permeability may be regulated by PKCβ1 activation (92), which is consistent with the preferential activation of PKCβ

isoforms in diabetes. Vascular permeability and neovascularization could be regulated by PKC activation via the expression of growth factors, such as the VEGF, which is increased in ocular fluids from diabetic patients and has been implicated in the neovascularization process of PD (92). PKC activation can increase the vascular permeability inducing structural abnormalities, such as thickening of capillary basement membrane and ECM accumulation mediated by TGFβ over expression. Since the basement membrane is involved in many functions, such as in structural support, vascular permeability, cell adhesion, proliferation, differentiation and gene expression, alteration in its components may cause vascular dysfunctions observed in diabetes (92).

FUNCTIONAL ALTERATIONS

Vascular permeability

Vascular permeability has been shown to be increased in target tissues of diabetic complications early in the course of the disease. The increased permeability occurring at the retinal level may be involved in the pathogenesis of retinopathy by favoring the accumulation of circulating macromolecules and cells within the tissue, ultimately resulting in retinal injury via several mechanisms.

Several factors participate in the regulation of vascular permeability under normal conditions: the Starling forces, i.e. the hydrostatic pressure and plasma oncotic pressure and the intrinsic barrier properties of the vessel wall determines the extent (and route) of transport of large solutes. The basement membrane contributes significantly to the barrier properties of the capillary wall, influencing both the size and charge selectivity towards macromolecules. However, the main determinant of the selectivity properties of the vessel wall is the endothelium. The transport of solutes across the endothelium occurs via two sets of pores, corresponding to a large population of small pores, which accounts for diffusion of small molecules, and a small population of large pores, which would be the only route for the limited exchange of macromolecules. While the small pores likely represent the interendothelial junctions, the anatomical identity of the large pore pathway remains to be clarified, although a growing body of evidence indicates that it may correspond to the vesicular system (96).

Although mechanisms regulating endothelial permeability are not completely understood, studies using pro-inflammatory cytokines have shown that the increased permeability occurring in response to these agents can occur via retraction or contraction of endothelial cells, resulting in shape change and formation of interendothelial gaps. Passive retraction of endothelial cells is regulated by the phosphorylation of actin-linking molecules by protein kinase C (PKC) and tyrosine kinases (TKs), whereas active cell contraction is dependent on the presence of Ca^{2+} and ATP and the phosphorylation of myosin light chain (MLC) by MLC kinase.

Increased transcapillary passage of macromolecules has been demonstrated to occur early in the course of human diabetes and vascular permeability has been shown to be enhanced in experimental diabetic animals, especially in tissue targets of long-term complications, i.e. kidneys, eyes, peripheral nerves and large vessels (97–99). Changes in any of the factors modulating vascular permeability have been implicated in the pathogenesis of increased permeability induced by diabetes. Peripheral blood flow and glomerular filtration rate (GFR) were shown to be enhanced in parallel with vascular permeation of radiolabeled albumin in experimental diabetic animals (and in the new granulation tissue chamber model), and interventions capable of preventing the increased leakage of macromolecules induced by hyperglycemia were demonstrated to be effective also in normalizing hemodynamics. Moreover, cross-linking of both ECM and circulating proteins resulting from non-enzymatic glycation with AGE formation has been demonstrated to increase the fiber radius of matrix, as analyzed using the fiber matrix theory, and the filtering of proteins through the matrix, respectively (100,101). However, a pivotal role in vascular permeability alterations has been attributed to the endothelial dysfunction induced by diabetes.

In order to investigate this phenomenon, in our laboratory an *in vitro* system has been developed for the assessment of endothelial cell permeability, using monolayers of bovine retinal endothelial cells (BREC) cultured on permeable membranes. Among the putative mechanisms implicated in the endothelial injury induced by the diabetic milieu, our preliminary data indicate the presence of functional changes of the endothelial cell barrier, possibly triggered by PKC activation. Moreover, both non-enzymatic glycation and, to a lesser extent, polyol pathway activation, seem to participate in the pathogenesis of increased permeability. Both these alterations result in increased free radical generation and oxidative stress, possibly leading to PKC activation and producing cytoskeletal changes.

Hemocoagulation

An hypercoagulable state has been implicated in the pathogenesis of diabetic vascular disease (102,103), due to alterations in the processes regulating hemostasis-coagulation, fibrinolysis, anticoagulant pathways and platelet aggregation. These abnormalities in hemostasis point to an adaptive/maladaptive replicative and biosynthetic program of vascular cells that endures the pathological process triggered by metabolic perturbation.

Dysregulated coagulation in diabetic patients is manifested by elevated plasma levels of fibrinogen (104), an independent risk factor for cardiovascular disease (105,106), correlated to increased platelet aggregability and increased thrombin formation (107) characteristic of the prethrombotic state. Moreover, human data suggest that hyperglycemia may cause thrombin activation also by inducing oxidative stress, because thrombin activation can be counterbalanced by GSH (108). An association between initial hyperfibrinogenemia and the subsequent occurrence of macroangiopathy (109,110) and microangiopathy has been reported in diabetic patients. One study found a positive relationship between fibrinogen and albumin excretion rate in insulin-dependent patients with retinopathy, but not in those without this complication (111). Another important issue is the relationship between fibrinogen levels and hyperglycemia, as evidenced by the with HbA_{1c} (112), as well as with insulin resistance (113). Plasma levels of activated factor VII have been found to be significantly increased in patients with type 1 diabetes (114), and some investigators have produced evidence that activated factor VII is affected directly by blood glucose levels (115,116). A central role for unmodulated hemostasis in diabetes is further supported by reports of increased concentration of factor Xa and prothrombin reaction products F1 and F2 in the blood of diabetic patients (117,118).

Several studies on the fibrinolytic system in diabetic patients have reported a decrease in fibrinolytic activity (106), partly attributed to an increased resistance of glycated fibrin to degradation by plasmin (113,119). The tissue-plasminogen activator (tPA):plasminogen activator inhibitor-1 (PAI-1) ratio may play a central role in this regard. In fact, an imbalance between tPA and PAI-1 has been consistently reported as the result of increased PAI-1 levels and tPA, whose absolute levels are still controversial (120). The net effect of increased PAI-1 is that both type 1 and type 2 diabetics have depressed t-PA-related fibrinolysis (121). In this regard, many studies have demonstrated an increased activity of this inhibitor in type 2 diabetics (122), and results of quantitative studies suggest a relationship between blood concentration of PAI-1, body mass index and plasma insulin concentration (123,124). Decreased fibrinolysis in diabetic patients may also be caused by glycosylation of plasminogen, rendering it less susceptible to activation by tPA (125). Increased plasma or plaque PAI-1 levels might contribute to aggravate the vessel injury by further promotion of thrombosis and matrix deposition (126). Epidemiological studies showed that impaired fibrinolysis and increased level of PAI-1 correlated with degree of coronary heart disease and the incidence of acute coronary syndrome including unstable angina, Q- and non-Q wave myocardial infarction, and sudden cardiac death (127,128). A possible explanation of the relationship between level of PAI-1 (in blood and in coronary plaques) and the incidence of the acute coronary syndrome in type 2 diabetes is given by Burton (129). Plaque surface expression of tPA contributes to vascular smooth muscle migration, neointimalization and activation of matrix metalloproteases. The increased level of PAI-1 and the consequent inhibition of tPA in atheroma and in vessel walls appear likely to potentiate the formation of atheroma plaques with lipid-laden cores and thin fibrous cap. That these remarkably acellular plaques are particularly prone to rupture would account for the high incidence of ACS and the adverse response to angioplasty (124,130). Previous studies have found, in fact, that plaques associated with acute coronary syndrome differ strikingly from those typically associated with stable angina by being lipid-laden, remarkably acellular and covered by thin fibrous caps prone to rupture (131,132).

Furthermore, diabetes is associated with functional impairment of the thrombomodulin natural anticoagulant pathway, as indicated by decreased protein C concentration in type 1 diabetics with poor metabolic control (133). High levels of soluble thrombomodulin have been found in patients with microalbuminuria (134), and Seigneur (135) reported the highest levels in diabetic patients with proliferative retinopathy. The appearance of the soluble form in plasma implies not only endothelial cell injury but also a change in hemostasis towards coagulopathy (136). Several data show a decreased function of antithrombin III in diabetics, possibly due to non-enzymatic glycosylation of its active site, inducing an impaired formation of thrombin–antithrombin III complexes. This finding correlates with reduced antithrombin III activity and increased fibrinopeptide A levels in normal and diabetic patients (137,138). Tissue factor pathway inhibitor (TFPI) is the most recently discovered inhibitor of blood coagulation. When the coagulation system is activated and activated factor X (X_a) is formed, TFPI binds X_a and neutralizes its activity. Moreover, the complex of TFPI and X_a inhibits the activity of the complex of activated factor VII and tissue factor, which triggers the coagulation cascade. In diabetic patients, the levels of TFPI in plasma were significanly higher than those in control subjects (138), with a positive correlation with glycated hemoglobin levels in type 1 diabetes, thus suggesting that elevated TFPI may be related to hyperglycemia (139).

CONCLUSIONS

Diabetic vascular disease is linked to a dysregulated process of tissue remodeling, involving both the ECM and cell compartment and sustained by an abnormal pattern of expression or local action of autocrine and paracrine factors normally regulating tissue homeostasis. These structural features are preceded and accompanied by functional abnormalities involving vascular permeability, hemodynamics and coagulation. Although no single factor has been so far identified as that playing a causative role in the development of diabetic vascular disease, TGFβ, IGF-1, VEGF, NO and others have been demonstrated to be involved in these changes. Multiple metabolic dysfunctions associated with hyperglycemia have been implicated in triggering changes in the local expression or action of cytokines. Despite the fact that these changes are the same in all the tissues, the features of the various target tissue diseases are quite different. Proliferative changes prevail at the macrovascular level and occur only later in the microvasculature of the retina, following an initial phase of ischemia. On the contrary, accumulation of matrix components, with negligible alterations in the cell compartment, is the main abnormality observed in the kidney glomerulus.

Efforts devoted to the explanation of the mechanisms underlying diabetic vasculopathy are crucial for the amelioration of morbidity and mortality of diabetic patients, who are still affected by invalidating syndromes.

REFERENCES

1. Walsh K, Isner JM: Apoptosis in inflammatory-fibroproliferative disorders of the vessel wall. *Cardiovasc Res* 45:756–765, 2000.
2. Ziyadeh FN: The extracellular matrix in diabetic nephropathy. *Am J Kidney Dis* 22:736–744, 1993.
3. Furness PN: Extracellular matrix and the kidney. *J Clin Pathol* 49:355–359, 1996.
4. Cagliero E, Maiello M, Boeri D., Roy S, Lorenzi M: Increased expression of basement membrane components in human endothelial cells cultured in high glucose. *J Clin Invest* 82:735–738, 1988.
5. Roy S, Sala R, Cagliero E, Lorenzi M: Overexpression of fibronectin induced by diabetes or high glucose: phenomenon with a memory. *Proc Natl Acad Sci USA* 87:404–408, 1990.
6. Berman A, Ledbetter S: Regulation of type IV collagen mRNA in retinal capillary endothelial cells and pericytes by glucose levels and aldose reductase inhibitor sorbinil. *Diabetes* 37(Suppl 1):96A, 1988.
7. Li W, Shen S, Khatami M, Rockey JH: Stimulation of retinal capillary pericyte protein and collagen synthesis in culture by high-glucose concentration. *Diabetes* 33:785–789, 1984.
8. Ayo SH, Radnik RA, Garoni JA, Glass WFII, Kreisberg JI: High glucose causes an increase in extracellular matrix proteins in cultured mesangial cells. *Am J Pathol* 136:1339–1348, 1990.
9. Pugliese G, Pricci F, Pugliese F, Menè P, Lenti L, Andreani D, Galli G, Casini A, Bianchi S, Rotella CM, Di Mario U: Mechanisms of glucose-enhanced extracellular matrix accumulation in rat glomerular mesangial cells. *Diabetes* 43:478–490, 1994.
10. Ljubimov AV, Burgeson RE, Butkowski RJ, Couchman JR, Zardi L, Ninomiya Y, Sado Y, Huang ZS, Nesburn AB, Kenney MC: Basement membrane abnormalities in human eyes with diabetic retinopathy. *J Histochem Cytochem* 44:1469–1479, 1996.
11. Roy S, Cagliero E, Lorenzi M: Fibronectin overexpression in retinal microvessels of patients with diabetes. *Invest Ophthalmol Vis Sci* 37:258–266, 1996.
12. Roy S, Maiello M, Lorenzi M: Increased expression of basement membrane collagen in human diabetic retinopathy. *J Clin Invest* 93(1):438–442, 1994.
13. Steffes MW, Osterby R, Chavers B, Mauer SM: Mesangial expansion as a central mechanism for loss of kidney function in diabetic patients. *Diabetes* 38:1077–1081, 1989.
14. Karttunen T, Risteli J, Autio-Harmainen H, Risteli L: Effect of age and diabetes on type IV collagen and laminin in human kidney cortex. *Kidney Int* 30:386–391, 1986.

15. Nerlich A, Schleicher E: Immunohistochemical localization of extracellular matrix components in human diabetic glomerular lesions. *Am J Pathol* 139:889–899, 1991.

16. Mohan PS, Carter WG, Spiro RG: Occurrence of type VI collagen in extracellular matrix of renal glomeruli and its increase in diabetes. *Diabetes* 39:31–37, 1990.

17. Shimomura H, Spiro RG: Studies on macromolecular components of human glomerular basement membrane and alterations in diabetes: decreased levels of heparan sulfate proteoglycan and laminin. *Diabetes* 36:374–381, 1987.

18. Wu VY, Wilson B, Cohen MP: Disturbances in glomerular basement membrane glycosaminoglycans in experimental diabetes. *Diabetes* 36:679–683, 1987.

19. Parthasarathy N, Spiro RG: Effect of diabetes on the glycosaminoglycan component of the human glomerular basement membrane. *Diabetes* 31:738–741, 1982.

20. Kanwar YS, Rosenweig LJ, Linker A, Jakubowski ML: Decreased *de novo* synthesis of glomerular proteoglycans in diabetes: biochemical and autoradiographic evidence. *Proc Natl Acad Sci USA* 80:2272–2275, 1983.

21. Ayo SH, Radnik RA, Glass WF II, Garoni JA, Rampt ER, Appling DR, Kreisberg JI: Increased extracellular matrix synthesis and mRNA in mesangial cells grown in high-glucose medium. *Am J Physiol* 260:F185–F191, 1991.

22. Pugliese G, Pricci F, Locuratolo N, Romeo G, Romano G, Giannini S, Cresci B, Galli G, Rotella CM, Di Mario U: Increased activity of the insulin-like growth factor system in mesangial cells cultured in high glucose conditions: relation to glucose-enhanced extracellular matrix production. *Diabetologia* 39:775–784, 1996.

23. Pugliese G, Pricci F, Pesce CM, Romeo G, Lenti E, Vetri M, Caltabiano V, Purrello F, Di Mario U: Early, but not advanced, experimental diabetic glomerulopathy is reversed by pancreatic islet transplants. Correlation with glomerular extracellular matrix mRNA levels. *Diabetes* 46:1198–1206, 1997.

24. Fukui M, Nakamura T, Ebihara I, Shirato I, Tomino Y, Koide H: ECM gene expression and its modulation by insulin in diabetic rats. *Diabetes* 41:1520–1527, 1992.

25. Lorenzi M, Cagliero E, and Toledo S: Glucose toxicity for human endothelial cells in culture: delayed replication, disturbed cell cycle, and accelerated death. *Diabetes* 34:621–627, 1985.

26. Podesta F, Romeo G, Liu WH, Krajewski S, Reed JC, Gerhardinger C, Lorenzi M: Bax is increased in the retina of diabetic subjects and is associated with pericyte apoptosis *in vivo* and *in vitro*. *Am J Pathol* 156:1025–1032, 2000.

27. Hirschi KK Rohovsky SA, Beck LH, Smith SR, D'Amore PA: Endothelial cells modulate the proliferation of mural cell precursors via platelet-derived growth factor-BB and heterotypic cell contact. *Circ Res* 84:298–305, 1999.

28. Mizutani M, Kern TS, Lorenzi M: Accelerated death of retinal microvascular cells in human and experimental diabetic retinopathy. *J Clin Invest* 97:2883–2890, 1996.

29. Gambaro G, Venturini AP, Noonan DM, Fries W, Re G, Gerbisa S, Milanesi C, Pesarini A, Borsatti A, Marchi E, Baggio B: Treatment with a glycosaminoglycan formulation ameliorates experimental diabetic nephropathy. *Kidney Int* 46:797–806, 1994.

30. Young BA, Johnson RJ, Alpers CE, Eng E, Gordon K, Floege J, Couser WG: Cellular events in the evolution of experimental diabetic nephropathy. *Kidney Int* 47:935–944, 1995.

31. Nakamura T, Fukui M, Ebihara I, Osada S, Nagaoka I, Tomino Y, Koide H: mRNA expression of growth factors in glomeruli from diabetic rats. *Diabetes* 42:450–456, 1993.

32. Zhang W, Khanna P, Chan LL, Campbell G, Ansari NH: Diabetes-induced apoptosis in rat kidney. *Biochem Mol Med* 61:58–62, 1997.
33. Ortiz A, Ziyadeh FN, Neilson EG: Expression of apoptosis-regulatory genes in renal proximal tubular epithelial cells exposed to high ambient glucose and in diabetic kidneys. *J Invest Med* 45:50–56, 1997.
34. Gibbons GH, Dzau VJ: The emerging concept of vascular remodeling. *N Engl J Med* 330:1431–1438, 1994.
35. Frenette PS, Wagner DD: Molecular medicine. Adhesion molecules — Part I. *N Engl J Med* 334:1526–1529, 1996.
36. Ruoslahti E, Obrink B: Common principles in cell adhesion. *Exp Cell Res* 227:1–11, 1996.
37. Border WA, Ruoslahti E: Transforming growth factor-β in disease: the dark side of tissue repair. *J Clin Invest* 90:1–7, 1992.
38. Border WA, Noble NA: Transforming growth factor-β in tissue fibrosis. *N Engl J Med* 1994; 331:1286–1292.
39. Ziyadeh FN, Sharma K, Eriksen M, Wolf G: Stimulation of collagen gene expression and protein synthesis in murine mesangial cells by high glucose in mediated by activation of transforming growth factor-β. *J Clin Invest* 93:536–542, 1994.
40. Sharma K, Ziyadeh FN: Renal hypertrophy is associated with upregulation of TGF-β1 experession in diabetic BB rat and NOD mouse. *Am J Physiol* 267:F1094–F1101, 1994.
41. Sharma K, Guo J, Jin Y, Ziyadeh FN: Neutralizing of TGF-β by anti-TGF-β antibody attenuates kidney hypertrophy and the enhanced extracellular matrix gene expression in STZ-induced diabetic mice. *J Am Soc Nephrol* 9:646A, 1998.
42. Hoffman BB, Sharma K, Zhu Y, Ziyadeh FN: Transcriptional activation of transforming growth factor-β1 in mesangial cells culture by high glucose concentration. *Kidney Int* 54:1107–1116, 1998.
43. Campistol J, Inigo P, Jimenez W, Lario S, Clesca P, Oppenheimer F *et al*: Losartan decreases plasma levels of TGF-beta 1 in transplant patients with chronic allograft nephropathy. *Kidney Int* 56:714–719, 1999.
44. Kagami S, Border WA, Mille DE, Noble NA: Angiotensin II stimulates extracellular matrix protein synthesis through induction of transforming growth factor-β expression in rat mesangial cells. *J Clin Invest* 93:2431–2437, 1994.
45. Sharma K, Mc Gowan TA: TGF-β in diabetic kidney disease: role of novel signaling pathways. *Cytokine Growth Factor Rev* 11:115–123, 2000.
46. Doi T, Striker LJ, Elliot SJ, Conti FG, Striker GE: Insulin-like growth factor-1 is a progression factor for human mesangial cells. *Am J Pathol* 134:395–404, 1989.
47. Olashaw NE, Van Wyk JJ, Pledger WJ: Control of late G_0G_1 progression and protein modification by SmC/IGF I. *Am J Physiol* 253:C575–C579, 1987.
48. Flyvbjerg A, Frystyk J, Marshall M: Additive increase in kidney insulin-like growth factor I and initial renal enlargement in uninephrectomized-diabetic rats. *Horm Metab Res* 22:516–520, 1990.
49. Flyvbjerg A, Bornfeldt KE, Marshall SM, Arnqvist HJ, Ørskov H: Kidney IGF-1 mRNA in initial renal hypertrophy in experimental diabetes in rats. *Diabetologia* 33:334–338, 1990.
50. Marshall SM, Flyvbjerg A, Frystyk J, Korsgaard L, Ørskov H: Renal insulin-like growth factor I and growth hormone receptor binding in experimental diabetes and after unilateral nephrectomy in the rat. *Diabetologia* 34:632–639, 1991.

51. Landau D, Chin E, Bondy C, Domene H, Roberts CT Jr, Gronbaek H, Flyvbjerg A, LeRoith D: Expression of insulin-like growth factor-binding proteins in the rat kidney: effects of long-term diabetes. *Endocrinology* 136:1835–1842, 1995.

52. Doi T, Striker LJ, Quaife C, Conti FG, Palmiter R, Behringer R, Brinster RL, Striker GE: Progressive glomerulosclerosis develops in transgenic mice chronically expressing growth hormone and growth hormone releasing factor but not in those expressing insulin-like growth factor-I. *Am J Pathol* 131:398–403, 1988.

53. Doi T, Striker LJ, Kimata K, Peten EP, Yamada Y, Striker GE: Glomerulosclerosis in mice transgenic for growth hormone Increased mesangial extracellular matrix is correlated with kidney mRNA levels. *J Exp Med* 173:1287–1290, 1991.

54. Jacot TA, Striker GE, Stetler-Stevenson M, Striker LJ: Mesangial cells from transgenic mice with progressive glomerulosclerosis exhibit stable, phenotypic changes including undetectable MMP-9 and increased type IV collagen. *Lab Invest* 75:791–799, 1996.

55. Sharp PS: Long-term follow up of patients who underwent yttrium-90 pituitary implantation for treatment of proliferative diabetic retinopathy. *Diabetologia* 30:199–207, 1987.

56. Meyer-Schwickerath R: Vitreous levels of the insulin-like growth factors I and II, and the insulin-like growth factor binding proteins 2 and 3, increase in neovascular eye disease. Studies in nondiabetic and diabetic subjects. *J Clin Invest* 92:2620–2625, 1993.

57. Hyer SL, Sharp PS, Brooks RA, Burrin JM, Kohner EM: A two year follow-up study of serum insulin-like growth factor-I in diabetics with retinopathy. *Metabolism* 38:586–589, 1989.

58. Stout RW: Hyperinsulinemia and atherosclerosis. *Diabetes* 45(Suppl 3):S45–S46, 1996.

59. Anderson PW, Zhang XY, Tian J, Correale JD, Xi XP, Yang D, Graf K, Law RE, Hsueh WA: Insulin and angiotensin II are additive in stimulating TGF-beta 1 and matrix mRNAs in mesangial cells. *Kidney Int* 50:745–753, 1996.

60. Pandolfi A, Iacoviello L, Capani F, Vitacolonna E, Donati MB, Consoli A: Glucose and insulin independently reduce the fibrinolytic potential of human vascular smooth muscle cells in culture. *Diabetologia* 39:1425–1431, 1996.

61. Schmetterer L, Muller M, Fasching P, Diepolder C, Gallenkamp A, Zanaschka G, Findl O, Strenn K, Mensik C, Tschernko E, Eichler HG, Wolzt M: Renal and ocular hemodynamic effects of insulin. *Diabetes* 46:1868–1874, 1997.

62. Chakravarthy U, Hayes RG, Stitt AW, McAuley E, Archer DB: Constitutive nitric oxide synthase expression in retinal vascular endothelial cells is suppressed by high glucose and advanced glycation endproducts. *Diabetes* 47:945–952, 1998.

63. Smith LEH, Shen W, Perruzzi C, Soker S, Kinose F, Xu X, Robinson G, Driver S, Bischoff J, Zhang B, Schaeffer JM, Senger DR: Suppression of retinal neovascularization *in vivo* by inhibition of vascular endothelial growth factor (VEGF) using soluble VEGF-receptor chimeric proteins. *Nature Med* 5:1390–1395, 1999.

64. Craven PA, Studer RK, DeRubertis FR: Impaired nitric oxide-dependent cyclic guanosine monophosphate in glomeruli from diabetic rats: evidence for protein kinase C-mediated suppression of the cholinergic responce. *J Clin Invest* 93:311–320, 1994.

65. Pieper GM, Moore-Hilton G, Roza AM: Evaluation of the mechanism of endothelial dysfunction in the genetically-diabetic BB rats. *Life Sci* 58:PL147–PL152, 1996.

66. Honing MLH, Morrison PJ, Banga JD, Stroes ESG, Rabelink TJ: Nitric oxide availability in diabetes mellitus. *Diab/Metab Rev* 14:26–42, 1998.
67. Sobrevia L, Cesare P, Yudilevich DL, Mann GE: Diabetes-induced activation of y^+ and nitric oxide synthase in human endothelial cells: association with membrane hyperpolarization. *J Physiol* 489:183–192, 1995.
68. Pieper GM: Acute amelioration of diabetic endothelial dysfunction with a derivate of the nitric oxide synthase cofactor, tetrahydrobiopterin. *J Cardiovasc Pharm* 29:8–11, 1997.
69. Cosentino F, Hishikawa K, Katusic ZS, Lüsher TF: High glucose increases nitric oxide synthase expression and superoxide anion generation in human aortic endothelial cells. *Circulation* 96:25–28, 1997.
70. Knowles RG: Nitric oxide biochemistry. *Biochem Soc Trans* 25:895–901, 1997.
71. Tischer E, Mitchell R, Hartman T, Silva M, Gospodarowicz D, Fiddes JC, Abraham JA: The human gene for vascular endothelial growth factor. Multiple protein forms are encoded through alternative exon splicing. *J Biol Chem* 266:11 947–11 954, 1991.
72. Ferrara N, Houck K, Jakeman L, Leung DW: Molecular and biological properties of the vascular endothelial growth factor family of proteins. *Endocr Rev* 13:18–32, 1992.
73. Alon T, Hemo I, Itin A, Pe'er J, Stone J, Keshet E: Vascular endothelial growth factor acts as a survival factor for newly formed retinal vessels and has implications for retinopathy of prematurity. *Nature Med* 1:1024–1028, 1995.
74. Adamis AP, Shima DT, Yeo KT, Yeo TK, Brown LF, Berse B, D'Amore PA, Folkman J: Synthesis and secretion of vascular permeability factor/vascular endothelial growth factor by human retinal pigment epithelial cells. *Biochem Biophys Res Commun* 193:631–638, 1993.
75. Aiello LP, Avery RL, Arrigg PG, Keyt BA, Jampel HD, Shah ST, Pasquale LR, Thieme H, Iwamoto MA, Park JE *et al*: Vascular endothelial growth factor in ocular fluid of patients with diabetic retinopathy and other retinal disorders. *N Engl J Med* 331:1480–1487, 1994.
76. Aiello LP, Pierce EA, Foley ED, Takagi H, Chen H, Riddle L, Ferrara N, King GL, Smith LE: Suppression of retinal neovascularization *in vivo* by inhibition of vascular endothelial growth factor (VEGF) using soluble VEGF-receptor chimeric proteins. *Proc Natl Acad Sci USA*; 92:10 457–10 461, 1995.
77. Hammes HP, Hammes HP, Lin J, Bretzel RG, Brownlee M, Breier G: Upregulation of the vascular endothelial growth factor/vascular endothelial growth factor receptor system in experimental background diabetic retinopathy of the rat. *Diabetes* 15:1219–1224, 1998.
78. Gerhardinger C, Brown LF, Roy S, Mizutani M, Zucker CL, Lorenzi M: Expression of vascular endothelial growth factor in the human retina and in nonproliferative diabetic retinopathy. *Am J Pathol* 152:453–462, 1998.
79. Ferrara N, Alitalo K: Clinical applications of angiogenic growth factors and their inhibitors. *Nature Med* 5:1359–1364, 1999.
80. Rivard A, Silver M, Chen D, Kearney M, Magner M, Annex B, Peters K, Isner JM: Rescue of diabetes-related impairment of angiogenesis by intramuscular gene therapy with adeno-VEGF. *Am J Pathol* 154:355–363, 1999.
81. Klein R, Klein BE: Diabetic eye disease. *Lancet* 350:197–204, 1997.
82. Antonetti DA Barber AJ, Khin S, Lieth E, Tarbell JM, Gardner TW: Vascular permeability in experimental diabetes is associated with reduced endothelial occludin content: vascular endothelial growth factor decreases occludin in retinal endothelial cells. Penn State Retina Research Group. *Diabetes* 47:1953–1959, 1998.

83. Gerhardinger C, McClure KD, Lorenzi M: Mechanisms of occludin overexpression in human diabetic retinopathy. *Diabetes* 49 (Suppl 1):A170, 2000.
84. Bek T: Immunohistochemical characterization of retinal glial cell changes in areas of vascular occlusion secondary to diabetic retinopathy. *Acta Ophthalmol Scand* 75:239–243, 1997.
85. Kuroki T, Inoguchi T, Umeda F, Ueda F, Nawata H: High glucose induces alteration of gap junction permeability and phosphorylation of connexin-43 in cultured aortic smooth muscle cells. *Diabetes* 47:931–936, 1998.
86. Morigi Angioletti S, Imberti B, Donadelli R, Micheletti G, Figliuzzi M, Remuzzi A, Zoja C, Remuzzi G: Leukocyte-endothelial interaction is augmented by high glucose concentrations and hyperglycemia in a NF-κB-dependent fashion. *J Clin Invest* 101(9):1905–1915, 1998.
87. Yerneni KK, Bai W, Khan BV, Medford RM, Natarajan R. Hyperglycemia-induced activation of nuclear transcription factor κB in vascular smooth muscle cells. *Diabetes* 48:855–864, 1999.
88. Brand K, Page S, Rogler G, Bartsch A, Brandl R, Knuechel R, Page M, Kaltschmidt C, Baeuerle PA, Neumeier D: Activated transcription factor nuclear factor-κB is present in the atherosclerotic lesion. *J Clin Invest* 97:1715–1722, 1996.
89. Nishizuka Y: Intracellular signaling by hydrolysis of phospholipids and activation of protein kinase C. *Science* 258:607–614, 1992.
90. Nishizuka Y: Protein kinase C and lipid signaling for sustained cellular responses. *FASEB J* 9:484–496, 1995.
91. Liacovitch M, Cantley LC: Lipid second messengers. *Cell* 77:329–334, 1994.
92. Daisuke Koya, King GL: Protein kinase C activation and the development of diabetic complication. *Diabetes* 47:859–866, 1998.
93. Vasilets LA, Schwarz W: Structure function relationships of cation binding in Na$^+$/K$^+$-ATPase. *Biochim Biophys Acta* 1154:201–222, 1993.
94. Takagi C, Bursell S-E, Lin Y-W, Takagi H, Duh E, Jiang Z, Clermont AC, King GL: Regulation of retinal hemodynamics in diabetic rats by increased expression and action of endothelin-1. *Invest Ophthalmol Vis Sci* 37:2504–2518, 1996.
95. Haneda M, Araki S-I, Togaea M, Sugimoto T, Isono M, Kikkawa R: Mitogen activated protein kinase cascade is activated in glomeruli of diabetic rats and glomerular mesangial cells cultured under high glucose conditions. *Diabetes* 46:840–853, 1997.
96. Dejana E: Endothelial adherent junctions: implications in the control of vascular permeability and angiogenesis. *J Clin Invest* 98(9):1949–1953, 1996.
97. Mogensen CE, Christensen CK, Vittinghus E: The stages in diabetic renal disease. With emphasis on the stage of incipient diabetic nephropathy. *Diabetes* 32(Suppl 2):64–78, 1983.
98. Cunha-Vaz JG, Fonseca JR, de Abreu JF, Ruas JF: Detection of early retinal changes in diabetes by vitreous fluorophotometry. *Diabetes* 28:16–19, 1979.
99. Chavers B, Etzwiler D, Barbosa J, Bach FH, Michael AF: Albumin deposition in dermal capillary basement membrane in parents of type 1 (insulin-dependent) diabetic patients. *Diabetologia* 26:415–419, 1984.
100. Walton HA, Byrne J, Robinson GB: Studies on the permeation properties of glomerular basement membrane: cross-linking renders glomerular basement membrane permeable to protein. *Biochim Biophys Acta* 1138:173–178, 1992.
101. Boyd-White J, Williams JC Jr: Effect of cross-linking on matrix permeability. A model for AGE-modified basement membranes. *Diabetes* 45:348–353, 1996.
102. Ostermann H, van de Loo J: Factors of the hemostatic system in diabetic patients. *Haemostasis* 16:386–416, 1986.

103. Karsten S: Blood vessel wall interactions in diabetes. *Diabetes* 46 (Suppl 2), 1997.

104. Ceriello A: Fibrinogen and diabetes mellitus: is it time for intervention trials? *Diabetologia* 40:731–734, 1997.

105. Ernest E, Resch KL: Fibrinogen as a cardiovascular risk factor: a meta-analysis and review of the litterature. *Ann Intern Med* 118:956–963, 1993.

106. Morale M, De Negri F, Carmassi F: Fibrin(ogen) and diabetes mellitus: don't forget fibrinolysis. *Diabetologia* 40:735–737, 1997.

107. Meade TW, Vickers MV: The effect of physiological levels of fibrinogen on platelet aggregation. *Thromb Res* 38:527–534, 1985.

108. Ceriello A, Giacomello R, Stel G, Motz E, Taboga C, Tonutti L, Pirisi M, Falletti E, Bartoli E: Hyperglycemia-induced thrombin formation in diabetes: the possible role of oxidative stress. *Diabetes* 44:924–928, 1995.

109. Juhan-Vague I, Alessi MC, Vague P: Thrombogenic and fibrinolytic factors and cardiovascular risk in non-insulin-dependent diabetes mellitus. *Ann Med* 28 (4):371–380, 1996.

110. Ganda OP, Arkin GH: Hyperfibrinogenemia. An important risk factor for vasular complications in diabetes. *Diabetes Care* 15:1245–1250, 1992.

111. Graves M, Malia RG, Goodfellow K, Mattock M, Stevens LK, Stephenson JM, Fuller JH, and the EURODIAB IDDM complications study: Fibrinogen and von Willebrand factor in IDDM: relationships to lipid vascular risk factors, blood pressure, glycaemic control and urinary albumin excretion rate: The EURODIAB IDDM complications study. *Diabetologia* 40:698–705, 1997.

112. Ceriello A, Taboga C, Giacomello R Falleti E, De Stasio G, Motz E, Lizzio S, Gonano F, Bartoli E: Fibrinogen plasma levels is a marker of thrombin activation in diabetes. *Diabetes* 43:430–432, 1994.

113. Cigolini M, Targher G, Desandra G, Muggeo M, Seidell JC: Plasma fibrinogen in relation to serum insulin, smoking habits and adipose tissue fatty acids in healthy men. *Eur J Clin Invest* 24:126–130, 1994.

114. Ibbotson SH, Walmsley D, Davies JA, Grant PJ: Generation of thrombin activity in relation to factor VIII:C concentrations and vascular complications in type 1 (insulin-dependent) diabetes mellitus. *Diabetologia* 35:863–867, 1992.

115. Ceriello A, Giuliano D, Quartaro A, Dello Russo P, Torella R: Blood glucose may condition factor VII levels in diabetic and normal subjects. *Diabetologia* 31:889–891, 1988.

116. Carmassi F, Morale M, Puccetti R, De Negri F, Manzani F, Navalese R, Mariani G: Coagulation and fibrinolytic system impairment in insulin dependent diabetes mellitus. *Thromb Res* 67:643–654, 1992.

117. Ceriello A, Giacomello R, Colatutto A, Taboga C, Gonano F: Increased prothrombin fragment 1 and 2 in type 1 diabetic patients. *Haemostasis* 22:50–51, 1992.

118. Myrp B, Rossing P, Jensen T, Gram J, Kluft C, Jesperson J: Procoagulant activity and intimal dysfunction in IDDM. *Diabetologia* 38:73–78, 1995.

119. Brownlee M, Vlassara H, Cerami A: Nonenzymatic glycosylation reduces the susceptibility of fibrin to degradation by plasmin. *Diabetes* 32:680–684, 1983.

120. Matsuda T, Morishita E, Jokaji H, Asakura H, Saito M, Yoshida T, Takemodo K: Mechanism on disorders of coagulation and fibrinolysis in diabetes. *Diabetes* 45 (Suppl 3), 1996.

121. Gram J, Jespersen J: Induction and possible role of fibrinolysis in diabetes mellitus. *Sem Thromb Haemost* 17:412–416, 1991.

122. Collier A, Rumley AG, Paterson JR, Leach JP, Lowe GDO, Small M: Free radical activity and hemostatic factors in NIDDM. *Diabetes* 41:909–913, 1992.

123. Calles-Escandon J, Mirza S, Sobel BE, Schneider DJ: Induction of hyperinsulinemia combined with hyperglycemia and hypertriglyceridemia increases plasminogen activator inhibitor type-1 (PAI-1) in blood in normal human subjects. *Diabetes* 47:290–293, 1998.
124. McGill JB, Schneider DJ, Arfken CL, Lucore CL, Sobel BE: Factors responsible for impaired fibrinolysis in obese subjects and NIDDM patients. *Diabetes* 43:104–109, 1994.
125. Geiger M: Plasminogen activation in diabetes mellitus. *Enzyme* 60:1169–1177, 1988.
126. Ribau JCO, Samis JA, Senis YA, Maurice DH, Giles AR, De Reske M, Absher PM, Hatton MWC, Richardson M: Aortic endothelial cell von Willebrand factor content, and circulating plasminogen activator inhibitor-1 are increased, but expression of endothelial leukocyte adhesion molecules is unchanged in insulin-dependent diabetic BB rats. *Atherosclerosis* 149:331–342, 2000.
127. Wiman B: Plasminogen activator inhibitor 1 (PAI-1) in plasma: its role in thrombotic disease. *Thromb Haemost* 74:71–76, 1995.
128. Sobel BE, Woodcock-Mitchell J, Schneider DJ, Holt RE, Marutsuka K, Gold H: Increased plasminogen activator inhibitor type-1 in coronary artery atherectomy specimens from type 2 diabetic compared with non-diabetic patients: a potential factor predisposing to thrombosis and its resistance. *Circulation* 97:2213–2221, 1998.
129. Burton E, Sobe L: Increased plasminogen activator inhibitor-1 and vasculopathy. *Circulation* 99:2496–1498, 1999.
130. BARI Investigators: Comparison of coronary bypass surgery with angioplasty in patients with multivessel disease. *N Engl J Med* 335:217–225, 1996.
131. Falk E: Unstable angina with fatal outcome: dynamic coronary thrombosis leading to infarction and/or sudden death: autopsy evidence of recurrent mural thrombosis with peripheral embolization culminating in total vascular occlusion. *Circulation* 71:609–708, 1985.
132. Davies MJ, Bland MJ, Hangartner WR, Angelini A, Thomas AC: Factors influencing the presence or absence of acute coronary thrombi in sudden ischemic death. *Eur Heart J* 10:203–208, 1989.
133. Jones DB, Wallace R, Frier BM: Vascular endothelial cell antibodies in diabetic patients. *Diabet Care* 15:552–555, 1992.
134. Galajda P, Martinka E, Mokan M, Kubisz P: Endothelial cell markers in diabetes mellitus. *Thromb Res* 85:63–65, 1997.
135. Seigneur M, Dufourc P, Gin H, Delafaye C, Amiral J, Pruvost A, Boisseau MR: Plasma thrombomodulin levels increase with the severity of the diabetic retinopathy. *Blood Coag Fibrin* 5:845–846, 1994.
136. Boffa MC: Considering cellular thrombomodulin distribution and its modulating factors can facilitate the use of plasma thrombomodulin as a reliable endothelial marker. *Haemostasis* 26 (Suppl 4):233–243, 1996.
137. Ceriello A, Giuliano D, Quatraro A, Marchi E, Barbanti M, Lefèbvre P: Evidence for a hyperglycaemia decrease of antithrombin III-thrombin complex formation in humans. *Diabetologia* 33:163–167, 1990.
138. Morishita E, Asakura H, Jokaji H, Saito M, Uotani C, Kumabashiri I, Yamazaky M, Aoshima K. Hashimoto T, Matsuda T: Hypercoagulability and high lipoprotein(a) levels in patients with type II diabetes mellitus: *Atherosclerosis* 120:7–14, 1996.
139. Leurs PB, van Oerle R, Wolffenbuttel BHR, Hamulyak K: Increased tissue factor pathway inhibitor (TFPI) and coagulation in patients with insulin-dependent diabetes mellitus. *Thromb Haemost* 77 (3):472–476, 1997.

22

Predictors of Cardiovascular Mortality in Type 2 Diabetes Background

MICHELE MUGGEO

Ospedale Civile Maggiore, Verona, Italy

Type 2 diabetes is one of the most prevalent diseases in the word, affecting more than 100 million people. This disease is associated with substantial morbidity and mortality rates, most notably relating to cardiovascular disease. The Framingham study has shown that the relative risk of ischaemic heart disease is about twice as great in male diabetics and four times greater in females in comparison with non-diabetic subjects of the same age. The risk of stroke is about three times as high in male diabetics and twice as high in female diabetics. The risk of *claudicatio intermittens* is about three times greater in male and almost nine times greater in female diabetics (1).

The increased incidence of cardiovascular diseases and death in diabetic subjects has been subsequently confirmed in a large number of recent studies, carried out in different populations (2–5). The Verona Diabetes Study, performed on more than 7000 diabetic patients and followed up for a period of 10 years, showed that about 40% of the patients died due to cardiovascular diseases, compared with 20% of deaths for tumour-related causes (6). Same results were obtained in another Italian study carried out in the north-west of the country (7).

From the anatomo-pathological point of view, what underlies the greater frequency of cardiovascular events in diabetic patients is the accelerated development of atherosclerosis and atherothrombosis. The Brunico study,

Diabetes in the New Millennium. Edited by U. Di Mario, F. Leonetti, G. Pugliese, P. Sbraccia and A. Signore.
© 2000 John Wiley & Sons, Ltd.

carried out in more than 800 subjects, all of whom were undergoing detailed carotid evaluation, showed that type 2 diabetes led to a five-fold greater risk of carotid stenosis than that observed in non-diabetic subjects. This increased risk remained in the multivariate analysis after adjustment for a considerable number of associated cardiovascular risk factors (8). This last finding is particularly important because type 2 diabetes is a condition in which hyperglycaemia is often associated with other confounding risk factors, such as insulin resistance, dyslipidaemia, obesity, hypertension and thrombophilia (9).

Besides the Brunico Study, the independent role of hyperglycaemia in the genesis of atherosclerosis and cardiovascular events was also demonstrated in a considerable number of prospective studies published so far, which revealed the independent association between cardiovascular events and the glycaemic control in patients with type 2 diabetes.

Over the last 10 years, a considerable number of studies have demonstrated that there is a strict relationship between cardiovascular diseases and glycaemic control in patients with type 2 diabetes. These studies have involved thousands of subjects, often newly diagnosed, followed up for periods ranging from 3.5 to 11 years and evaluated on the basis of various cardiovascular endpoints (10). It is necessary to underline that the majority of these studies considered a single fasting glycaemic value and a single value of glycosylated haemoglobin measured at baseline to predict cardiovascular events occurring many years later. Therefore, other studies were designed in order to have serial follow-up measurements of glycaemia and/or glycosylated haemoglobin levels.

The observational version of the UKPDS showed that the mean glycosylated haemoglobin value during follow-up was a good predictor of the occurrence of ischaemic heart disease (11). In particular, the multivariate analysis demonstrated that every 1% increase in glycosylated haemoglobin levels is associated with an approximately 10% increase in the risk of cardiovascular disease. This is in line with the results of other observational studies (12,13), and confirmed by the interventional version of the UKPDS, which showed that intensive treatment leading to an approximately 1% reduction in glycosylate haemoglobin levels led to a 16% reduction in the occurrence of myocardial infarction (14).

The recognition of the predictors of cardiovascular mortality is the first step in planning an intervention aimed at reducing mortality. Predictors can be divided in biological and modifiable factors. The biological factors, such as age, gender and family history, are not changeable. The modifiable predictors are cigarette smoking, high blood pressure, high blood glucose, elevated total and low density lipoprotein (LDL)-cholesterol, obesity, diabetes treatment, model of diabetes care and so on.

The purpose of this chapter is to discuss the risk factors for cardiovascular diseases that are specific for type 2 diabetes, as they are related to its natural history, mode of treatment, duration of the disease, level of metabolic control and complications.

The excess of cardiovascular mortality in type 2 diabetes is only partially explained by the classic risk factors, which include age, gender, high blood pressure, smoking, high LDL-cholesterol, low HDL-cholesterol, obesity, life-style, etc. Other factors specifically related to the natural history of diabetes strongly affect survival of diabetic subjects. Age of onset, duration of the disease, long-term glucose control, severity of the disease and presence of chronic complications, mode of therapy and model of care all contribute to patient survival.

Duration of diabetes is computed from the time of diagnosis, which does not coincide with the biological onset of the disease. There is a latency period of 4–7 years between the biological onset of type 2 diabetes and its clinical recognition (15). During this latency period the mortality risk is similar or even higher than the mortality risk of known diabetic patients, as hyperglycaemia and other risk factors remain untreated (16). This can explain why, in the Verona Diabetes Study (VDS), patients with duration of disease of 0–4 years already showed a 23% increase of mortality risk (SMR = 1.23, 95% CI 1.19–1.27) (17). In univariate analysis, mortality risk increases with the duration of diabetes, but when the changes in therapy over time are taken into account, the effect of diabetes duration loses its predictive value in relation to mortality. This suggests that the progression of diabetes and its severity are better described by the changes of therapy rather than by the time elapsed since diagnosis. When the risk of mortality is computed accounting only for age and duration, the latter is a predictor of mortality. However, when other confounders are accounted for, the effect of duration is no longer significant. By increasing duration of diabetes, the proportion of patients treated with diet progressively decreases, as both observed in the VDS. Conversely, the proportion of patients requiring insulin treatment increases four-fold from the first to the third tertile of duration. Mortality is significantly associated with therapy: use of oral agents and, even more strikingly, use of insulin is associated with a significant increase in mortality and this result further supports the concept that mode of treatment is a potent marker of severity of the disease. Severity of the disease includes not only the degree of hyperglycaemia, but also the clustering of other risk factors (4), as well as the presence of chronic complications. In the VDS the prevalence of diabetic complications at baseline was significantly higher in patients who died in the following 5 years as compared with diabetic patients still alive after 5 years.

Duration of diabetes in Finnish subjects aged 65–74 years was found as being a strong predictor of cardiovascular events (18). This study, due to the high (40.2%) prevalence of newly detected type 2 diabetic patients at the baseline, allowed a better evaluation of the importance of the duration of the disease with respect to cardiovascular risk. It is reasonable to think that mechanisms associated with long-lasting hyperglycaemia underlay this relation. These findings on cardiovascular events, along with the above-reported evidence strongly suggest that diabetic patients should be identified and treated at the earliest stages of the disease in order to reduce the incidence of complications and, hence, mortality.

In studies on general populations including also diabetic patients (19,20) it has been clearly shown that glycaemia and, of course, diabetes are associated with increased risk of mortality, primarily from cardiovascular diseases. There is a strong relationship between the degree of metabolic control, as measured by a single determination of fasting plasma glucose or HbA_{1c} at baseline, and the incidence of microvascular complications. A poor metabolic control also amplifies the effect of other powerful diabetes specific risk factors, such as duration of diabetes (18) and microalbuminuria (12). However, intensive treatment of hyperglycaemia, resulting in a reduction of HbA_{1c} from 7.9% to 7%, was associated with an impressive decrease in microvascular complications, with a moderate reduction in cardiovascular events, such as fatal and non-fatal myocardial infarction (11).

The weaker association between HbA_{1c} and cardiovascular mortality could be due to the fact that the assessment of long-term glucose control by fasting plasma glucose (FPG) or HbA_{1c} does not fully reflect the complex interrelation between everyday glucose control and outcomes. For instance, a frequent recurrence of hyperglycaemic and hypoglycaemic spikes could disproportionately increase the overall glycaemic risk. This additional risk, related to the 'valley and peak phenomenon', is not detected by a single determination of fasting plasma glucose or HbA_{1c}. The latter correlates with the mean glucose level of a given patient and does not reveal the excursions of plasma glucose over time.

To detect 'glycaemic variability' we have suggested computation of a coefficient of variation ($CV = SD/mean \times 100$) of a time series of FPG determinations. This parameter, obtained by serial measurements of fasting plasma glucose, offers additional information on the impact of long-term glucose control on mortality. In fact, in type 2 diabetic patients, grouped in tertiles of coefficient of variation of FPG during a 3 year period (1984–1986), the subsequent 10-year mortality was greater in patients of the third tertile of CV-FPG. This association was stronger than that between the mean of fasting plasma glucose (M-FPG) and mortality. Interestingly, the higher mortality experienced by the patients of the third tertile of CV-FPG was explained by cardiovascular mortality. These patients showed a longer duration of diabetes, a more frequent use of insulin, a higher M-FPG and a higher number of hypoglycaemic events than patients belonging to the first and the second tertiles (21).

Further, as shown by Figure 22.1, the CV-FPG during 1984–1986 was a stronger predictor of 10 year mortality (1987–1996) than M-FPG. Of course,

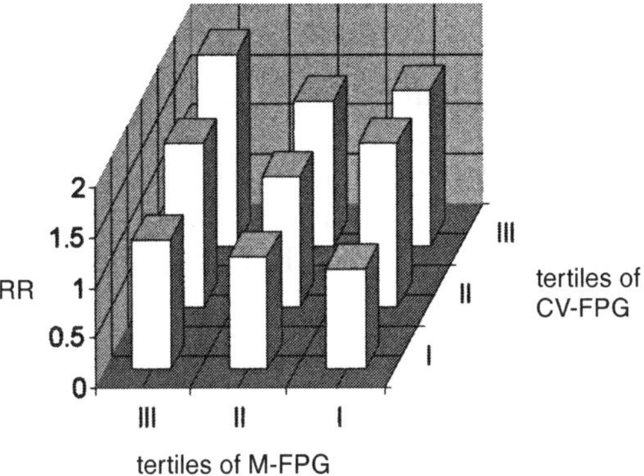

Figure 22.1. Relative risks of all-cause mortality during 1987–1996 in 1800 type 2 diabetic patients aged 40–80 years from the Verona Diabetes Study. The patients were included in the study if they had at least two fasting plasma glucose determinations per year during 1984–1986. Patients were grouped into tertiles of mean (M) and coefficient of variation (CV) of fasting plasma glucose (FPG) during 1984–1986

these results do not necessarily mean that the severity of hyperglycaemia is not important in determining the outcome in type 2 diabetes, but indicate that the prognostic value of M-FPG is lower than that of CV-FPG. Indeed, these data suggest that CV-FPG might be more reliable than M-FPG in assessing the relationship between long-term glucose control and survival. On the other hand, CV-FPG might be a feature of glucose control 'variability' distinct from hyperglycaemia.

All these data underlie the importance of glycaemic peaks occurring in diabetic patients, especially after meals. In the Diabetes Intervention Study, carried out in 1139 type 2 diabetic patients by Hanefeld *et al* (22), the cumulative incidence of cardiovascular events during 11 years of follow-up was significantly correlated with post-prandial blood glucose, rather than with fasting blood glucose at baseline, thus suggesting that post-prandial glucose levels could better describe the glycaemic risk for cardiovascular diseases. Recent population studies, carried out in Europe (23) and in the USA (24) have demonstrated that in both non-diabetic and type 2 diabetic patients 2 hour OGTT plasma glucose, and not fasting plasma glucose, is a strong predictor of mortality. On the contrary, in a 10 year prospective study of patients with newly diagnosed type 2 diabetes, cardiovascular mortality increased three-fold in patients included in the highest blood glucose tertile at baseline when compared with patients included in the lowest blood glucose tertile (25). The 8–10 year follow-up study of the Wisconsin cohort reported that glycated haemoglobin (HbA_{1c}) was associated with increased mortality, mainly due to vascular causes, in people with younger-onset diabetes and in older-onset diabetic people after controlling for other risk factors (26)

Several studies of type 1 diabetic patients have shown the beneficial effects of tight control of blood glucose on the initiation and progression of diabetic retinopathy, nephropathy, microalbuminuria and neuropathy. In the Diabetes Control and Complications Trial, cardiovascular events were also reduced, although not significantly, by 41% in the group of patients aged 13–39 years with good glycaemic control (27). Intensive glucose control in patients with newly diagnosed type 2 diabetes in the UK Prospective Diabetes Study, who had a low risk of microvascular complications, had a beneficial effect on aggregate diabetes-related endpoints (i.e. any diabetes-related endpoint, diabetes-related deaths, all-cause mortality, myocardial infarction, stroke, amputation or death from peripheral vascular disease, microvascular complications), and significantly reduced the rate of progression from normoalbuminuria to microalbuminuria (14). The University Group Diabetes Program, the Kumamoto Study, and the Veterans Affairs Cooperative Study did not show significant beneficial effects due to improved glycaemic control on macrovascular disease and cardiovascular mortality (28–30). The UKPDS found a borderline significant reduction in the number of myocardial infarctions with intensive blood glucose control, but significantly fewer diabetes-related deaths and strokes were seen only with tight blood pressure control. A recent study, conducted on microalbuminuric type 2 diabetic patients aged 40–65 years, showed that nearly 4 years of intensive multi-factorial treatment slowed the progression leading to nephropathy, retinopathy and autonomic neuropathy (31).

Type of treatment in type 2 diabetes changes over time, and usually the proportion of diet-treated patients declines with increasing age, whereas the proportion of those treated with oral agents and insulin increases. As previously observed, there is a strong association between therapy and mortality risk, but it is difficult to discriminate the effect of therapy itself from the effect of the severity of diabetes. In everyday clinical practice the therapy of type 2 diabetes is approached stepwise and the decision to treat patients with insulin is based on the level of hyperglycaemia and/or the presence of chronic complication or associated diseases. In multivariate analysis, even accounting for level of glucose control (mean FPG or HbA_{1c}), the association between therapy and mortality is affected by other confounders, such as complications and comorbidities.

Thus, mode of therapy remains a marker of disease severity and increased mortality risk, rather than the cause. These changes may reflect a progressive increase of severity of diabetes, as well as the effect of complications and comorbidity over time. Several studies have consistently reported an increased mortality rate in diabetic subjects treated with hypoglycaemic agents compared with those on diet (21,32). The highest rate of mortality is observed in patients treated with insulin (21). The association between insulin and mortality does not increase with the dose, further supporting the absence of a cause–effect

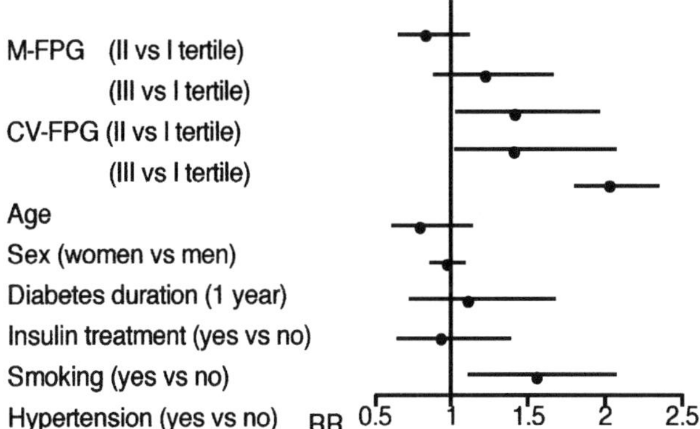

Figure 22.2. Relative risk (with 95% confidence intervals) of cardiovascular mortality during 1987–1996 in 1800 type 2 diabetic patients aged 40–80 years from the Verona Diabetes Study. Multivariate analysis was carried out by the Cox model

relationship. Indeed, in some studies severity of diabetes predicted mortality among diabetic patients (32).

The impact of the model of diabetes care on mortality has been attracting more attention over the recent years (33). So far, there are some indirect evidences that demonstrate that patients attending specialized clinics experience lower mortality chances than patients who do not attend such clinics. Recently, it has been reported that patients cared for by physicians at a Diabetes Centre receive better quality diabetes care than patients cared for by physicians at a general medicine clinic (34). In the frame of the VDS, the impact on mortality from all and specific causes of attending the Diabetes Centre was evaluated by comparing 4047 type 2 diabetic patients regularly attending the Verona Diabetes Centre with 3101 who did not. The patients were followed-up for 10 years in order to ascertain life status and the causes of death. Patients attending the Diabetes Centre were periodically examined by an experienced diabetologist to assess metabolic control, to re-evaluate ongoing therapy and to screen for diabetic complications and cardiovascular risk factors. Educational courses concerning diabetes and its complications, as well as the control of cardiovascular risk factors, were organized either for individual patients or for small groups of patients. Moreover, patients attending the Centre received advice from a professional dietician. As a result, patients attending the Verona Diabetes Centre experienced a reduction of risk of mortality from all causes of about 20%, independently of the contribution of other variables (35). In the Verona Diabetes Study the beneficial effects of attending the Diabetes Centre in patients aged 56–74 years and older patients (75 years and over) were compared with age-matched type 2 patients not attending the clinic (75). In the former group, the RR of all cause mortality was 0.9 (95% CI = 0.82–0.99), while in the latter RR was 0.91 (95% CI = 0.81–1.02), no longer statistically significant (35).

CONCLUSION

Diabetes is an important contributor to cardiovascular mortality and reduces life expectancy in type 2 patients. Figure 22.2 shows the main predictors of mortality found in the Verona Diabetes Study: age, sex, hypertension and variability of both glycaemia and BMI. Among the parameters of long-term glucose control, mean fasting glucose is a predictor of mortality only when in the multivariate analysis the variability (i.e. coefficient of variation) is not included in the model. When the long-term glucose instability is considered, in type 2 diabetic patients the coefficient of variation of FPG becomes the strongest predictor of mortality. The patients with the highest variability also experience the greatest rate of hypoglycaemic events, and this exposes the patients to adjunctive risk of cardiovascular mortality. These data suggest that the stability of glycaemia and BMI, along with a global control of risk factors, would prevent many unnecessary cardiovascular deaths.

REFERENCES

1. Kannel WB, McGee DL: Diabetes and cardiovascular diseases. The Framingham Study. *J Am Med Assoc* 241:2035–2038, 1979.
2. Kleinman JC, Donahue RP, Harris MI, Finucane FF, Madans JH, Brock DB: Mortality among diabetics in a national sample. *Am J Epidemiol* 128:389–401, 1988.
3. Manson JE, Colditz GA, Stampfer MJ, Willett WC, Krolewski AS, Rosner B, Arky RA, Speizer FE, Hennekens CH: A prospective study of maturity-onset diabetes mellitus and risk of coronary heart disease and stroke in women. *Arch Intern Med* 151:1141–1147, 1991.
4. Stamler J, Vaccaro O, Neaton JD, Wentworth D for the Multiple Risk Factor Intervention Trial Research Group: Diabetes, other risk factors, and 12-yr cardiovascular mortality for men screened in the Multiple Risk Factor Intervention Trial. *Diabet Care* 16:434–444, 1993.
5. Haffner SM, Lehto S, Ronnemaa T, Pyorala K, Laakso M: Mortality from coronary heart disease in subjects with type 2 diabetes and in nondiabetic subjects with and without prior myocardial infarction. *N Engl J Med* 339:229–234, 1998.
6. De Marco R, Locatelli F, Zoppini G, Verlato G, Bonora E, Muggeo M: Cause-specific mortality in type 2 diabetes mellitus. *Diabet Care* 22:756–761, 1999.
7. Bruno G, Merletti F, Boffetta P, Cavallo-Perin P, Bargero G, Gallone G, Pagano G: Impact of glycemic control, hypertension, and insulin treatment on general and cause-specific mortality: an Italian population-based cohort of type II (non-insulin-dependent) diabetes mellitus. *Diabetologia* 42:297–301, 1999.

8. Bonora E, Kiechl S, Oberhollenzer F, Egger G, Bonadonna RC, Muggeo M: Impaired glucose tolerance, type 2 diabetes mellitus and carotid atherosclerosis. Prospective results from the Bruneck Study. *Diabetologia* 43:156–164, 2000.

9. Barrett-Connor E: Does hyperglycemia really cause coronary heart disease? *Diabet Care* 20:1620–1623, 1997.

10. Laakso M: Hyperglycemia and cardiovascular disease in type 2 diabetes. *Diabetes* 48:937–942, 1999.

11. Turner RC, Millns H, Neil HAW, Stratton IM, Manley SE, Matthews DR, Holman RR for the United Kingdom Prospective Diabetes Study Group: Risk factors for coronary heart disease in non-insulin-dependent diabetes mellitus: United Kingdom prospective diabetes study (UKPDS: 23). *Br Med J* 316:823–828, 1998.

12. Gall MA, Borch-Johnsen K, Hougaard P, Nielsen FS, Parving HH: Albuminuria and poor glycemic control predict mortality in NIDDM. *Diabetes* 44:1303–1309, 1995.

13. Moss SE, Klein R, Klein BEK, Meuer SM: The association of glycemia and cause-specific mortality in a diabetic population. *Arch Intern Med* 154:2473–2479, 1994.

14. UK Prospective Diabetes Study Group: Intensive blood-glucose control with sulphonylureas or insulin compared with conventional treatment and risk of complications in patients with type 2 diabetes (UKPDS 33). *Lancet* 352:837–853, 1998.

15. Harris MI: Undiagnosed NIDDM: clinical and public health issue. *Diabet Care* 15:815–819, 1992.

16. Wingard DLW, Barrett-Connor E: Hearth disease and diabetes. In *Diabetes in America*. 2nd edn. Bethesda, MD: National Institutes of Health, National Institute of Diabetes and Digestive and Kidney Diseases, 1995, pp. 423–440.

17. Brun E, Nelson RG, Bennett PH, Imperatore G, Zoppini G, Verlato G, Muggeo M: Diabetes duration and cause specific mortality in the Verona Diabetes Study (submitted for publication).

18. Kuusisto J, Mykkaken L, Pyorala K, Laasko M: NIDDM and its metabolic control predict coronary heart disease in elderly subjects. *Diabetes* 43:960–967, 1994.

19. Haffner SM, Stern MP, Hazuda HP, Mitchell BD, Patterson JK: Cardiovascular risk factors in confirmed prediabetic individuals: does the clock for coronary disease start ticking before the onset of clinical diabetes? *J Am Med Assoc* 263: 2893–2898, 1990.

20. Balkau B, Shipley m, Jarrett RJ, Pyorala K, Pyorala M, Forhan A, Eschwege E: High blood glucose concentration is a risk factor for mortality in middle-aged nondiabetic men: 20-year follow-up in the Whitehall Study, The Paris Prospective Study, and the Helsinki Policemen Study. *Diabet Care* 21:360–367, 1998.

21. Muggeo M, Zoppini G, Bonora E, Brun E, Bonodonna RC, Moghetti P, Verlato G: Fasting plasma glucose variability predicts 10-year survival of type 2 diabetic patients. *Diabet Care* 23:45–50, 2000.

22. Hanefeld M, Fisher S, Julius U, Schulze J, Schwanenbeck U, Schmechel H, Ziegelash HJ, Lindner J: Risk factors for myocardial infarction and death in newly detected NIDDM: the Diabetes Intervention Study, 11-year follow-up. *Diabetologia* 39:1577–83, 1996.

23. The DECODE study group: Glucose tolerance and mortality: comparison of WHO and American Diabetes Association diagnostic criteria. *Lancet*, 354:617–621, 1999.

24. Sievers ML, Bennett PH, Nelson RG: Effect of glycemia on mortality in Pima Indians with type 2 diabetes. *Diabetes* 48:896–902, 1999.
25. Uusitupa MIJ, Niskanen LK, Siitonen O, Voutilainen E, Pyorala K: Ten-year cardiovascular mortality in relation to risk factors and abnormalities in lipoprotein composition in type 2 (non-insulin-dependent) diabetic and non-diabetic subjects. *Diabetologia* 36:1175–1184, 1993.
26. Moss SE, Klein R, Klein BEK, Meuer SM: The association of glycemic control and cause-specific mortality in a diabetic population. *Arch Intern Med* 154:2473–2479, 1994.
27. The Diabetes Control and Complications Trial Research Group. The effect of intensive treatment of diabetes on the development and progression of long-term complications in insulin-dependent diabetes mellitus. *N Engl J Med* 329:977–986, 1993.
28. University Group Diabetes Program: A study of the effects of hypoglycemic agents on vascular complications in patients with adult onset diabetes. *Diabetes* 25:1129–1253, 1975.
29. Abraira C, Colwell JA, Nuttall FQ, Sawin CT, Nagel NJ, Comstock JP, Emanuele NV, Levin SR, Henderson W, Sook Lee H, VA CSDM Group: Veterans Affairs Cooperative Study on Glycemic Control and Complications in Type II Diabetes (VA CSDM). Results of the feasibility trial. *Diabet Care* 8:1113–1123, 1995.
30. Shichiri M, Kishikawa H, Ohkubo Y, Nakayasu W: Long term results of the Kumamoto Study on Optimal Diabetes Control in Type 2 Diabetic patients. *Diabet Care* 23:B21-B29, 2000.
31. Gaede P, Vedel P, Parving HH, Pedersen O: Intensified multifactorial intervention in patients with type 2 diabetes mellitus and microalbuminuria: the Steno type 2 randomised study. *Lancet* 353:617–622, 1999.
32. Knuiman MW, Werlborn TA, Whittal DE: An analysis of excess mortality rates for persons with type 2 diabetes mellitus in Western Australia using the Cox proportional hazards regression model. *Am J Epidemiol* 135: 638–648, 1992.
33. Griffin S: Diabetes care in general practice: meta-analysis of randomized controlled trials. *Br Med J* 317:390–395, 1998.
34. Hayes TM, Harries J: Randomized controlled trial of routine hospital clinic care vs. routine general practice care for type 2 diabetics. *Br Med J* 289:728–730, 1994.
35. Zoppini G, Verlato G, Bonora E, Muggeo M: Attending the diabetes center is associated with reduced cardiovascular mortality in type 2 diabetic patients: the Verona Diabetes Study. *Diabet Metab Res Rev* 15:170–174, 1999.

23

The Pathophysiology of Hypertension in Diabetes: Microvascular Complications

S.M. THOMAS, G. GRUDEN and G.C. VIBERTI
Division of Medicine, Guy's, King's and St Thomas's School of Medicine, London, UK

Diabetes and hypertension are common conditions, frequently co-exist and both are risk factors for vascular diseases, stroke, coronary artery disease and peripheral vascular diseases (1). Further, it is increasingly recognized that hypertension is an important risk factor for several 'diabetic microvascular complications'. There is therefore a complex interaction between diabetes and blood pressure. Both have 'multifactorial' causes and presumably represent an outcome of a gene–environment interaction.

Arterial hypertension is more prevalent in diabetes as compared to the non-diabetic population and is more common in type 2 diabetes than in type 1 diabetes, where it often is a consequence of diabetic kidney disease (DKD).

HYPERTENSION AND DIABETIC KIDNEY DISEASE

The development of DKD is accompanied in both type 1 and type 2 diabetes by a rise in arterial blood pressure.

Diabetes in the New Millennium. Edited by U. Di Mario, F. Leonetti, G. Pugliese, P. Sbraccia and A. Signore.
© 2000 John Wiley & Sons, Ltd.

Type 1 diabetes

In those with normal albumin excretion rates, the prevalence of arterial hypertension, defined as SBP $\geqslant$ 160 or DBP $\geqslant$ 95 is between 6% and 15%. In type 1 diabetes there is a close link between the development and progression of DKD and the rise in arterial pressure. Even in 'normotensive' patients with microalbuminuria, both systolic and night-time diastolic ambulatory 24 hour blood pressure (BP) levels are higher than in patients with normoalbuminuria (2–4). The sitting blood pressure rises in the phase of microalbuminuria by an average of 3–4 mmHg/year, as compared to 1 mmHg/year in long-term normoalbuminuric and health controls (2186). The level of blood pressure correlates with both the rate of development of DKD (Viberti, unpublished data) and with the rate of progression of established DKD (5).

Thus, arterial hypertension and DKD develop in parallel in type 1 diabetes, and the rise in arterial pressure and possibly abnormalities in diurnal BP rhythm are the major determinant, not only of the rate of progression of the diabetic renal disease but also of associated cardiovascular comorbidity and mortality.

There is some debate as to whether a rise in arterial pressure may precede the development of microalbuminuria. In a 7 year longitudinal study of 137 patients in the UK, mean arterial pressures (MAP) were higher in those who developed microalbuminuria as compared to those who remained normoalbuminuric (6). The mean MAP at the start of the study was 138/82, as compared to 124/73 in those who maintained normal albumin excretion rate (AER). In multiple regression analysis, initial, blood pressure and smoking were significant determinants of the development of persistent microalbuminuria. This finding did not confirm a previous study of 205 patients during a 5 year follow-up period where with less accurate measurements blood pressure tended to rise after the development of microalbuminuria (7). A longitudinal study of 24 hour BR monitoring showed a parallel rise in BP and AER before the development of microalbuminuria (8). Thus, that hypertension is merely a consequence of renal disease in type 1 diabetes is open to serious question, with the suggestion that pre-existing raised arterial pressure may be a risk factor for the development of the renal lesion. It is also possible that this close relationship between DKD and hypertension may lie in the existence of common antecedents (9).

Separate independent studies in different cohorts have established that patients with type 1 diabetes who develop DKD have a familial predisposition to hypertension. In a study of 26 surviving parents of 17 patients with type 1 diabetes and nephropathy, mean systolic pressures were 15 mmHg higher and diastolic pressures 8 mmHg higher than in the parents of non-proteinuric diabetic controls (10). This was later confirmed in a series of other studies (11,12). Similarly, in the EURODIAB IDDM study, a cross-sectional study of

3250 patients with type 1 diabetes from 16 European centres, both albuminuria and hypertension in the diabetic offspring was associated with hypertension in the parents (13).

Thus, the suggestion is that common factors may link the risk of essential hypertension and the development of DKD in type 1 diabetes. This has prompted a search for common genetic risk factors but to date no conclusive evidence has been obtained (14).

Type 2 diabetes

Hypertension is more common in type 2 diabetes than in both the non-diabetic population and in type 1 diabetes, particularly in women, even when adjusted for age and body mass index (BMI). Using the WHO BP criteria, the prevalence of hypertension in type 2 diabetes was 29% in men and 25% in women. There was a marked effect of age, particularly on SBP, and in patients older than 55 years there is a prevalence of 43% in males and 52% in females.

Similarly, in the hypertension in diabetes study, an arm of the UK Prospective Diabetes Study (UKPDS), where hypertension was defined as SBP$\geqslant$160 or DBP$\geqslant$90 mmHg in patients not on treatment or SBP$\geqslant$150 mmHg, DBP$\geqslant$85 mmHg, in those on anti-hypertensives the prevalence of hypertension was 39% (35% in men, 46% in women) (1).

Hypertension in both diabetic and non-diabetic populations is more common in certain ethnic groups. In the UKPDS there was a prevalence of hypertension in blacks of 49%, and in whites of 38%, with people of Asian origin, largely from the Indian sub-continent, having the lowest prevalence (35%).

There remains a strong association between DKD and hypertension at least in some populations.

In the UKPDS Hypertension in Diabetes study, intensive treatment of blood pressure (mean 144/82 mmHg) resulted in a 29% reduction in the risk of microalbuminuria and a 39% reduction in the risk of clinical proteinuria, as compared with less tight control (mean 154/87 mmHg) after 6 years (15). The importance of blood pressure in the development of the renal lesion in type 2 diabetes is clear in the Pima Indians. This race of native Americans have a very high prevalence of type 2 diabetes and elevated blood pressure before the onset of diabetes predicts albuminuria after the development of type 2 diabetes (16).

MECHANISMS OF DIABETIC INJURY

Therefore for a number of reasons hypertension is common in both type 1 and type 2 diabetes. The mechanism by which hypertension may promote macrovascular disease in diabetes is similar to that in non-diabetic subjects, thus we shall focus on the mechanism by which hypertension may promote diabetic microvascular complications. To explore this we shall use the glomerulus as a model. The association between arterial hypertension and the glomerular lesion is the best described, although the processes may apply to other microvascular circulations.

The importance of hypertension in the development of diabetic glomerular injury is demonstrated clearly in models of renal artery stenosis. If diabetic rats have a renal artery unilaterally clipped — the two-kidney, one-clip Goldblatt model — there is the development of much more severe glomerular lesions in the unclipped kidney (17). Consistent with this, autopsy findings in diabetic patients with unilateral renal artery stenosis showed nodular glomerulosclerotic lesions to be confined to the kidney with the patent renal artery (18,19).

Intraglomerular pressure is maintained by the resistance in the afferent and efferent arterioles which relates to the tone in the myocytes within the vessel walls. Following the development of diabetes there is vasodilatation of both the afferent and efferent arterioles. The degree of vasodilatation of the afferent arteriole is, however, significantly greater than that seen in the efferent arteriole. Overall, this results in an increase in renal blood flow but the imbalance between the afferent and the efferent vasodilatation results in a marked increase in the intraglomerular transcapillary pressure (Figure 23.1). In both animal models of diabetes and in type 1 diabetes in humans, this results in elevated glomerular filtration rate (GFR) levels early in the disease which is associated with increased glomerular and renal volume.

An elevation of renal plasma flow of 9%–14% is reported in type 1 diabetes and the distribution of GFR in type 1 diabetes is shifted to the right, as compared with non-diabetic controls (20). The hypothesis is that those with the highest GFRs are those at most risk of DKD. This, however, remains controversial. Two retrospective studies demonstrated that the initial rate of glomerular hyperfiltration positively correlated with the development of DKD (21,22). This was not confirmed by a prospective 10-year case–control study, which found no association between early hyperfiltration and the subsequent development of DKD, although there was a higher rate of GFR decline in the groups with initial hyperfiltration prior to the development of proteinuria (23).

Studies in the Munich Wistar rat have demonstrated that diabetes results in an increase in whole kidney and single nephron GFR (24). After the onset of diabetes there is an increase in single nephron plasma flow and in the glomerular transcapillary hydraulic pressure. The more severe degrees of structural glomerular damage in these rats were associated with the higher rates of single nephron GFR (25). The loss of afferent arteriolar tone also results in a loss of renal autoregulation, and even small rises in systemic arterial pressure are transmitted directly to the glomerulus (26). Thus, it may be expected that

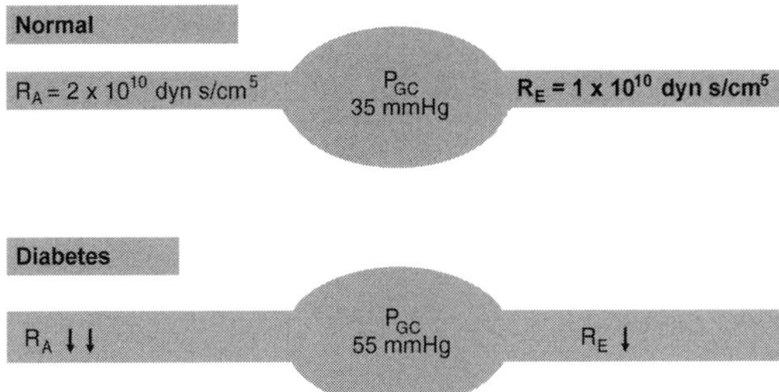

Figure 23.1. Regulation of intraglomerular pressure. R_A = resistance afferent; R_E = resistance efferent > ; P_{GC} = pressure glomerular capillary

the development of raised arterial pressure may be more deleterious to the kidney in diabetes than in those without diabetes.

MECHANISMS OF HAEMODYNAMIC DAMAGE

The key clinicopathological features of DKD are an increase in glomerular permeability, which is associated with increases in mesangial matrix volume, eventually leading to sclerosis of the glomerulus and capillary occlusion.

In vitro models simulating the effect of this haemodynamic insult in the glomerulus have been developed. Mesangial cells are connected to the capillary wall via cytoplasmic projections and rises in capillary pressure are therefore associated with a stretching of the mesangial cell (Figure 23.2). Recent calculations suggest that the typical rise in glomerular pressure in type 1 diabetes is associated with an *in vitro* mesangial cell stretching of

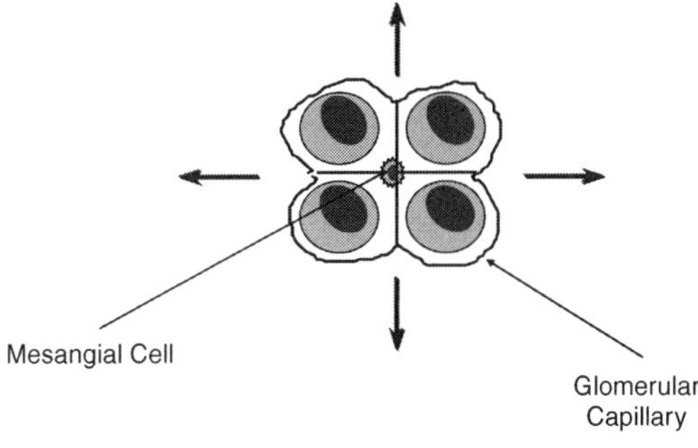

Figure 23.2. Mesangial cell stretching as a result of haemodynamic insult in the glomerulus causing rises in capillary pressure

approximately 10% as compared to around 4% at normal levels of intraglomerular pressure (27).

The application of mechanical stretch to cultured mesangial cells induces the production of both human matrix components, such as fibronectin (28), and of pro-sclerotic growth factors, such as TGFβ1(29,30). This matrix induction appears to be, at least initially, a direct effect of stretch, as in rat mesangial cells stretch-induced a1 (I) collagen gene expression precedes that of TGFβ1 and is unchanged by TGFβ1 inhibition (31).

This, however, does not exclude a late, indirect effect whereby stretch-induced TGFβ1 may augment matrix production. Recently Gruden *et al* (32) have shown that stretch can directly induce fibronectin production which occurs early and is TGFβ1-independent. This increase in matrix production was perpetuated by late stretch induced TGFβ1 production, resulting in a substantial and prolonged TGFβ1-dependent fibronectin production.

A number of intracellular mediators of stretch induced matrix production have been identified. The application of mechanical stretch to in rat mesangial cells activates several members of the mitogen-activated protein (MAP) kinase family, such as extracellular-regulated kinases 1 and 2 (Erk1–2) and c-Jun N-terminal kinase 1 and 2 (Jnk1–2) (33). Another important intra-cellular kinase, that has been implicated is p38 MAP kinase, the human homologue of the yeast, which is activated in response to various extracellular stresses, such as hyperosmolar and oxidative stress and TGFβ1 and inflammatory cytokines.

P38 MAP kinase activates transcription factors enhancing extracellular matrix gene expression. Studies in human mesangial cells showed a significant increase in activated p38 MAP kinase levels, with an activation time course different from that of other MAP kinases activated by stretch, such as Jnk1–2 and Erk1–2 (32,33). Stretch-induced activation of JnK-1 and ERK1–2 returns to basal within 60 and 120 minutes, whereas that of p38 MAP kinase was still sustained after 33 hours.

P38 MAP kinase activation is protein kinase C (PKC)-dependent, which is of importance as stretch is known to activate PKC, and PKC activation is thought to be of importance in the pathogenesis of many diabetic vascular lesions (34).

In this study, stretch-induced fibronectin was p38 MAP kinase-dependent, as was TGFβ1 induced fibronectin production. P38 MAP kinase phosphorylates the activation domain of c-fos and c-jun, increasing their transcriptional activity. c-fos and c-jun combine to form the AP1 transcription complex, which activates genes with a TPA-response element (TRE) in their promoter region, such as TGFβ1 and fibronectin.

These stretch-induced effects, importantly, do not occur at 'physiological' degrees of mesangial stretch of around 4% and appear to be a consequence of higher intraglomerular pressures, producing abnormal degrees of cell stretch.

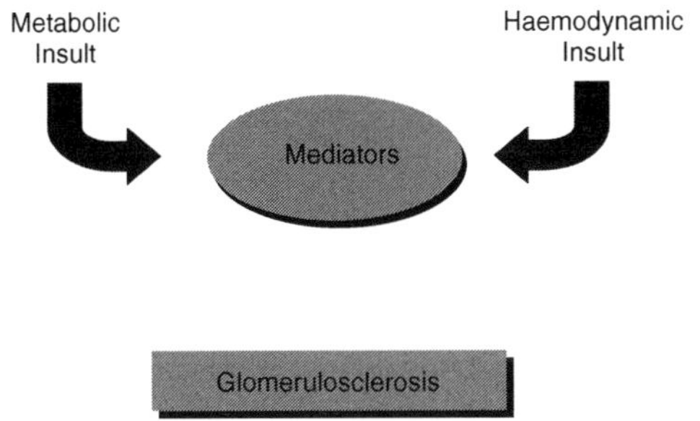

Figure 23.3. Mechanisms of diabetic nephropathy

They also appear to be relatively specific, as no increase in matrix production is seen in fibroblasts when a mechanical stretch is applied.

There is an important interaction between the metabolic insult of diabetes and the haemodynamic one (Figure 23.3). Clinically, the progression of DKD is associated with both higher arterial pressures and worse glycaemic control (35). At the cellular level, exposure to high glucose concentrations can induce the production of TGFβ1 and matrix production (36), as well as important intracellular mediators such as PKC and P38 MAP kinase (34,37). The metabolic and haemodynamic insults interact also at the cellular level. The application of mechanical stretch augments glucose-induced matrix production in mesangial cells (38), suggesting important synergy between the haemodynamic and the metabolic insults. It will be appreciated that this synergy may operate at a number of levels, with several of the intracellular mediators such as PKC and P38 MAP kinase being potential sites where the two processes may interact.

The application of mechanical stretch to human mesangial cells also induces other important cytokines, such as VEGF (39), a potent permeability factor, which is highly expressed in the glomerular capillary wall and may be important in glomerular permeability and in the regulation of arteriolar tone via induction of nitric oxide production (40).

Stretch also interacts with the renin–angiotensin system (RAS) in mesangial cells. *In vitro*, angiotensin II (Ang II) and stretch independently induce human mesangial cell production of VEGF (41). Ang ll-induced VEGF, but not stretch induced VEGF, is completely inhibited by the AT1 receptor antagonist losartan. Thus, Ang II is not the mediator of stretch-induced VEGF. Importantly, though, the application of stretch to human mesangial cells upregulates the AT1 receptor, resulting in an augmentation of Ang II-induced VEGF production.

This complex interaction between Ang II and the haemodynamic insult raises the interesting possibility that the pre-existent intraglomerular pressure level modulates the Ang II effects on mesangial cells.

CONCLUSION

At the clinical level, not only is hypertension common in diabetes but the diabetic microcirculation is more vulnerable to fluctuations in systemic arterial pressure. At the cellular level, many of the pathways by which altered haemodynamics may lead to the pathological features of excess permeability and sclerosis are being discovered. In addition, complex interactions between the haemodynamic setting and the metabolic mediators of diabetic injury are becoming apparent.

REFERENCES

1. UKPDS Prospective Diabetes Study (UKPDS) Group: Hypertension in Diabetes Study (HDS): II. Increased risk of cardiovascular complications in hypertensive type 2 diabetic patients [published erratum appears in *J Hypertens* 11(6):681, 1993]. *J Hypertens* 11:319–325, 1993.
2. Hansen KW, Christensen CK, Andersen PH, Pedersen MM, Christiansen JS, Mogensen CE: Ambulatory blood pressure in microalbuminuric type 1 diabetic patients. *Kidney Int* 41:847–854, 1992.
3. Hansen KW, Mau Pedersen M, Marshall SM, Christiansen JS, Mogensen CE: Circadian variation of blood pressure in patients with diabetic nephropathy. *Diabetologia* 35:1074–1079, 1992.
4. Voros P, Lengyel Z, Nagy V, Nemeth C, Rosivall L, Kammerer L: Diurnal blood pressure variation and albuminuria in normotensive patients with insulin-dependent diabetes mellitus. *Nephrol, Dialysis Transpl* 13:2257–2260, 1998.
5. Rossing P, Hommel E, Smidt UM, Parving HH: Impact of arterial blood pressure and albuminuria on the progression of diabetic nephropathy in IDDM patients. *Diabetes* 42:715–719, 1993.
6. Microalbuminuria Collaborative Study Group United Kingdom. Predictors of microalbuminuria in Type 1 diabetes mellitus. *Diabet Med* 16 918–16 925, 1999.
7. Mathiesen ER, Ronn B, Jensen T, Storm B, Deckert T: Relationship between blood pressure and urinary albumin excretion in development of microalbuminuria. *Diabetes* 39:245–249, 1990.
8. Poulsen PL, Ebbehoj E, Hansen KW, Mogensen CE: 24-h blood pressure and autonomic function is related to albumin excretion within the normoalbuminuric range in IDDM patients. *Diabetologia* 40:718–725, 1997.
9. Viberti GC, Earle K: Predisposition to essential hypertension and the development of diabetic nephropathy. *J Am Soc Nephrol* 3:S27–33, 1992.
10. Viberti GC, Keen H, Wiseman MJ: Raised arterial pressure in parents of proteinuric insulin dependent diabetics. *Br Med J Clin Res Ed* 295:515–517, 1987.
11. Barzilay J, Warram JH, Bak M, Laffel LM, Canessa M, Krolewski AS: Predisposition to hypertension: risk factor for nephropathy and hypertension in IDDM. *Kidney Int* 41:723–730, 1992.
12. Fagerudd JA, Tarnow L, Jacobsen P, Stenman S, Nielsen FS, Pettersson-Fernholm KJ, Gronhagen-Riska C, Parving HH, Groop PH: Predisposition to essential hypertension and development of diabetic nephropathy in IDDM patients. *Diabetes* 47:439–444, 1998.

13. Roglic G, Colhoun HM, Stevens LK, Lemkes HH, Manes C, Fuller JH: Parental history of hypertension and parental history of diabetes and microvascular complications in insulin-dependent diabetes mellitus: the EURODIAB IDDM Complications Study. *Diabet Med* 15:418–426, 1998.
14. Doria A: Genetic markers of increased susceptibility to diabetic nephropathy. *Horm Res* 50(Suppl 1):6–11, 1998.
15. UKPDS Prospective Diabetes Study (UKPDS) Group: Efficacy of atenolol and captopril in reducing risk of macrovascular and microvascular complications in type 2 diabetes: UKPDS 39. UK Prospective Diabetes Study Group. *Br Med J* 317:713–720, 1998.
16. Nelson RG, Pettitt DJ, Baird HR, Charles MA, Liu QZ, Bennett PH, Knowler WC: Pre-diabetic blood pressure predicts urinary albumin excretion after the onset of type 2 (non-insulin-dependent) diabetes mellitus in Pima Indians. *Diabetologia* 36:998–1001, 1993.
17. Mauer SM, Steffes MW, Azar S, Sandberg SK, Brown DM: The effects of Goldblatt hypertension on development of the glomerular lesions of diabetes mellitus in the rat. *Diabetes* 27:738–744, 1978.
18. Berkman J, Rifkin H: Unilateral nodular diabetic glomerulosclerosis (Kimmelstiel Wilson). Report of a case. *Metabolism* 22:715–722, 1973.
19. Beroniade VC, Lefebvre R, Falardeau P: Unilateral diabetic glomerulosclerosis recurrence of an experiment of nature. *Am J Nephrol* 7:55–59, 1987.
20. Barnes DJ, Pinto J, Viberti GC, Cameron S, Davison AM, Grunfeld J, Kerr D, Ritz E, Winearls C. Eds. The patient with diabetes mellitus. In *Oxford Textbook of Clinical Nephrology*. 2nd edn. Oxford: Oxford Medical, pp. 723–777, 1998.
21. Mogensen CE: Early glomerular hyperfiltration in insulin-dependent diabetics and late nephropathy. *Scand J Clin Lab Invest* 46:201–206, 1986.
22. Mogensen CE, Christensen CK: Predicting diabetic nephropathy in insulin-dependent patients. *N Engl J Med* 311:89–93, 1984.
23. Yip JW, Jones SL, Wiseman MJ, Hill C, Viberti GC: Glomerular hyperfiltration in the prediction of nephropathy in IDDM: a 10-year follow-up study. *Diabetes* 45:1729–1733, 1996.
24. Hostetter TH, Troy JL, Brenner BM: Glomerular hemodynamics in experimental diabetes mellitus. *Kidney Int* 19:410–415, 1981.
25. Hostetter TH, Rennke HG, Brenner BM: The case for intrarenal hypertension in the initiation and progression of diabetic and other glomerulopathies. *Am J Med* 72:375–380, 1982.
26. Zatz R, Mayer TW, Rennke HG, Brenner BM: Predominance of haemodynamic rather than metabolic factors in the pathogenesis of diabetic glomerulopathy. Proc *Natl Acad Sci USA* 82:5963–5967, 1985.
27. Cortes P, Riser BL, Zhao X, Narins RG: Glomerular volume expansion and mesangial cell mechanical strain: mediators of glomerular pressure injury. *Kidney Int* 45(Suppl):S11–16, 1994.
28. Riser BL, Cortes P, Zhao X, Bernstein J, Dumler F, Narins RG: Intraglomerular pressure and mesangial stretching stimulate extracellular matrix formation in the rat. *J Clin Invest* 90:1932–1943, 1992.
29. Gruden G, Thomas SM, Sacks S, Burt D, Chusney GD, Viberti GC: Mechanical stretching induces TGF-β1 gene expression and protein secretion in human mesangial cells. [Abstract] *Diabet Med* 13(4)(Suppl 3):96, 1995.
30. Riser BL, Cortes P, Heilig C, Grondin J, Ladson-Wofford S, Patterson, D, Narins RG: Cyclic stretching force selectively upregulates transforming growth factor-beta isoforms in cultured rat mesangial cells. *Am J Pathol* 148:1915–1923, 1996.

31. Riser BL, Cortes P, Yee J: Modelling the effects of vascular stress in mesangial cells. *Curr Opin Nephrol Hypertens* 9:43–47, 2000.
32. Gruden G, Zonca S, Hayward A, Thomas S, Gnudi L, Viberti GC. P38 Mitogen activated protein kinase is central to the sclerotic process elicited by mechanical stretch in human mesangial cells. *Diabetes* 49(4):655–661, 2000.
33. Ishida T, Haneda M, Maeda S, Koya D, Kikkawa R: Stretch induced overproduction of fibronectin in mesangial cells is mediated by the activation of mitogen activated protein kinase. *Diabetes* 48:595–602, 1999.
34. Ishii H, Koya D, King GL: Protein kinase C activation and its role in the development of vascular complications in diabetes mellitus. *J Mol Med* 76:21–31, 1998.
35. Alaveras AE, Thomas SM, Sagriotis A, Viberti GC: Promoters of progression of diabetic nephropathy: the relative roles of blood glucose and blood pressure control. *Nephrol Dialysis Transpl* 12(Suppl 2):71–74, 1997.
36. Ziyadeh FN, Sharma K, Ericksen M, Wolf G: Stimulation of collagen gene expression and protein synthesis in murine mesangial cells by high glucose is mediated by autocrine activation of transforming growth factor-beta. *J Clin Invest* 93:536–542, 1994.
37. Igarashi M, Wakasaki H, Takahara N, Ishii H, Jiang ZY, Yamauchi T, Kuboki K, Meier M, Rhodes CJ, King GL: Glucose or diabetes activates p38 mitogen-activated protein kinase via different pathways. *J Clin Invest* 103:185–195, 1999.
38. Cortes P, Zhao X, Riser BL, Narins RG: Role of glomerular mechanical strain in the pathogenesis of diabetic nephropathy. *Kidney Int* 51:57–68, 1997.
39. Gruden G, Thomas S, Burt D, Lane S, Chusney G, Sacks S, Viberti G: Mechanical stretch induces vascular permeability factor in human mesangial cells: mechanisms of signal transduction. *Proc Natl Acad Sci USA* 94:12112–12116, 1997.
40. Brenchley P. VEGF/VPF: a modulator of microvascular function with potential roles in glomerular pathophysiology. *J Nephrol* 9(1):10–17, 1996.
41. Gruden G, Thomas S, Burt D, Zhou W, Chusney G, Gnudi L, Viberti G: Interaction of angiotensin II and mechanical stretch on vascular endothelial growth factor production by human mesangial cells. *J Amer Soc Nephrol* 10:730–737, 1999.

24

Distal By-pass and Endoluminal Revascularization in Diabetic Patients with Limb-threatening Ischemia

GIOVANNI GHIRLANDA and FRANCO CITTERIO
Policlinico Universitario A. Gemelli, Università Cattolica, Rome, Italy

Diabetes is the leading cause of amputations in peacetime. These are generally performed for uncontrolled sepsis, for extensive osteomyelitis and above all for critical ischemia of legs due to peripheral vascular disease (1–2). Many reports have pointed out the severity of this disease. It is estimated that 16–58% of diabetics have an ischemic leg and 15% of patients at some point in their disease have ischemic ulcers on their feet, with a 0.5% annual incidence of gangrene. About 3% of all diabetics will undergo an amputation because of gangrene and half of them will need a second amputation within 2–3 years of the first (3). Therefore, ischemic leg represents an important social problem, considerably contributing to morbidity, mortality and health care costs of diabetics. In the USA, the costs of an amputation have been estimated as $20 000 and, moreover, the impact on quality of life is very profound (4–5). The first step in reducing amputations is prevention through an intensive educational programme. In many centers an intensive educational programme has reduced amputations by 50% (6–8). WHO and most diabetic associations have proposed reduction by 50% of amputations in diabetics as one the main goals in the management of diabetes for subsequent years (9). Intervention on known risk factors, such as metabolic control, smoking, hypertension and

Diabetes in the New Millennium. Edited by U. Di Mario, F. Leonetti, G. Pugliese, P. Sbraccia and A. Signore.
© 2000 John Wiley & Sons, Ltd.

dyslipidemia, is very important (10). Another goal should be to increase revascularization procedures as much as possible, which are often refused to diabetics due to a supposed small vessel disease responsible for the trophic lesions and not suitable for surgical intervention (11–12).

For several years the only proposed therapy has been demolitive: the frequent and often indiscriminated indication for amputation was due to reluctance to perform limb revascularization in these patients. Indeed, widespread opinion was that necrotic foot lesions were caused by micro-angiopathy, similar to that present in the kidney and the retina. So diabetics were often given the impression that amputation was part of their disease, and many doctors also accepted this fate. Recent data derived by light and electron microscopy, vascular casting of freshly amputated limbs and physiological studies on capillary permeability, performed with labelled albumin, did not confirm the view that diabetic patients have more occlusive vascular disease in the foot than non-diabetics (10).

Diabetic patients indeed have a peculiar pattern of arterial obstruction, which consists of a precocious and preferential involvement of infrapopliteal arteries that spares more proximal sites and distal vessels, such as the dorsalis pedis and plantar arches (Table 24.1). It is possible that infrapopliteal vascular occlusion without the possibility of an efficient collateral circulation brings about precocious ischemic damage without a serious involvement of the iliac and pedal vessels (13). In diabetes there are many functional alterations of microcirculation: loss of autoregulation, reduced hyperemic response to different stimuli (thermal, pain), abnormal rheological properties of blood cells. Endothelial function is then disturbed in a thrombophilic way and, if neuropathy is also present, neurogenic flow regulation is lacking. When ischemia due to femoropopliteal occlusive disease is superimposed, the effects of these alterations are amplified and we observe the well-known clinical picture of diabetic trophic foot lesions (14–15).

This new biological knowledge, together with recent advances in imaging technology, such as intra-arterial digital subtraction angiography, improvement in surgery of vascular anastomosis, better metabolic and intensive care and progress in anesthesia management, have all contributed to prompting surgeons to perform distal revascularization in diabetics as well as non-diabetics (12,16).

Table 24.1.　Rate of significant stenosis or occlusion in different districts of arterial tree in our series of diabetic patients with limb ischemia

Region	(%)
Aortoiliac	35
Femoral	68
Popliteotibial	80
Dorsoplantar	15

Prosthetic vascular grafts in low flow segments tend to occlude rapidly. Better results are achieved with autologous saphenous vein, reversed to allow blood flow, or *in situ* after valvulotomy. The *in situ* technique is particularly suitable for longer bypasses because of lesser incidence of torsion, but it does not lack complications, such as thrombosis due to intimal damage or incomplete valvulotomy, hemorrhages due to the rupture of a fissurated vein and A–V fistulas that may cause intratissular hematoma or ischemia by diversion of the blood. Recent use of angioscopy has significantly reduced these complications. The use of the reversed saphenous vein remains a good surgical technique for short bypasses or when arterial and vein sites of anastomosis are distant from each other. Both techniques have a deleterious effect on endothelial cells, which mainly lose their fibrinolytic function, which is then fully restored after a month.

As the femoral superficial and popliteal arteries are often sites of arteriosclerotic stenosis, concerns have been raised over the choice of these arteries as inflow sites for distal bypasses. Several reports have demonstrated that bypasses with more distal graft origin sites compared favorably with those of common femoral origin, and also that the presence of a stenosis with a diameter of less than 35% does not influence the graft patency rate. Preoperative percutaneous transluminal angioplasty is effective in improving the patency rate when a stenosis proximal to the inflow site significantly reduces blood flow. Stenoses shorter than 3 cm are usually suitable for the PTA treatment.

Also, outflow quality influences bypass patency: a good run-off is defined by the continuity of the outflow vessels with the foot and, in the case of the peroneal artery, direct communication between one of the terminal branches and a pedal vessel. For the dorsalis pedis, a good outflow is defined as continuity with a patent pedal arch and with most visible interdigital arteries. Moreover, in distal bypasses with a popliteal origin, the length of vein graft needed is shorter, allowing better choice of the portion of the vein to be used, and it is then possible to easily discard small-diameter segments or diseased areas.

Two subgroups of patients deserve further comment about the opportunity to perform a distal bypass: patients with type 1 diabetes and a severe microangiopathy at renal and ocular level, and patients with a pedal dorsal artery not in continuity with any sural vessel. The Boston group, directed by Dr LoGerfo (17) presented data on a group of patients with type 1 diabetes with severe ischemia and retinopathy in 92% of cases and renal failure in 45%. The graft patency rate and limb salvage were acceptable when compared with other series of distal bypasses performed on ischemia in type 2 diabetes. Moreover, no patients in this study lost the limb while the grafts were patent; this confirms that occlusive large vessel disease is the leading cause for limb loss also in these patients with severe microangiopathy in other areas (17).

Some patients have a peculiar pattern of arterial occlusion that affects all three tibial vessels without a continuity with the reconstituted dorsal pedal artery below the ankle. Bypasses were performed also in patients where the artery was not visualized but where there was an audible Doppler signal at its anatomic location. In several instances an active infection of the foot was also present, and this was treated with intravenous antibiotics and an accurate wound debridement. After a mean of 10 days, the local situation was considered suitable for the intervention. The overall results in this kind of patient are comparable with other series of diabetic patients in terms of patency graft rate (80% at 18 months), mortality and limb salvage (17).

Finally it is noteworthy that in some instances, if the bypass failed, limb salvage was equally achieved. Because the increased metabolic demands of active infections and extensive tissue loss may overcome the healing possibilities of an ischemic limb with otherwise sufficient circulation, a temporary good blood flow may be crucial to obtain the definitive healing of a lesion.

We studied a series of 89 consecutive diabetic patients (55 men, 34 women) referred to our hospital for trophic damage of limbs (ischemic lesions, limited necrosis or gangrene). Their mean age was 65 ± 10 years; mean duration of diabetes was 12 ± 4 years. Ulcers of different severity were the indication for surgery in 56 patients; in 22 cases distal revascularization was indicated for limited gangrene involving one or more toes. All patients underwent preoperative traditional or digital angiography; Doppler flowmetry and measurement of brachial–ankle index were performed. In cases with angiographic evidence of unsatisfactory distal vessels, intraoperative angiography and direct run-off exploration were performed. Bypass procedures were performed when one of the three arteries of the lower limb or one of the two arteries of the foot was demonstrated to be patent and when peripheral vasculature was judged adequate (evidence of plantar arch and most metatarsal and digital arteries) (Table 24.2).

Sixty-seven infrapopliteal bypasses were performed. Autologous reversed saphenous vein was used in 64 cases; two patients received a composite graft of polytetrafluoroethylene (PTFE) plus saphenous vein, and in 1 patient a prosthetic graft (PTFE) was implanted. Forty-six grafts originated from the common or superficial femoral and 21 from the popliteal artery.

Distal anastomosis was found in the tibioperoneal artery in nine cases, the posterior tibial artery in 32 cases, the anterior tibial artery in six cases, the

Table 24.2 Indication for revascularization

Ischemic lesions
Nonhealing neuropathic ulcers
Rest pain
Severe claudicatio
Rapidly ingravescent claudicatio

dorsalis pedis artery in 16 cases and the peroneal artery in four cases. Because of poor run-off, four distal arteriovenous fistulas and four sequential bypasses with intermediate anastomosis to the popliteal artery were performed (in two cases, both procedures were carried out). Owing to concomitant aorto-iliac disease, six patients also required an adjunctive femoral revascularization, performed by axillo-femoral bypass. Additional vascular procedures (one profundoplasty and one endarterectomy of the superficial femoral artery) were performed in two of the patients receiving a simple distal bypass. Minor amputation (digital or transmetatarsal) was performed concomitantly in 30 cases and postponed in 37. Peridural anesthesia was always employed; in cases of adjunctive axillofemoral bypass, proximal surgical procedures were done under local anesthesia. Antibiotic prophylaxis was routinely used. After the operation, anti-aggregant and oral anticoagulant drugs were administrated.

Follow-up consisted of clinical visits and Doppler examinations every month for at least 1 year and every 6 months thereafter. When indicated, control angiography was performed. According to the established criteria, 67 patients of 89 patients (75%), were found suitable for reconstructive surgery; 19% did not qualify for surgery after preoperative angiography; and 6% were excluded after intraoperative angiography and exploration. Out of the 67 operated patients, two died in the postoperative period from myocardial infarction and cardiac arrest. Other postoperative complications were reversible acute renal failure in two cases, pulmonary embolism with good outcome in one case, and gas gangrene in one case, which required lower limb amputation. Early graft thrombosis occurred in six cases (9%), but in four of them immediate graft revision was successful.

No late deaths occurred and no patients were lost to follow-up in the 5 year period. Altogether, the 1 year actuarial patency rate was 75% and the 5 year actuarial patency rate 65%. Causes of failure were amputation for gas gangrene (1.5%), early thrombosis (3%) and late thrombosis (9%). Only in one case of late thrombosis was intervention attempted, but it was not successful.

Good functional rehabilitation of the foot (with complete integrity or minor amputation) was obtained in every case of surgical success. The limb salvage rate was 85% at 1 year and 80% at 5 years. At present, in none of the six cases of late thrombosis has lower limb or foot amputation been necessary. In our group of diabetic patients with trophic limb lesions, distal revascularization was possible in 75% of cases. Good results in terms of graft patency, limb salvage and postoperative complications justify this surgical indication. Mortality was lower than that observed for major amputations.

More recently, new technologies have been applied to vascular surgery with the use of catheter-based techniques that allow endoluminal recanalization procedures. The use of thrombolysis to open occluded vessels, in association with percutaneous transluminal angioplasty, stenting and atherectomy to remove and treat critical stenosis, has brought us into a new era in the treatment of peripheral vascular disease.

The advantages of endovascular procedures include the possibility of performing interventions under local or peridural anesthesia, minor traumatization, quick recovery and early discharge of the patient. Disadvantages are the limited long-term success rate vs. classical bypass surgery and the high rate of restenosis. Nevertheless, considering that the diabetic patient has a high risk for cardiovascular accidents, minor surgical procedures also achieving limited results may better apply to patients whose life expectancy is less than 50% after 10 years (3,18,19).

Recently, endovascular revascularization by mechanical atherectomy using Auth's rotational device (Rotablator) has been advocated in the treatment of the occlusion of peripheral arteries. New atherotomes, which are provided with a rotating head, cause minor damage in the arterial wall and result in a more rapid endothelialization of the inner surface.

We studied 74 patients with type 2 diabetes: the mean duration of disease was 15 years and mean age was 64 years. All of them showed ischemic trophic lesions and were referred to our department for distal revascularization or below-knee amputation. All underwent intra-arterial digital subtraction angiography: 19 patients showed extended occlusion of the femoral superficial artery, while the popliteal and tibial arteries were occluded in 39 patients and stenotic in 16 patients. Mechanical atherectomy was performed in 66 patients without any significant side-effects and resulted in immediate patency of the treated arteries. During the first week after revascularization, the patients were treated with heparin and were subsequently discharged with anticoagulant therapy. Two patients had occlusion of the treated segment after 3 months, while in 64 patients the vessels have been patent for a mean follow-up period of 16 months (range 2–96 months). The limb salvage rate was 93%. We conclude that mechanical atherectomy with the Rotablator is a safe and effective endoluminal recanalization procedure in diabetic patients, mainly in those presenting with general or local contraindications to bypass surgery.

In conclusion, we think that in the future diabetic ischemic lesions should be managed with the same basic principles used in vascular reconstructive surgery in non-diabetic patients, and that no patients should be any longer denied a distal revascularization for limb salvage because of their diabetes (12,20).

REFERENCES

1. The LEA Study Group: Comparing the incidence of lower extremity amputations across the world: the global lower limb extremity amputation study. *Diabet Med* 12:14–18, 1995.

2. Reiber GE, Lipsky BA, Gibbons GW: The burden of diabetic foot ulcer. *Am J Surg* 176:5–10, 1998.
3. Larsson J, Agard CD, Apelqvist P: Long term prognosis after amputation in diabetic patient. *Clin Orthop* 350:149–158, 1998.
4. Apelqvist J, Larsson J, Ragnarsson-Tennvall G, Persson U: Long term costs in diabetic patients with foot ulcers. *Foot Ankle* 16:388–394, 1995.
5. Holzer SE., Camerota A, Marteus L, Cuerdon T, Crystal-Peters J, Zagari M: Costs and duration of care for lower extremity ulcers in patient with diabetes. *Clin Ther* 1:169–181, 1998.
6. Edmonds ME, Blundell MP, Morris ME, Thomas EM, Cotton LT, Watkins PJ: Improved survival of the diabetic foot: the role of a specialised foot clinic. *Q J Med* 60:763–771, 1986.
7. Holstein P, Ellitsgaard N, Sorensen S, Bornefeldt Olsen B, Black E, Ellitsgaard V, Perrild H: The number of amputations has decreased. *Nord Med* 11:142–144, 1996.
8. Larsson J, Apelqvist J, Agard CD, Stenstrom A: Decreasing incidence of major amputation in diabetic patients: a consequence of a multidisciplinary foot care team approach? *Diabetic Medi* 12: 770–776, 1995.
9. Edmonds ME, Boulton A, Buckenham T, Every N, Foster A *et al*: Saint Vincent and improving diabetes care. Report of the diabetic foot and amputation group. *Diabet Med* 13(Suppl 1):S27–S42, 1996.
10. Falkenberg M: Metabolic control and amputations among diabetics in primary health care. A population based intensified program governed by patient education. *Scand Prim Health Care* 8:96–102, 1990.
11. LoGerfo FW, Colman JD: Vascular and microvascular disease of the foot in diabetes. Implications for foot care. *N Engl J Med* 311:1615–1619, 1984.
12. LoGerfo FW, Gibbons GB, Pomposelli FB: Trends in the care of the diabetic foot. Expanded role of arterial reconstruction. *Arch Surg* 125:617–621, 1992.
13. Faglia E, Favales F, Quarantiello A *et al*: Angiographic evaluation of peripheral arterial occlusive disease and its role as a prognostic determinant for major amputation in diabetic subjects with foot ulcers. *Diabet Care* 4:625–630, 1998.
14. Ubbink DT, Kitslaar PH, Tordoir JH, Reneman RS, Jacobs MJ: Skin microcirculation in diabetic and non-diabetic patients at different stages of lower limb ischemia. *Eur J Vasc Surg* 7:659–666, 1993.
15. Tooke JE, Brash PD: Microvascular aspects of diabetic foot disease. *Diabet Med* 13:26–29, 1996.
16. Estes JM, Pomposelli FB Jr: Lower extremity arterial reconstruction in patients with diabetes. *Diabet Med* 13:43–57, 1996.
17. Pomposelli FB Jr, Jepsen SJ, Gibbons GW, Campbell DR, Freeman DV, Miller A, LoGerfo FW: Efficacy of the dorsal pedal bypass for limb salvage in diabetic patients: short-term observations. *J Vasc Surg* 11(6):745–751, 1990.
18. Boyko EJ, Davignon D, Smith DG, Ahroni JH: Increased mortality associated with diabetic foot ulcer. *Diabet Med* 13:967–972, 1996.
19. Apelqvist J, Larsson J, Agardh CD: Long term prognosis for diabetic patients with foot ulcers. *J Int Med* 233:485–491, 1993.
20. Akbari CM, Pomposelli FB Jr, Gibbons GW, Campbell DR, Pulling MC, Mydlarz D, LoGerfo FW: Lower extremity revascularization in diabetes: late observations. *Arch Surg* 135(4):452–456, 2000.

25

New and Conventional Therapeutic Measures in Diabetic Complications Studies in Nephropathy, Cardiovascular Disease and Hypertension

CARL ERIK MOGENSEN
Department of Diabetes and Endocrinology, University Hospitals, Aarhus, Denmark

Modulation of hyperglycemia and blood pressure in diabetes has over the years emerged more and more strongly as a core issue in preventing long-term complications, both of a somewhat different genesis, although the complications may in fact be similar. In type 1 diabetes elevated blood pressure is closely linked to diabetic renal disease, initially detectable in terms of microalbuminuria. Here, increasing blood pressure is a key component of a vicious circle and is a major risk factor for later nephropathy. Antihypertensive treatment has been documented to be a pivotal measure to prevent these complications, as is treatment of hyperglycemia by any standard strategy available.

In type 2 diabetes we have a similar scenario as regards microvascular complications but, due to the aging of many of the patients, macrovascular and cardiac complications are obviously more prominent. In these cases, hypertension is a clear vascular risk factor and its reversal by a variety of antihypertensive treatment modalities is crucial. This is recently further documented in many large-scale clinical trials. Although diabetic angiopathy has specific elements, as originally described by Lundbaek (1), hypertension

Diabetes in the New Millennium. Edited by U. Di Mario, F. Leonetti, G. Pugliese, P. Sbraccia and A. Signore.
© 2000 John Wiley & Sons, Ltd.

seems to be an important modulating risk factor, even for the rather specific vascular complications related to diabetes. The blood vessels in diabetes seem clearly to be more susceptible not only to 'diabetic' lesions but to pressure-induced damage and deterioration of organ function (2,3).

A novel concept is crucial: even with so-called normal blood pressure, treatment may be indicated, namely in the presence of microalbuminuria or proteinuria (2). An important point is difficulties in defining the cut-off point for abnormal blood pressure, especially in diabetes. Several trials have documented the beneficial effect of antihypertensive treatment, including ACE-inhibitors, even without well-defined hypertension. The basis for the diabetic-related lesions is, however, hyperglycemia and related abnormalities. Therefore, treatment of high blood glucose must have equally high priority (3).

From a historical point of view, the beneficial effect of antihypertensive treatment was first seen in type 1 diabetes in patients with overt renal disease (2). Over the past few decades there has, however, been an explosion in the number of clinical trials related to antihypertensive treatment in diabetic vascular and renal disease. Almost all trials have been unequivocally positive, most recently the HOPE study (4,5), in which the blood pressure reduction from ACE-I was rather minimal, just as in microalbuminuric type 1 patients (2–4 mmHg) (2). It is also clear that best possible glycemic control is a key factor in renal complications, both for type 1 and type 2 diabetes (3,6). Thus, from a clinical view-point there is a main focus on the key risk factors: hypertension and hyperglycemia, the double jeopardy, and its amelioration by multiple treatment regimens (3).

INTENSIVE ANTIHYPERTENSIVE TREATMENT PREVENTS CARDIOVASCULAR COMPLICATIONS IN TYPE 2 DIABETES

The UKPDS (3,7) showed that the effect of antihypertensive treatment on several diabetes-related complications was observed sooner and was more pronounced than the effect of glycemic treatment. It is highly exciting that we now see results of several other trials published around or after the UKPDS in complete accordance with these British results. This is important because hypertensive diabetic patients have at least a two-fold increase of risk for cardiovascular disease compared to non-diabetics. Optimizing treatment of both hypertension and hyperglycemia gives, however, a clearly more beneficial result. The concept of the deleterious effect of several other risk factors is important in this respect, including smoking and dyslipidemia (3).

For instance, in the calcium antagonist-based HOT Study (8) as many as 1501 diabetic patients were stratified according to various blood pressure levels, e.g. with diastolic lower than 80 compared to diastolic lower than 90 as the goal (85 mmHg being the intermediary goal). With a blood pressure of 144/81 obtained in the first group there was significantly fewer cardiovascular complications in diabetic people as compared to a somewhat higher mean blood pressure (BP) of 148/85. Additional treatment, including ACE inhibitors, was given in surprisingly many patients. Especially with diastolic BP at 80 and lower, the authors documented a clear-cut risk reduction. The BP values fit well with the intensively treated patients in the UKPDS where this group had a mean BP of 144/82 compared to 154/87 in the standard group. In the Steno Type 2 Study (9), a multifactorial design (BP, glycemia, lipids and life-style) was used with respect to intervention. BP in the intensively treated group at the Steno, using mainly ACE inhibitors, was 138/78 compared to the less intensively treated group, where the blood pressure was 144/81. Table 25.1 is a list of recent studies on antihypertensive treatment in type 2 diabetes (2).

Thus, in general the goal for antihypertensive treatment in most type 2 diabetics may be set at 135–140/80–85 or lower. In fact this was also recommended in recent guidelines (10), but this goal is not always easy to achieve. However, life-threatening and discomforting complications can be prevented by effective treatment. Obviously, very old age and other confounding factors should be borne in mind. There may still be some doubt about which type of antihypertensive treatment should be preferred, but generally in most trials ACE inhibitors have a favorable effect (11,12). In the UKPDS a similar effect was found comparing ACE inhibitors and β-blockers (3). In the CAPP Study (7), the ACE inhibitor captopril was more effective than other drugs in type 2 diabetes. Interestingly, in the recently published Syst-Eur Studies, calcium channel blockers in older patients with diabetes also seem to be effective in patients with systolic hypertension (13). In the Stop-2 Study (14), antihypertensive treatment was equally important in type 2 diabetes. The HOPE Study documented beneficial effect by an ACE inhibitor in at-risk patients, including diabetes, and patients with microalbuminuria (4,5).

Table 25.1. Recent studies on antihypertensive treatment in type 2 diabetes

	Favours:
SHEP	Diuretics vs. placebo
ABCD	ACE-I vs. CCB
Facet	ACE-I vs. CCB
HOT	Strict control (CCB-based)
UKPDS	Strict control (ACE-I + β-bl-based)
SYST-EUR	CCB (often with ACE-I) vs. placebo
CAPPP	ACE-I vs. conventional
HOPE	ACE-I vs. placebo
STOP-2	AHT, β-bl and ACE-I vs. CCB
ALLHAT* ACE-I and CCB	Chlorothalidone vs. Doxazosin**

*ALLHAT expected to end year 2002.
**Doxazosin arm stopped.
AHT, antihypertensive treatment; CCB, calcium channel blockers; β-bl, beta-blockers [modified from (2)].

The conclusion is unambigous: more aggressive antihypertensive treatment is strongly recommended in the treatment of type 2 diabetes with respect to both cardiovascular and microvascular complications. It should be noted that a combination of various drugs, including low-dose diuretics, are quite common and may indeed be useful from both a BP and a mechanistic point of view. Only UKPDS focuses on elimination of the double jeopardy (3). Combination of ACE inhibitors and angiotensin-receptor blockers has a strong theoretical background and this combination is producing interesting results in type 2 microalbuminuric patients (15).

OPTIMIZED GLYCEMIC CONTROL

Originally, the UKPDS was carried out to document that optimal glycemic control had a beneficial effect on development of cardiovascular and renal complications in diabetes. This concept originated from the University Group Study from the USA, suggesting that there may be a deleterious effect by intervention by certain antihyperglycemic agents, such as sulphonylureas, insulin and possibly metformin. These observations partially paralyzed optimal treatment of diabetes for many years, especially in the USA, since it was not completely clear that improved metabolic control would ameliorate complications. However, by now it is clear that better treatment of glycemia reduces complications, especially microvascular complications but possibly also to some extent macrovascular complications, although this is less clear. What is, however, crystal clear is that treatment of both known risk factors, namely hypertension and hyperglycemia, provides the best prevention of diabetic complications, both micro- and macrovascular complications in type 2 diabetes. The effect of antihypertensive treatment, however, usually occurs earlier in the course of treatment compared to antihyperglycemic treatment (3).

In type 1 diabetes, optimized glycemic control is on a long-term basis able to ameliorate development of microvascular disease (6), although this is more difficult to prove in the area of macrovascular disease. Usually these patients are not subject to development of macrovascular complications so early in the course of diabetes and at their relatively young age.

EARLY RENAL DISEASE: MICROALBUMINURIA

Microalbuminuria is the straightforward and well-established sign of renal damage, predicting the future progression of renal disease unless effective intervention is undertaken. This has recently been confirmed with new follow-up data from the DCCT (6,16) (Table 25.2). Development and progression of microalbuminuria is clearly correlated to the degree of glycemia (6), but soon after the development of microalbuminuria in type 1 diabetes increasing BP can be documented (17). Without intervention, microalbuminuria will increase

Table 25.2. *N Engl J Med*: IDDM prediction of worsening nephropathy

Publication	Mogensen (1984) (16)	Post-DCCT (2000) (6)
Initial microalbuminuria	14 Patients	64 patients
Percentage to proteinuria	8.5%/year	8%/year**

**2% with intensive therapy.

by 15–20% every year, again depending on both BP level and glycemia (6,16). This has been observed for both types of diabetes, and as a consequence many studies have been conducted to define an optimized diabetes care regimen, including early antihypertensive treatment, in patients with borderline hypertension or in patients with normal BP.

As may be predicted from studies on the natural history of the disease, improved metabolic control as well as antihypertensive treatment is able to stabilize or reduce microalbuminuria for long periods of time. A combined comprehensive approach is the logical programme for such patients. Interestingly, patients with microalbuminuria still have well-preserved glomerular filtration rate (GFR) (2). Therefore, microalbuminuria (as early in the course as possible) is an ideal stage for intervention, because loss of organ function (decline in GFR) has not yet been inflicted (Table 25.3).

As a consequence, it is now widely recommended to screen patients for microalbuminuria, an inexpensive and easy procedure (18). This is most readily done by monitoring the urinary albumin:creatinine ratio in an early morning urine sample and following this value longitudinally. Also, albumin concentration alone may be used, but this is more uncertain. This approach may be used not only for screening, but also for intervention strategies. An early increase in albuminuria can most clearly be documented by a regular longitudinal follow-up.

Confounders are very poor metabolic control, urinary tract infection, exercise, cardiac failure, fever, very high blood pressure, and certain stress situations. However, such conditions are easily recognized in the clinical setting (19). Lower creatinine production and urinary excretion is seen in females. Increasing age and loss of muscle mass is a general confounder.

PROTEINURIA OR OVERT RENAL DISEASE IN DIABETES

It has been well documented that antihypertensive treatment can reduce the fall rate of renal function considerably (20–23). Without treatment, the mean fall rate of GFR is around 10 ml/min/year, but treatment can reduce this by more than 50%. ACE inhibitors in combination with diuretics is an important intervention strategy, but any effective BP-lowering intervention seems to be beneficial. Patients with blood pressure close to normal, with or without intervention, usually progress slowly but still depending on the level of HbA_{1c}. However, usually the fall

Table 25.3. 10 Controlled studies of IDDM microalbuminuric patients (duration of study ≥ 2 years)

Study	Drugs	Base-line no of patients.	Mean Age (y)	Mean BP	Duration of study (y)	DD (y)	Mean or median UAE (μg/min)	Effect on UAE of drug	Effect on BP	Effect of GFR	Note
European Captopril Study (1994) (24)	Cap/ Pla	46/46	32	124/77	2	17	55	↘	↘	No	European arm
North American Captopril Study (1995) (25)	Cap/Pla	70/73	33	120/77	2	18	62	↘	↘	Creatinine cl. stable	North American arm
EUCLID (1997) (26)	Lis/Pla	32/37	33	122/80	2	13	~42	↘	↘?	?	Little/no effect on normo-albuminuria
PRIMA (1997) (27)	Ram/Ram/ Pla 1,25/5,0/-	18/19	–	?	2	24	61	No	No	No	HbA$_{1C}$ = 7.4
Italian Micro-albuminuria (1998) (28)	Lis/Nif/Pla	33/26/34	37	129/83	3	18	71	Lis ↘ ↘/ Nif ↘	L ↘ ↘/ Nif ↘	S-crea: No	Effect with Nif
Mathiesen, Steno (1999) (29)	Cap + Diu/ Con	21/23	~29	126/77	8	18	93	↘	?	Stable with Cap + Diu, Diu	Preservation of GFR by ACE-I

ATLANTIS Paul O'Hare (personal communication, 1999).	Ram/Pla 1,25/ 5,0/-	44/44/46	40	132/76	2	20	53	Ram 1,25+5 mg ↘	↘	No	Not dose-dependent $HbA_{1c}=11.0$
Melbourne DNSG (30)	Per/Nif/Pla	13/10/10	~30	132/77	2.5	16	62	Per↘/ Nif-	Tendency by Per/ Nif↘	No	No effect with Nif
Padua/Aarhus (low grade micro) (1998) (31)	Lis/Pla	32/28	41	124/83 131/81	2	13.5 15.1	36 (range 20–70)	↘	↘(24h)	No	Effect in low micro-albuminuria related to FF
Rudberg (1999) (32)	Ena/ Meto/ Ref	7/6/9	~19	125/81	~3	11	~31	E↘/ M↘/ ref.-	No	No	Preservation of structure by Ena/Meto
Europe 9/ North-American (1)	Mostly ACE-I	All 727 pts	19–40	127/79	2.8	16.7	Mainly ACE-I ↘	Mostly ↘			

Cap = captopril, Lis = lisinopril, Ram = ramipril, Per = perindopril, Ena = enalapril, Meto = metoprolol, Nif = nifedipine, Con = control group, Pla = placebo, Ref = reference group, DD = diabetes duration.

of GFR cannot be completely stopped. Therefore, new intervention approaches are being developed, such as combination therapy with various antihypertensive agents, e.g. ACE inhibitors in combination with β-blockers, diuretics and other agents (22). However, the fall rate in GFR can rarely be completely blunted, and therefore early treatment in patients with microalbuminuria is advocated, because GFR fall seems to be prevented by this early intervention. Good metabolic control is essential for slowing down progression (2).

However, when diabetic complications are evolving, increasing BP remains a decisive factor in promoting organ damage in the kidney, and antihypertensive treatment, including new drugs (15,23), seems to be the therapeutic cornerstone in ameliorating deterioration in organ function, along with good glycemic control. Strict antihypertensive therapy may limit the need for any dramatic reduction of the protein content of the diet (2). Thus, a unique opportunity exists for the clinician: normalizing or reducing BP by any treatment is very likely to prevent or postpone many diabetic complications, both microvascular and macrovascular.

NEW DEVELOPMENT

New antihypertensive trials have recently been completed or are in progress, as seen in Table 25.4. The HOPE Study, already concluded, documented clearly that treatment with ACE inhibitors in the presence of two or more risk factors was

Table 25.4.   Trial in diabetes and microalbuminuria and proteinuria

		Principal investigator	Completion
Microalbuminuria	DIABHYCAR (ramipril, small doses)	Marre	2001
	HOPE*, MICROHOPE (ramipril, moderate to high dose)	Yusuf/Gerstein	1999
	CALM** (lisinopril and/or candesartan)	Mogensen	2000
	DETAIL (telmisartan)	Barnett	2003
	Perindopril/indapamide	Mogensen/ Viberti	2001
Macroalbuminuria	Renaal (losartan)	Brenner	2001
	IDNT (ibesartan)	Lewis	2000/2001
	ABCD2C (valsartan)	Schrier	2003
Non-diabetic (microalbuminuria)	PREVEND*** (fosinopril)	DeJong	2003

*Already published.
**Dual blockade.
*** + Statin treatment in a factorial design.
Reproduced from Morgensen (2) by permission of Kluwer Academic Publishers.

Table 25.5. Proposed and potential strategies for the prevention and treatment of diabetic complications, with focus on nephropathy

Strategy	Helpful in diagnosis	Helpful in treatment
Analysis of genetic factors (33,34)	No, but studies are needed	At risk patients cannot yet be found. No genetic modulation possible
Familial factors (34)	To some extent (early diagnosis of hypertension)	No
Antiglycemic treatment (6,35)	Yes (HBA$_{1C}$ monitoring)	Yes clearly demanding and sometimes not feasible
Various types of ACE inhibitors (36,37)	No	Some renal studies stopped. Other studies started
Aldose reductase inhibitor (38)	No	No, renal studies stopped (?)
Growth factor inhibition (39)	No	Needs investigation
Protein kinase C inhibitors (40)	No	Needs investigation
Antihypertensive treatment (41,42)	Yes, often along with microalbuminuria and albuminuria or high BP	Yes, mainly ACE-I as basis for combination therapy
ACE inhibitors and blocking in the RAS system (2,4,5,15)	No (genotyping not useful)	Yes, profoundly, especially in microalbuminuric patients
Lipid-lowering (43)	Yes, dyslipidemia	Probably, but needs further confirmation
Aspirine (8)	No	Probably (only for macrovascular disease)
C-peptide (44,45)	Sometimes	Further studies planned
Endothelial and endo-peptidase inhibitors (46,47)	No	Under investigation
Glycosaminoglycans (48)	No	Under investigation
Metalloproteinase (49)	No(+)	Under investigation
Low protein diet (50)	No	New studies awaited (Parving HH *et al*, in preparation)

clearly beneficial. This was also the case for patients, diabetics or non-diabetics, with microalbuminuria, a parameter which has been established as a main risk indicator. In this study it was documented that microalbuminuria was a strong risk marker for advanced cardiovascular disease and mortality, as seen in earlier studies. The most important point was, however, that treatment with an ACE inhibitor was able to prevent these advanced complications. We are still awaiting results from other important studies related to diabetes and microalbuminuria or macroalbuminuria and risk markers, as seen in Tables 25.4 and 25.5.

New treatment strategies, such as combining ACE inhibitors with angiotensin receptor blockers, has a rationale and can produce positive results (15). Table 25.5 is a review of new treatment concepts and strategies, possibly helpful in diagnosis and in planning treatment, but further studies are requested in most strategies (2).

REFERENCES

1. Lundbæk K: Diabetic angiopathy, a specific vascular disease. *Lancet* 1:377–379, 1954.
2. Mogensen CE: Microalbuminuria, blood pressure and diabetic renal disease: Origin and development of ideas. In Mogensen CE (Ed.) *The Kidney and Hypertension in Diabetes Mellitus*, 5th edn. Boston, MA: Kluwer Academic, 2000, pp. 655–706.
3. Mogensen CE: Combined high blood pressure and glucose in type 2 diabetes: double jeopardy. *Br Med J* 317:693, 1998.
4. The Heart Outcomes Prevention Evaluation Study Investigators. Effects of an angiotensin-converting-enzyme inhibitor, ramipril, on death from cardiovascular causes, myocardial infarction and stroke in high-risk patients. *N Engl J Med* 342:145–153, 2000.
5. Heart Outcomes Prevention Evaluation (HOPE) Study Investigators: Effects of ramipril on cardiovascular and microvascular outcomes in people with diabetes mellitus: results of the HOPE study and MICRO-HOPE substudy. *Lancet* 355:253–259, 2000.
6. The Diabetes Control and complications Trial Research Group: Retinopathy and nephropathy in patients with type 1 diabetes four years after a trial of intensive therapy. *N Engl J Med* 342:381–389, 2000.
7. UK Prospective Diabetes Study Group: Tight blood pressure control and risk of macrovascular and microvascular complications in type 2 diabetes: UKPDS 38. *Br Med J* 317:703–713, 1998.
8. Hansson L, Zanchetti A, Carruthers SG, Dahlöf B, Julius S *et al*: Effects of intensive blood-pressure lowering and low-dose aspirin in patients with hypertension: principal results of the hypertension optimal treatment (HOT) randomised trial. *Lancet* 13:1755–1762, 1998.
9. Gæde P, Vedel P, Parving H-H, Pedersen O: Intensified multifactorial intervention in patients with type 2 diabetes mellitus and microalbuminuria: the Steno type 2 randomised study. *Lancet* 353:617–622, 1999.
10. Guidelines subcommittee: 1999 World Health Organization–International Society of Hypertension guidelines for the management of hypertension. *J Hypertens* 17:151–183, 1999.
11. Hansson L, Lindholm LH, Niskanen L *et al*: Effect of angiotensin-converting-enzyme inhibition compared with conventional therapy on cardiovascular morbidity and mortality in hypertension: the captopril Prevention Project (CAPP) randomised trial. *Lancet* 353:611–616, 1999.
12. Estacio RO, Jeffers BW, Hiatt WR, Biggerstaff SL, Gifford N *et al*: The effect of nisoldipine as compared with enalapril on cardiovascular outcomes in patients with non-insulin-dependent diabetes and hypertension. *N Engl J Med* 338:645–653, 1998.
13. Toumilehto J, Rastenyte D, Birkenhäger W *et al*: Effects of calcium-channel blockade in older patients with diabetes and systolic hypertension. *N Engl J Med* 340:677–684, 1999.
14. Hansson L, Lindholm LH, Ekbom T, Dahlöf B, Lanke J, Scherstén B, Wester P-O, Hedner T, de Faire U for the STOP-Hypertension-2 study Group: Randomised trial of old and new antihypertensive drugs in elderly patients: cardiovascular mortality and morbidity the Swedish Trial in Old Patients with Hypertension-2 study. *Lancet* 354:1751–1756, 1999.

15. Mogensen CE, Neldam S, Tikkannen I, Oren S, Viskoper R, Watts RW, Cooper ME for the CALM Study Group: Role of dual blockade of the renin–angiotensin system in hypertensive, microalbuminuric, non-insulin dependent diabetes: the CALM Study. *Br Med J* 2000 (submitted).
16. Mogensen CE, Christensen CK: Predicting diabetic nephropathy in insulin-dependent patients. *N Engl J Med* 311:89–93, 1984.
17. Mogensen CE, Østerby R, Hansen KW, Damsgaard EM: Blood pressure elevation vs. abnormal albuminuria in the genesis and prediction of renal disease in diabetes. *Diabet Care* 15:1192–1204, 1992.
18. Mogensen CE, Keane WF, Bennett PH *et al*: Prevention of diabetic renal disease with special reference to microalbuminuria. *Lancet* 346:1080–1084, 1999.
19. Mogensen CE, Vestbo E, Poulsen PL *et al*: Microalbuminuria and potential confounders. A review and some observations on variability of urinary albumin excretion. *Diabet Care* 18:572–581, 1995.
20. Mogensen CE: Systemic blood pressure and glomerular leakage with particular reference to diabetes and hypertension. *J Intern Med* 235:297–316, 1994.
21. Lewis EJ, Hunsicker LG, Bain RP, Rohde RD: The effect of angiotensin converting enzyme inhibition on diabetic nephropathy. *N Engl J Med* 118:577–581, 1993.
22. Mogensen CE, Mau Pedersen M, Ebbehøj E *et al*: Combination therapy in hypertension-associated diabetic renal disease. *Int J Clin Pract* 90(Suppl):52–58, 1997.
23. Mogensen CE: Long-term antihypertensive treatment inhibiting progression of diabetic nephropathy. *Br Med J* 285:685–688, 1982.
24. Viberti GC, Mogensen CE, Groop L, Pauls JF, for the European Microalbuminuria Captopril Study Group: Effect of captopril on progression to clinical proteinuria in patients with insulin-dependent diabetes mellitus and microalbuminuria. *J Am Med Assoc* 271:275–279, 1994.
25. Laffel LMB, McGill JB, Gans DJ, on behalf of the North American Microalbuminuria Study Group: The beneficial effect of angiotensin-converting-enzyme inhibition with captopril on diabetic nephropathy in normotensive IDDM patients with microalbuminuria. *Am J Med* 99:497–504, 1995.
26. The Euclid Study Group: Randomised placebo-controlled trial of lisinopril in normotensive patients with insulin-dependent diabetes and normoalbuminuria or microalbuminuria. *Lancet* 349:1787–1792, 1997.
27. Bojestig M, Karlberg B, Verho M, and the Prima Study Group (1997): ACE inhibition during two years did not improve urinary excretion in normotensive microalbuminuric patients. *Diabetologia* 41:A544, 1998.
28. Crepaldi G, Carta Q, Deferrari G, Mangili R, Navalesi R, Santeusanio F, Spalluto A, Vanasia A, Villa GM, Nosadini R, for the Italian Microalbuminuria Study Group in IDDM: Effects of lisinopril and nifedipine on the progression to overt albuminuria in IDDM patients with incipient nephropathy and normal blood pressure. *Diabet Care* 21:104–110, 1998.
29. Mathiesen ER, Hommel E, Hansen HP, Smidt UM, Parving H-H: Randomised controlled trial of long term efficacy of captopril on preservation of kidney function in normtensive patients with insulin dependent diabetes and microalbuminuria. *Br Med J* 319:24–25, 1999.
30. Jerums G, on behalf of the Melbourne Diabetic Nephropathy Study Group, Melbourne, Australia: Ace inhibition vs. calcium-channel blockade in normotensive type 1 and type 2 diabetic patients with microalbuminuria. *Nephrol Dialysis Transpl* 13:1065–1066, 1998.
31. Ebbehøj E, Poulsen PL, Nosadini R, Fioretto R, Fioretto P, Crepaldi C, Mogensen CE: Early ACE-I intervention in microalbuminuria: 24 h BP, renal function and exercise changes. Abstract of the 34th Annual Meeting of the EASD, Barcelona, Spain, 8–12 September 1998. *Diabetologia* 41(1), 1998.

32. Rudberg S, Østerby R, Bangstad H-J, Dahlquiest G, Persson B. Effect of angiotensin converting enzyme inhibitor or beta blocker on glomerular structural changes in young microalbuminuric patients with type 1 (insulin-dependent) diabetes mellitus. *Diabetologia* 42:589–595, 1999.

33. Doria A, Warram JH, Krolewski AS: Genetic susceptibility to nephropathy in insulin-dependent diabetes: from epidemiology to molecular genetics. *Diabet Metab Rev* 11:287–314, 1995.

34. Fogarty DG, Rich SS, Hanna L, Warram JH, Krolewski AS: Urinary albumin excretion in families with type 2 diabetes is heritable and genetically correlated to blood pressure. *Kidney Int* 57:250–257, 2000.

35. Schichiri M, Kishikawa H, Ohkubo Y, Wake N: Long-term results of the Kumamoto Study on optimal diabetes control in type 2 diabetic patients. *Diabet Care* 23(s2):B21–B30, 2000.

36. Friedman EA: Advanced glycation end-products in diabetic nephropathy. *Nephrol Dial Transpl* 14 (s3):1–9, 1999.

37. Khalifah RG, Baynes JW, Hudson BG: Amadorins: novel post-Amadori inhibitors of advanced glyaction reactions. *Biochem Biophys Res Commun* 257:251–258, 1999.

38. Oates J, Mylari BL: Aldose reductase inhibitors: therapeutic implications for diabetic complications. *Exp Opin Invest Drugs* 8:2095–2119, 1999.

39. Flyvbjerg A, Hill C, Logan A: Pathophysiological role of growth factors in diabetic kidney disease: focus on innovative therapy. *Trends Endocrinol Metab* 10:267–272, 1999.

40. King GL, Ishii H, Koya D: Diabetic vascular dysfunction: a model of excessive activation of protein kinase C. *Kidney Int* 52:S77–S85, 1997.

41. Breyer J, Berl T, Bain RP, Rohde RD, Lewis EJ, and the Collaborative Study Group: Effect of intensive blood pressure control on the course of type 1 diabetic nephropathy. *Am J Kidney Dis* 34:809–817, 1999.

42. Lièvre M, Gueyffier F, Ekbom T, Fagard R, Cutler J, Schron E, Marre M, Boissel J-P for the INDANA Steering Committee: Efficacy of diuretics and beta-blockers in diabetic hypertensive patients: results from a meta-analysis. *Diabet Care* 23(s2):B65–B72, 2000.

43. Steiner G: Lipid intervention trials in diabetes. *Diabet Care* 23(s2):B49–B54, 2000.

44. Wahren J, Johansson BL: Ernst-Friedrich-Pfeiffer Memorial Lecture. New aspects of C-peptide physiology. *Horm Metab Res* 30:A2–A5, 1998.

45. Johansson B-L. Borgt K, Fernqvist-Forbes E, Kernell A, Odergren T, Wahren J: Beneficial effects of C-peptide on incipient nephropathy and neuropathy in patients with type 1 diabetes mellitus. *Diabet Med* 17:1–9, 2000.

46. Tikkane T, Tikkanen I, Rockell MD *et al*: Dual inhibition of neutral endopeptidase and angiotensin-converting enzyme in rats with hypertension and diabetes mellitus. *Hypertension* 32:778–785, 1998.

47. Turner AJ, Murphy LJ: Molecular pharmacology of endothelin converting enzyme. *Biochem Pharmacol* 51:91–102, 1996.

48. Gambaro G, Van der Woude FJ: Glycosaminoglycans: use in treatment of diabetic nephropathy (review). *J Am Soc Nephrol* 11:359–368, 2000.

49. Ebihara S, Nakamura T, Shimada N, Koide H: Increased plasma metalloproteinase-9 concentrations precede development of microalbuminuria in non-insulin-dependent diabetes mellitus. *Am J Kidney Dis* 32:544–550, 1998.

50. Walker JD: Non-glycaemic intervention in diabetic nephropathy: the role of dietary protein intake. In Mogensen CE (Ed.). *The Kidney and Hypertension in Diabetes Mellitus*, 5th edn. Boston, MA: Kluwer Academic, 2000, pp. 473–486.

26

Pathophysiology of Diabetic Retinopathy

MARA LORENZI and CHIARA GERHARDINGER

Schepens Eye Research Institute and Department of Ophthalmology,
Harvard Medical School, Boston, MA, USA

The retinal microangiopathy that develops almost universally in patients with 15 or more years of type 1 or type 2 diabetes becomes sight-threatening when it leads to macular edema and/or retinal ischemia. When retinal ischemia triggers unregulated angiogenesis, diabetic retinopathy is said to have entered the proliferative stage. Thus, proliferative diabetic retinopathy is an ischemic retinopathy, the manifestations of which are similar to those encountered in other ischemic conditions of the retina, and it is the early, non-proliferative microangiopathy that constitutes the specific sequela of poorly controlled diabetes.

To be able to describe, cohesively and accurately, the pathophysiology of this early microangiopathy, from which all the clinical manifestations of diabetic retinopathy proceed, would represent a major accomplishment. It would imply that essential pathogenetic events have been identified, their sequence reconstructed, and their mechanisms and implications fully revealed. Specifically, we would have identified which metabolic abnormalities induce the discrete cellular and molecular changes that are in turn necessary and sufficient to drive the processes that result in the clinically important features of diabetic retinopathy. The reality is that such a fresco cannot yet be painted. We are toiling instead at a mosaic that is beginning to reveal images in the background, but neither the details of the images nor their reciprocal relationships are yet sharply defined.

The theme emerging from recent work is that diabetic retinopathy is a complex disease of the retina as well as of retinal vessels, in so far as multiple retinal cell types are affected by diabetes and multiple processes are likely to be operative in the causation of the microangiopathy. We will review briefly how this work is advancing the understanding of the two sight-threatening lesions of diabetic retinopathy (capillary permeability, leading to macular edema, and capillary closure and obliteration, leading to retinal ischemia and unregulated angiogenesis) and identify along the way key issues that require additional work.

CAPILLARY PERMEABILITY AND MOLECULES OF TIGHT JUNCTIONS

Macular edema develops when abnormal permeability of retinal capillaries causes passive influx of plasma or blood into the retina of such magnitude that it overwhelms the active reabsorbing transport. Normally, retinal and brain vascular endothelium functions as a selective barrier through three mechanisms: presence of specific transporters or enzymes; minimal or absent pinocytosis, which limits transcellular passage of solutes; and presence of continuous interendothelial tight junctions, which prevents paracellular diffusion of solutes (1). Both transcellular and paracellular permeability appear to be increased in diabetic retinal vessels, but the latter may be the key contributor to leakage. Schlingemann *et al.* (2) have provided indirect evidence for increased endothelial transcytosis by documenting in the retinas of diabetic eye donors a spatial correlation between the vascular expression of the PAL-E antigen (which is associated with the endothelial plasmalemmel vesicles and normally absent from barrier endothelium) and leakage of plasma proteins (2). Also, Gardiner *et al.* (3) have noted increased endocytosis by retinal vascular endothelial cells in rats with short duration of diabetes (6 weeks) infused with horseradish peroxidase (3). However, the tracer present in endocytotic vesicles was not transported outside the endothelium. A similar finding had been reported by Wallow and Engerman almost two decades previously in dogs with 5 years duration of diabetes (4). In the diabetic dogs, the infused horseradish peroxidase was present in pinocytotic vesicles within the cytoplasm of retinal endothelium, but did not identify leaky vessels. Leakage of the tracer with infiltration of the vessel wall and extravascular parenchyma was instead observed in spatial correlation with gaping interendothelial tight junctions (4). It is thus possible that increased pinocytosis is an early and sustained abnormality of the retinal endothelial cells in diabetes, which may or may not, however, translate into increased permeability. Retinal vessels appear to become abnormally permeable when tight junctions are altered and permit paracellular flux of macromolecules and other solutes.

The complex molecular architecture of tight junctions is rapidly becoming known (5), and work in progress addresses how diabetes impacts on the regulation of tight junction proteins. Tight junctions seal the paracellular space through a continuous network of intermembrane fibrils formed by the transmembrane proteins claudins and occludin. Occludin binds to the cytosolic plaque proteins ZO-1 and ZO-2, which, in turn, bind actin filaments, thus anchoring the tight junction to the cytoskeleton. Occludin was the first integral transmembrane protein of tight junctions to be identified (6), and its behavior in diabetes has now been investigated in two studies. Antonetti *et al.* (7) have reported a 35% decrease in retinal occludin content in rats with 3 months duration of streptozotocin diabetes, concomitant with increased vascular leakage of fluoresceinated albumin (7). However, in retinas obtained post mortem from human subjects with type 2 diabetes of 5–10 years duration and showing albumin permeation of the vascular walls, we have actually detected a four-fold increase in occludin content (8). The reasons for this discrepancy may be several. One possibility is that the experimentally diabetic rats did not accurately model chronically treated human diabetes in so far as they were severely catabolic, showing a 22% loss in body weight (7). A second reason may relate to the modulatory role of vascular endothelial growth factor (VEGF), which *in vitro* decreases the occludin content of retinal endothelial cells (7). VEGF expression has been reported to increase at early stages of experimental diabetes in the rat (9), but has been found unchanged in the human diabetic retina (10). A third reason may be the different stage of diabetic retinopathy at which the rat and human observations were obtained. The human diabetic donors had evidence of characteristic lesions of microangiopathy, and it is conceivable that the endothelial response to diabetes may be a function of the overall status of the cells. It is of note that overexpression of occludin in cultured epithelial cells, if increasing on the one hand transepithelial electrical resistance (an index of the strength of the tight junction seal), is on the other hand associated with increased paracellular flux (11). If this scenario pertains to occludin function in vascular endothelium, occludin overexpression could affect the physiology and permeability of retinal capillary tight junctions as much as occludin underexpression. Much additional work is clearly required in order to ascertain how the molecular composition of tight junctions is altered in diabetes, and which changes are necessary and sufficient to compromise the seal.

The mechanisms responsible for the compromised barrier properties of retinal capillaries should also be clarified, and the investigation will need to address events both within and outside the endothelial cells. Within, because transcellular transport relies on endothelial structures and tight junction proteins are synthesized and assembled by endothelial cells; outside, because the unique barrier properties of retinal and brain endothelium reflect the inductive influence of the surrounding glial elements (1,12). There is currently no evidence that the increased permeability of diabetic retinal capillaries is to be attributed to glial dysfunction, but there is mounting evidence of glial abnormalities in the diabetic retina. We describe briefly below such abnormalities and the range of consequences that may be worthy of exploration.

GLIAL CELL ABNORMALITIES IN DIABETIC RETINOPATHY

Retinal vessels are intimately enveloped by glial processes (13). We have recently noted that glial processes are so inextricably enmeshed in the outer basement membrane of retinal microvessels, that it is practically impossible to isolate retinal capillaries free of glial contamination (14). The macroglia of the retina is constituted by astrocytes, present only in the nerve fiber layer, and Müller cells which span the entire depth of the neural retina and surround with their processes neuronal cell bodies, axons, and vessels. Müller cells subserve the critical housekeeping functions of removing from the extracellular space potassium ions, CO_2 and neurotransmitters released during neural activity (13). The subsequent release of potassium and acid equivalents at the endfeet of Müller cells (known as the 'spatial buffering system') is thought to be the mechanism coupling neuronal activity to blood flow regulation. Being the only cells in the retina endowed with enzyme glutamine synthetase (13), Müller cells transform the glutamate taken up via high-affinity carriers into glutamine, which is then returned to the neural cells for glutamate resynthesis (13). In the retina as in the brain, glial cells provide the inducing influences for the acquisition of barrier properties by the vascular endothelium (1,12).

A suggestion that Müller cells may be affected by diabetes came from the observation of b-wave abnormalities in the electroretinogram of diabetic subjects (15), and we thus tested human diabetic retinas for the pattern of Müller cell changes observed after retinal insults or in retinal degenerations: increased expression of the anti-apoptotic molecule Bcl-2 and of the intermediate filament protein glial fibrillary acidic protein (GFAP), and decreased expression of glutamine synthetase. Neither the levels of Bcl-2 nor of glutamine synthetase were altered in the retinas of diabetic donors; there was however, a marked upregulation of GFAP expression (15). Whereas in non-diabetic retinas GFAP immunoreactivity was confined to the proximal retina, in most diabetic retinas the GFAP-positive filaments within the Müller cell processes appeared greatly thickened and extended the length of the entire Müller cell, throughout the outer retina (15). Leith *et al.* confirmed this finding in the rat retina, and showed that marked induction of GFAP is evident as early as 3 months after induction of diabetes (16). These investigators also detected in the diabetic rat retinas decreased ability to convert glutamate into glutamine and increased levels of glutamate, when compared with retinas of normal rats, and proposed that glutamate excitotoxicity may occur in the diabetic retina as a consequence of Müller cell dysfunction.

In so far as increased expression of GFAP is the hallmark of 'reactive astrocytosis' (17), these findings pose the question of whether retinal glial cells do acquire a reactive phenotype in diabetes. Best studied in relation to events in the central nervous system, reactive astrocytes upregulate the expression of a multitude of molecules, including molecules involved in cell adhesion and migration, tissue repair and scar formation, inflammation and neuroprotection (17). Such an altered local environment would magnify tremendously the number of abnormal signals received by vascular cells early in the course of diabetes. On the other hand, GFAP overexpression may simply reflect an effect of high glucose on the transcriptional regulation of this molecule. Müller cells are likely targets of hyperglycemia, being endowed with GLUT-1 (15), which permits unregulated transport of glucose, aldose reductase (18,19), which exposes them to the consequences of polyol pathway activation, and having an elevated rate of glycolysis (20). Definition of the extent to which exposure to high glucose alters Müller cell homeostasis will provide insights highly relevant to the pathophysiology of diabetic retinopathy.

CAPILLARY CLOSURE, APOPTOSIS AND PRO-INFLAMMATORY EVENTS

Retinal ischemia and attendant neovascularization develop when a critical number of capillaries becomes occluded and obliterated. The obliterative process is first observed (21) in isolated capillaries or small groups of capillaries scattered about the retinal vasculature, and advances centripetally to involve the arterioles and their branches. Capillaries lose both endothelial cells and pericytes, thus becoming acellular tubes of basement membrane. As acellular capillaries begin to appear, other capillaries show only the scattered loss of pericytes, identified by the appearance of 'ghosts' (the protruding pockets of basement membrane from which the pericyte nuclei have disappeared).

Many theories have been advanced over the years to explain the process leading to capillary obliteration in the diabetic retina, and we see at this time three leading contenders. The first, chronologically, is the 'shunt' theory proposed many decades ago by Cogan and Kuwabara (22), and centered on the early loss of pericytes. The theory proposes that loss of pericyte contractile function leads to distension of some channels, with subsequent 'drying up' of alternate capillary pathways. There is then the 'occlusive' theory, based on evidence of microthrombosis (23) and leukostasis (24,25) observed in experimental diabetes, in turn facilitated by increased expression of adhesion molecules by retinal vascular cells (26). The third theory, which could be called the 'suicide' theory, is based on our observations of accelerated apoptosis of both retinal pericytes and endothelial cells in diabetic retinal vessels (27). These theories need not be mutually exclusive, and recent studies have begun to identify possible points of intersection or convergence of the processes emphasized in each theory.

Accelerated apoptosis of microvascular pericytes and endothelial cells is a likely prodrome to capillary obliteration. We have documented that it precedes, by many months, the appearance of acellular capillaries and pericyte ghosts (27); and, more recently, that it predicts these histological outcomes in two animal models of diabetic retinopathy (28). It may be noted that apoptosis is increasingly becoming identified as a sequela of diabetes/hyperglycemia across different tissues and circumstances, having also been detected in the neural retina of diabetic humans and rats (29), and in the pre-implantation embryos of pregnant diabetic rodents (30). Hence, reconstruction of its molecular mechanisms should provide clues to key pathogenic events. We have begun the investigation of such mechanisms in the retina by addressing whether diabetes changes the levels, and thus the balance, of endogenous regulators of apoptosis. We found that, in the adult human retina, Bcl-2, the best known pro-survival member of the Bcl-2 family of endogenous regulators of apoptosis, is almost exclusively present in Müller glial cells, cannot be detected in vessels, and its levels are not modified by diabetes (15). Similarly, in the study of 18 diabetic and 20 non-diabetic donors, we found that retinal levels of the pro-survival (Bcl-X_L) and proapoptotic (Bcl-X_S) isoforms of Bcl-X were not altered by diabetes (14). Diabetes did instead change the levels of proapoptotic Bax (14). In both diabetic and non-diabetic retinas, Bax immunoreactivity was almost exclusively present in the inner retina, with specific staining detected in cells of the inner nuclear layer, ganglion cells and the endothelial and medial layers of blood vessels. Bax levels were slightly, but significantly, greater in the retina of diabetic than non-diabetic donors. When we examined the pattern of Bax expression in retinal microvessels using trypsin digests, we observed frequent localization of intense Bax staining around the fragmented (apoptotic) nuclei of pericytes. Exposure of retinal pericytes to high glucose *in vitro* for several weeks recapitulated both increased Bax expression and accelerated apoptosis (14). A sequence of events may thus be proposed, where some effects of high glucose alter the regulation of Bax levels and the ensuing mitochondrial membrane permeabilization (31) results in pericyte apoptosis. Pericyte apoptosis would, in turn, be a sufficient event to explain the appearance of ghosts, because pericytes replicate little if at all in the adult retina (32); and the loss of their contractile control on retinal capillary blood flow could certainly generate the conditions for the shunts theorized by Cogan and Kuwabara.

Less straightforward is the reconstruction of the mechanisms leading to the completely acellular vessels from which endothelial cells have also disappeared, and which are non-perfused. We have previously proposed that apoptosis of retinal endothelial cells may lead to their increased turnover [endothelial cells maintain the capability to replicate in the adult retina (32)], and eventually to acellular capillaries because of exhaustion of their replicative life-span (27). There is morphological evidence for regenerating endothelial cells in diabetic retinal vessels (4), and their increased labeling index confirms increased turnover (33). Additional mechanisms linking endothelial cell apoptosis to acellular capillaries are the hyperadhesive (34) and procoagulant (35) properties that apoptotic endothelial cells can acquire. These could precipitate leukostasis and microthrombosis, compromise perfusion, and thus result in the hypoxic demise of a stretch of capillary. Human diabetic retinal vessels have been reported to exhibit increased expression of intercellular adhesion molecule-1 (ICAM-1) (26), and we have recently documented an increased number and extension of microthrombi in the vessels of human diabetic donors when compared with age-matched non-diabetic donors (36). A recent intriguing finding is that increased retinal expression of ICAM-1 and leukostasis can be detected as early as 1 week after induction of streptozotocin diabetes (25), at a time when our detection methods do not as yet show evidence of apoptotic endothelial cells. These observations may well indicate that upregulated expression of ICAM-1 and leukostasis precede, and may eventually cause, endothelial cell apoptosis, rather than being solely its consequences. On the other hand, events occurring in the context of the large changes in plasma glucose and osmolarity that follow the acute onset of experimental diabetes may or may not reflect events sustained under more chronic and treated conditions.

An additional observation proposes that mechanisms for the development of acellular capillaries may also be linked to events primarily occurring in the pericytes. We have recently observed that pericytes, but not endothelial cells, of human diabetic retinal vessels show activation of the transcription factor nuclear factor–κB (NF–κB). Of note, the diabetic donors exhibiting an elevated number of NF–κB-positive pericyte nuclei also had an increased prevalence of apoptotic microvascular cells and acellular capillaries when compared with diabetic donors with a minimal count of NF–κB-positive pericytes, similar to the count of non-diabetic donors (37). Because the program of gene expression activated by NF–κB can include pro-inflammatory mediators (38), studies are currently in progress to ascertain whether NF–κB activation in retinal pericytes does in fact result in the synthesis and secretion of cytokines that may reach neighboring endothelial cells and compromise their non-adhesive and non-thrombogenic properties.

CONCLUSIONS AND PERSPECTIVE

Important, albeit not definitive, knowledge has been gained during the last few years on pathophysiological events operative in diabetic retinopathy. The

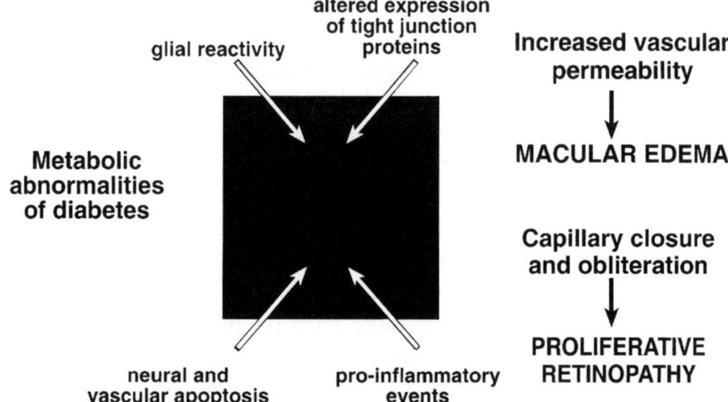

Figure 26.1. Recently identified cellular and molecular processes that occur in the diabetic retina and may link the metabolic abnormalities with sight-threatening features of retinal diabetic microangiopathy

Diabetes Control and Complications Trial and the UK Prospective Diabetes Study have unequivocally affirmed the value of tight metabolic control in the prevention and slowing of diabetic retinopathy. The content of the 'black box' that for decades has hidden the nature of the connections between the metabolic abnormalities and the clinically important functional and histological features of retinal diabetic microangiopathy is beginning to be revealed (Figure 26.1).

The involvement of multiple cell types and the contribution of multiple processes to a given event is not surprising in a disease such as diabetes, which is known to affect multiple cell types. Just as diabetic neuropathy is the consequence of diabetes-induced damage to neural cells and fibers, glia and blood vessels of the peripheral nervous system, diabetic retinopathy may come to be viewed as a result of damage to the corresponding cell types in the retina. The challenge ahead is to obtain a more cohesive picture of the plurality of effects exerted by diabetes on the retina while sorting out the molecular pathways that explain the microangiopathy. This work has obvious relevance to the development of rationally targeted adjunct interventions.

ACKNOWLEDGEMENTS

The authors' work was supported by National Institutes of Health Grant EY-09122 and grants from the American Diabetes Association and Juvenile Diabetes Foundation International.

REFERENCES

1. Risau W: Induction of blood–brain barrier endothelial cell differentiation. *Ann NY Acad Sci* 633:405–419, 1991.
2. Schlingemann RO, Hofman P, Vrensen GFJM, Blaauwgeers HGT: Increased expression of endothelial antigen PAL-E in human diabetic retinopathy correlates with microvascular leakage. *Diabetologia* 42:596–602, 1999.
3. Gardiner TA, Stitt AW, Archer DB: Retinal vascular endothelial cell endocytosis increases in early diabetes. *Lab Invest* 72:439–444, 1995.
4. Wallow IHL, Engerman RL: Permeability and patency of retinal blood vessels in experimental diabetes. *Invest Ophthalmol Vis Sci* 16:447–461, 1977.
5. Fanning AL, Mitic LL, Anderson JM: Transmembrane proteins in the tight junction barrier. *J Am Soc Nephrol* 10:1337–1345, 1999.
6. Furuse M, Hirase T, Itoh M, Nagafuchi A, Yonemura S, Tsukita S, Tsukita S: Occludin: a novel integral membrane protein localizing at tight junctions. *J Cell Biol* 123:1777–1788, 1993.
7. Antonetti DA, Alistair JB, Khin S, Lieth E, Tarbell JM, Gardner TW, Penn State Retina Research Group: Vascular permeability in experimental diabetes is associated with reduced endothelial occludin content. *Diabetes* 47:1953–1959, 1998.
8. Gerhardinger C, Podestà F, Lorenzi M: Retinal levels of occludin are increased in background diabetic retinopathy and are associated with overexpression of glial fibrillar acidic protein. *Diabetes* 48(Suppl 1):A20, 1999.
9. Hammes H-P, Lin J, Bretzel RG, Brownlee M, Breier G: Upregulation of the vascular endothelial growth factor/vascular endothelial growth factor receptor system in experimental background diabetic retinopathy of the rat. *Diabetes* 47:401–406, 1998.
10. Gerhardinger C, Brown LF, Roy S, Mizutani M, Zucker CL, Lorenzi M: Expression of vascular endothelial growth factor in the human retina and in nonproliferative diabetic retinopathy. *Am J Pathol* 152:1453–1462, 1998.
11. Balda MS, Whitney JA, Flores C, González S, Cereijido M, Matter K: Functional dissociation of paracellular permeability and transepithelial electrical resistance and disruption of the apical-basolateral intramembrane diffusion barrier by expression of a mutant tight junction membrane protein. *J Cell Biol* 134:1031–1049, 1996.
12. Tout S, Chan-Ling T, Hollander H, Stone J: The role of Müller cells in the formation of the blood–retinal barrier. *Neuroscience* 55:291–301, 1993.
13. Newman E and Reichenbach A: The Müller cell: a functional element of the retina. *Trends Neurosci* 19:307–312, 1996.
14. Podestà F, Romeo G, Liu W-H, Krajewski S, Reed JC, Gerhardinger C, Lorenzi M: Bax is increased in the retina of diabetic subjects and is associated with pericyte apoptosis *in vivo* and *in vitro*. *Am J Pathol* 156:1025–1032, 2000.
15. Mizutani M, Gerhardinger C, Lorenzi M: Müller cell changes in human diabetic retinopathy. *Diabetes* 47:445–449, 1998.
16. Leith E, Barber AJ, Xu B, Dice C, Ratz MJ, Tanase D, Strother JM, and the Penn State Retina Research Group: Glial reactivity and impaired glutamate metabolism in short-term experimental diabetic retinopathy. *Diabetes* 47:815–820, 1998.
17. Eddleston M, Mucke L: Molecular profile of reactive astrocytes — Implications for their role in neurologic disease. *Neuroscience* 54:15–36, 1993.
18. Akagi Y, Yajima Y, Kador PF, Kuwabara T, Kinoshita JH: Localization of aldose reductase in the human eye. *Diabetes* 33:562–566, 1984.
19. Ludvigson MA, Sorenson RI: Immunohistochemical localization of aldose reductase. II. Rat eye and kidney. *Diabetes* 29:450–459, 1980.

20. Poitry-Yamate CL, Poitry S, Tsacopoulos M: Lactate released by Müller glial cells is metabolized by photoreceptors from mammalian retina. *J Neurosci* 15:5179–5191, 1995.
21. Engerman RL, Kern TS: Retinopathy in animal models of diabetes. *Diabet Metab Rev* 11:109–120, 1995.
22. Cogan DG, Kuwabara T: Capillary shunts in the pathogenesis of diabetic retinopathy. *Diabetes* 12:293–300, 1963.
23. Sima AAF, Chakrabarti S, Garcia-Salinas R, Basu PK: The BB-rat — an authentic model of human diabetic retinopathy. *Curr Eye Res* 4:1087–1092, 1985.
24. Schroder S, Palinski W, Schmid-Schonbein GW: Activated monocytes and granulocytes, capillary nonperfusion, and neovascularization in diabetic retinopathy. *Am J Pathol* 139:81–100, 1991.
25. Miyamoto K, Khosrof S, Bursell SE, Rohan R, Murata T, Clermont AC, Aiello LP, Ogura Y, Adamis AP: Prevention of leukostasis and vascular leakage in streptozotocin-induced diabetic retinopathy via intercellular adhesion molecule-1 inhibition. *Proc Natl Acad Sci USA* 96:10836–10841, 1999.
26. McLeod DS, Lefer DJ, Merges C, Lutty GA: Enhanced expression of intracellular adhesion molecule-1 and P-selectin in the diabetic human retina and choroid. *Am J Pathol* 147:642–653, 1995.
27. Mizutani M, Kern TS, Lorenzi M: Accelerated death of retinal microvascular cells in human and experimental diabetic retinopathy. *J Clin Invest* 97:2883–2891, 1996.
28. Kern TS, Tang J, Mizutani M, Kowluru R, Nagaraj R, Romeo G, Podestà F, Lorenzi M: Response of capillary cell death to aminoguanidine predicts the development of retinopathy: comparison of diabetes and galactosemia. *Invest Ophthalmol Vis Sci*, 2000 (in press).
29. Barber AJ, Lieth E, Khin SA, Antonetti DA, Buchanan AG, Gardner TW, and the Penn State Retina Research Group: Neural apoptosis in the retina during experimental and human diabetes. *J Clin Invest* 102:783–791, 1998.
30. Moley KH, Chi MM-Y, Knudson CM, Korsmeyer SJ, Mueckler MM: Hyperglycemia induces apoptosis in pre-implantation embryos through cell death effector pathways. *Nature Med* 4:1421–1424, 1998.
31. Kroemer G and Reed, JC: Mitochondrial control of cell death. *Nature Med* 6:513–519, 2000.
32. Engerman RL, Pfaffenbach D, Davis MD: Cell turnover of capillaries. *Lab Invest* 17:738–743, 1967.
33. Sharma NK, Gardiner TA, Archer DB: A morphologic and autoradiographic study of cell death and regeneration in the retinal microvasculature of normal and diabetic rats. *Am J Ophthalmol* 100:51–60, 1985.
34. Hebert MJ, Gullans SR, Mackenzie HS, Brady HR: Apoptosis of endothelial cells is associated with paracrine induction of adhesion molecules. *Am J Pathol* 152:523–532, 1998.
35. Bombeli T, Karsan A, Tait JF, Harlan JM: Apoptotic vascular endothelial cells become procoagulant. *Blood* 89:2429–2442, 1997.
36. Boeri D, Maiello M, Lorenzi M: Increased prevalence of microthrombosis in retinal capillaries of diabetic individuals. *Diabetes* 49(Suppl 1):A169 (Abstr), 2000.
37. Romeo G, Podestà F, Kern TS, Lorenzi M: Activated nuclear factor-β (NF-β) in pericytes is associated with early lesions of human diabetic retinopathy. *Diabetes* 48(Suppl 1):A154 (Abstr), 1999.
38. Pahl HL: Activators and target genes of Rel/NF-β transcription factors. *Oncogene* 18:6853–6866, 1999.

27

Pathophysiology of Diabetic Nephropathy: Role of Estrogens

GARY E. STRIKER[1,2], MYLENE POTIER[2], SHARON J. ELLIOT[2], MICHAEL KARL[1,3], and LILIANE J. STRIKER[2]

[1]Vascular Biology Institute; [2]Renal Cell Biology Laboratory; [3]Division of Diabetes, Endocrinology and Metabolism, University of Miami School of Medicine, PO Box 016960 (R126), Miami, FL 33101, USA

Aging women have a disproportionately high incidence of vascular diseases, including endstage renal disease. Whereas women are relatively protected prior to menopause, after menopause the incidence of diabetic nephropathy, the major cause of end-stage renal disease, rises, especially in minority women. Epidemiological data from the US Renal Data System (USRDS) provide strong evidence for a causal relationship between estrogen deficiency and increased risk of diabetic nephropathy. These data show that the incidence of end-stage renal disease increases with age in women, and that the increase is exaggerated among minority women, especially diabetics. Women with non-insulin dependent diabetes mellitus (NIDDM) and insulinopenia have a diminished ovarian capacity to synthesize estrogens, suggesting a relative estrogen deficiency (1). There is an age-dependent increase in NIDDM, making aging and estrogen deficiency an important public health issue.

Estrogen action is mediated via estrogen receptor (ER) subtypes, ERα and β. We found that both ER subtypes were expressed and functional in human and mouse mesangial cells. In the presence of 17β-estradiol (estradiol) (10^{-10}–10^{-8} M), there was an increase in the steady-state mRNA levels of both ERα and ERβ. ERα protein levels increased $\sim$three-fold after 24 hours and up to $\sim$8.5-fold after 72 hours. ERβ protein levels increased $\sim$1.6-fold in the presence of estradiol (10^{-9} M) after 72 hours. Thus, the regulation of ER expression in

Diabetes in the New Millennium. Edited by U. Di Mario, F. Leonetti, G. Pugliese, P. Sbraccia and A. Signore.
© 2000 John Wiley & Sons, Ltd.

mesangial cells was estrogen-dependent and estrogens may maintain or even increase the estrogen responsiveness of mesangial cells. The effect(s) of estrogens may account for their protective role in progressive glomerular disease. Glomerulosclerosis is largely due to excess of extracellular matrix and/ or decrease of matrix metalloproteinases (MMPs) in mesangial cells. Estradiol increased MMP-9 mRNA and activity, which may partly account for the protective role of estrogens in diabetic nephropathy.

INTRODUCTION

Mesangial cells are vascular smooth muscle cells which play a central role in maintaining the structure and function of the renal glomerulus (2). Mesangial cells contribute to the glomerular synthesis and degradation of extracellular matrix (ECM) components, including the synthesis of type IV collagen and the ECM-degrading matrix metalloproteinases (MMPs) (3). This suggests that mesangial cells have many characteristics in common with macrovascular smooth muscle cells. Recently, vascular smooth muscle cells have been recognized as an important estrogen target tissue in which the direct effects of estrogens make a substantial contribution to protection against cardiovascular disease (4). The US Renal Data System provides strong evidence for a causal relationship between estrogen deficiency and an increased risk for diabetic glomerulosclerosis (Table 27.1) (5). Thus, the impact of estrogen deficiency on ECM turnover in the development and/or progression of atherosclerotic lesions may be similar to that on glomerulosclerosis in postmenopausal women. Furthermore, this suggests that mesangial cells could be an important estrogen target in the glomerulus and that estrogen replacement may play a preventive role in the progression of diabetic nephropathy after menopause. Estrogen action is mediated via estrogen receptors. Two estrogen receptor subtypes have been characterized, ERα and β, which belong to the superfamily of nuclear receptors (6–9). While both ERα and β, as well as estrogen receptor splice variants, have been identified in vascular smooth muscle cells (10–15), expression of estrogen receptors has not been reported in mesangial cells. Furthermore, little is known about the regulation of ER subtypes by estrogens in vascular smooth muscle cells. Mesangial cells are believed to be the major site of ECM biosynthesis in the glomerulus (2). 17β-estradiol has been shown to decrease TGFβ1-mediated collagen synthesis by mesangial cells (16). The effects of 17β-estradiol on MMPs, which could affect ECM accumulation, is unknown.

We found that mesangial cells expressed both ERα and β and that estrogens regulated the expression of these ERs in mesangial cells. In addition, estrogens and anti-estrogens regulated the expression of MMP-9 in mesangial cells. These findings may have important implications for diabetic nephropathy.

Table 27.1. Incidence of ESRD (rate/10 million) (USRDS, FY 1995 data)

Sex	Age	White	F/M	African-American	F/M	Asian/Pacific Islander	F/M	Native American	F/M
Women	35–39	299	0.7	723	0.8	84	0.4	969	0.8
Men	35–39	460		880		224		1190	
Women	65–69	2961	1.0	14268	1.5	6013	0.9	23559	1.6
Men	65–69	3046		9819		6754		14533	

EXPERIMENTAL PROCEDURES

Cell culture

Human glomeruli were microdissected from kidneys not suitable for transplantation. Mesangial-like glomerular outgrowths were patch-cloned, propagated and grown in Waymouth's medium supplemented with 20% FBS. Mesangial cells were characterized by their stellate morphology and positive staining for α-smooth muscle actin (17). Experiments were performed with cells at passages 3–6. Mesangial cells from C57BL/6J, NOD (before and after the onset of diabetes mellitus) and ROP$^{+/+}$ female mice have been previously described (18–20). Cells were used at passages when we showed that they retained their phenotype. They were maintained in DMEM/F12, supplemented with 20% FBS.

Cell culture conditions

Estrogen receptor regulation was studied in cells cultured in Phenol Red-free medium supplemented with charcoal-stripped FBS, since a lipophilic impurity contained in the phenol red has been described as a weak estrogen agonist (21). Growth curves were performed in this medium and in standard medium. For most experiments, cells were cultured in Phenol Red-free medium supplemented with 20% charcoal-stripped FBS in presence of increasing concentrations of estradiol (10^{-10} M–10^{-8} M) for 5 days and cells were plated at a cell density to obtain similar cell numbers under each condition at day 1 and day 3. Transfection experiments were performed to assess endogenous estrogen receptor function. Cells were plated as previously described and medium was replaced by Phenol Red-free medium supplemented with 0.1% charcoal-stripped FBS.

Mesangial cells were initially grown for 3 days in Phenol Red-free medium supplemented with 20% charcoal-stripped FBS in six-well plates and the medium was replaced with Phenol Red-free medium supplemented with 0.1% charcoal-stripped FBS and increasing concentrations of estradiol (10^{-10} M–10^{-8} M) for 24 and 72 hours to assess the regulation of ERs mRNA and protein expression, as well as the regulation of MMP-9 expression and activity. Cell layers were harvested for RNA and/or protein collection, and the supernatants were used to measure MMP-9 activity.

Isolation of mRNA and RT–PCR

Total RNA was extracted from confluent cell cultures using the guanidium thiocyanate–phenol–chloroform method (22). RT was performed on $2\,\mu g$ of total RNA in a total volume of $20\,\mu l$. The specificity of each amplification reaction was monitored in control reactions in which the RT had been omitted. Amplification of human ER subtypes α and β in human mesangial cells were performed using primer pairs described by Enmark *et al* (6), which resulted in amplicons of 344 bp and 392 bp length, respectively.

Western blots

Cell layers were washed with PBS, collected in presence of lysis buffer, homogenized and the homogenate was centrifuged for 30 minutes at 15 000 rpm at 4°C. Supernatant protein concentrations were measured and the samples were diluted in Laemmli buffer, boiled, and equal amounts of protein from each experimental condition were run on a 10% polyacrylamide gel. Prestained markers were electrophoresed in parallel to estimate molecular weight. After electrotransfer to the nitrocellulose, immunoblotting was performed with either human or mouse ERα and ERβ antisera. Immunoreactive bands were determined by exposing the nitrocellulose blots to a chemiluminescence solution, followed by exposure to a Hyperfilm^{TM} ECL^{TM} film. Control experiments included ERα and ERβ human recombinant peptides as positive controls and specificity of signal was demonstrated by incubating blots with excess immunizing peptide.

Transfection and luciferase assays

Mesangial cells cultured in phenol red-free medium supplemented with 20% charcoal-stripped FBS were transfected with the reporter construct, pVitA2-ERE-TKLuc $(0.25\,\mu g/\text{well})$, using TransFast. To adjust for transfection efficiency, mesangial cells were cotransfected with pRSV-βgal $(0.25\,\mu g/\text{well})$, a gift of Drs G. Tremblay and V. Giguere (8). After 1 hour, phenol red-free medium supplemented with 10% charcoal-stripped FBS was added to the transfected cells. Cells were incubated for additional 24 hours in the presence of $10^{-8}\,M$ estradiol or vehicle (ethanol). For luciferase and galactosidase assays, cells were lysed in $100\,\mu l$ reporter lysis buffer at room temperature. Light emission was detected using a luminometer. Values were expressed as arbitrary light units normalized to the β-galactosidase activity.

MMP-9 activity

Cell supernatants were collected 24 and 72 hours following treatment, counted for the purpose of adjusting medium volume to cell number for MMP-9 assays. MMP-9 activity in the medium was measured using 10% zymogram gels, as described previously (23).

RESULTS

Response of MMP levels in sclerosis-prone mesangial cells to 17β-estradiol

C57 Bl/6 and prediabetic NOD mesangial cells were found to be more responsive to physiologic concentrations of 17β-estradiol than were ROP$^{+/+}$ or post-diabetic mesangial cells (Figure 27.1).

Expression of ERα and ERβ in human mesangial cells

We detected both ERα and ERβ transcripts in the human mesangial cells (Figure 27.2). Using ERα and ERβ antisera, there were signals at $\sim$66 and $\sim$53 kDa, respectively, by Western analysis. The estimated molecular weight of these bands corresponds to the size predicted for human ERα and ERβ (6,7). Recombinant peptides of the human ERα and ERβ served as positive controls. Preincubation of the ER antisera with their respective immunizing peptides completely abrogated these signals, confirming the specificity of the bands for ERα and ERβ. Thus, human mesangial cells express both ERα and ERβ. We found 408 bp and 409 bp amplicons corresponding to mouse ERα and ERβ transcripts in C57BL/6J female mouse mesangial cells (8,9).

Transcriptional activity of estrogen receptors in mouse mesangial cells

17β-estradiol (10^{-8} M) induced a $\sim$two-fold increase in luciferase activity in the transfected mesangial cells. Thus, the endogenous estrogen receptors maintain their function as ligand-regulated transcription factors in mesangial cells. When mesangial cells were cultured for 1 or 3 days in Phenol Red-free medium containing 20% charcoal-stripped FBS, there were changes in the levels of ERα and ERβ mRNA, but they were not coordinately regulated (Figure 27.3). There was a decrease in the steady levels of ERα mRNA, ($p < 0.01$), while ERβ mRNA levels increased ($p < 0.01$). In addition, the changes were not of the same magnitude. ERα mRNA decreased to a level of 46.9$\pm$8.1% after 1 day and this decrease persisted to day 3. ERβ mRNA levels increased at day 1 and reached a $\sim$2.7-fold increase after 3 days. After 3 days of culture, the addition of 17β-estradiol (10^{-10}–10^{-8} M) led to a progressive increase in both ERα and ERβ mRNA levels. ERα mRNA levels reached a

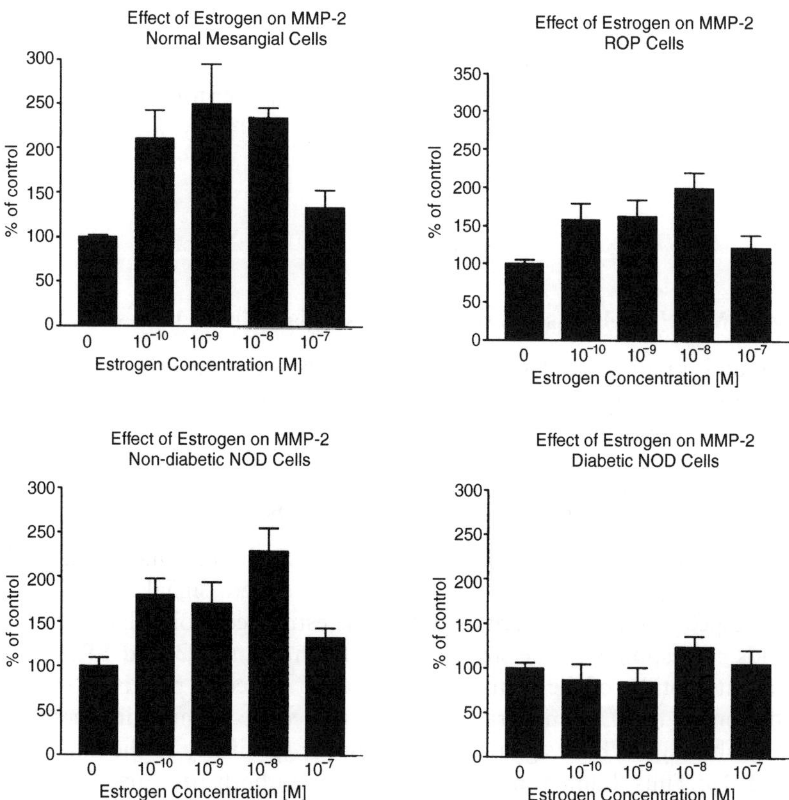

Figure 27.1. *Estrogens increase MMP-2 synthesis.* There was a concentration-dependent (dose–response) increase in MMP-2 synthesis by mesangial cells from sclerosis-resistant mice (top left panel). This was also true for sclerosis-prone mesangial cells, except that the response was considerably blunted (top right panel). The response in mesangial cells isolated from non-obese diabetic mice prior to the onset of diabetes mellitus (bottom left panel) resembled that in ROP cells. However, cells isolated from non-obese diabetic mice after the onset of diabetes (bottom right panel) had little response to added estrogen

$\sim$1.8-fold increase after 24 hours and a $\sim$2.7-fold ($p < 0.01$) increase after 72 hours after exposure to 10^{-9} M 17β-estradiol. The increase in ERβ mRNA levels peaked at 10^{-9} M 17β-estradiol. There were $\sim$1.3-fold (after 24 hours) and $\sim$2.1-fold ($p < 0.05$) (after 72 hours) increases. In summary, these studies demonstrated that mesangial cell ERα and ERβ mRNA levels changed in opposite directions when cultured in Phenol Red-free medium supplemented with charcoal-stripped FBS. In the presence of physiological concentrations of 17β-estradiol the mRNA levels of both estrogen receptor subtypes increase in mesangial cells.

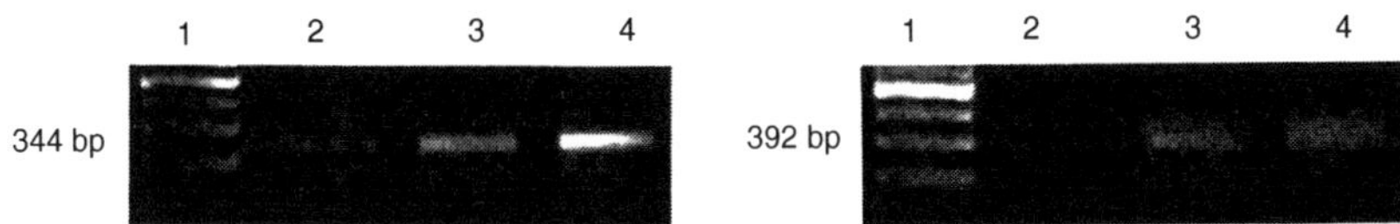

Figure 27.2. *Human mesangial cells express ER.* Total RNA and protein were collected from human mesangial cells grown in Waymouth's medium supplemented with 20% FBS. The presence of ERα and ERβ transcripts was analysed by RT–PCR using specific primer sequences, as described in 'Experimental Procedures'. Representative 344 bp amplicons of ERα (*Left*, lane 4) and 392 bp amplicons of ERβ (*Right*, lane 4) are shown after agarose gel electrophoresis. Molecular weight standard in lane 1, negative RT reactions in lane 2 and positive control in lane 3 were run in parallel

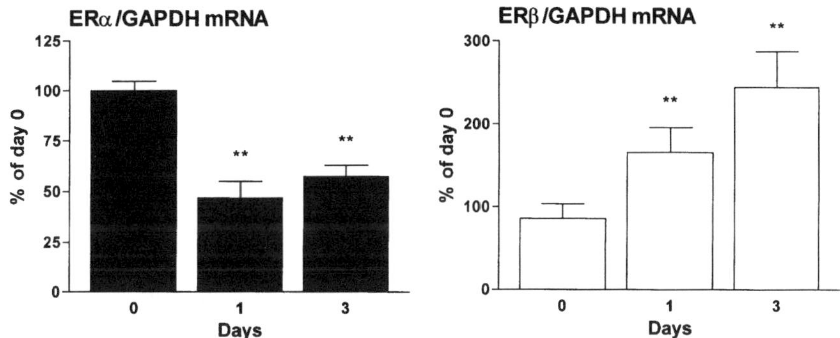

Figure 27.3. *Culture conditions change ERα (left) and ERβ (right) mRNA expression.* Mesangial cells isolated from C57BL/6J mouse glomeruli were grown for 1 and 3 days in Phenol Red-free DMEM/F12 supplemented with 20% charcoal-stripped FBS. ERα and ERβ mRNA expression, normalized to GAPDH. Data are expressed as percentage of day 0. Shown are means±SE of three independent experiments. Statistical significance ($p < 0.01$), compared to day 0, indicated by **

Regulation of ERα and ERβ protein expression

Estrogens accelerate ER protein turnover by a proteasome-mediated process, which affects ER protein levels (24). After 3 days of culture in Phenol Red-free medium supplemented with 20% charcoal-stripped FBS, there was a ~2.2-fold increase in ERα protein and a decrease in ERβ protein levels, by Western analysis. The levels of estrogen receptor proteins and the levels of their mRNAs were discordant. When 17β-estradiol (10^{-10}–10^{-8} M) was added, 3 days after culture under these conditions, there was an increase in ERα protein levels. We observed a ~three-fold increase in ERα protein after 24 hours (17β-estradiol 10^{-10} M). After 72 hours, the maximal increase (~8.5-fold) was seen at 10^{-9} M of 17β-estradiol ($p < 0.05$). There was a ~2.4-fold increase in ERα level in the control cells treated with vehicle after 72 hours. ERβ protein levels increased ~1.6-fold in the presence of 10^{-9} M 17β-estradiol ($p < 0.05$) after 72 hours of treatment and decreased $\sim$0.6-fold in the control cells treated with vehicle. Thus, estrogens affected estrogen receptor protein levels in mesangial cells and increased their estrogen responsiveness.

MMP-9 activity

Following 3 days of culture, the presence of 17β-estradiol (10^{-10}–10^{-8} M) resulted in an increase in MMP-9 mRNA expression and activity after 24 hours. There was a significant $\sim$1.7-fold (175.4$\pm$25.0% of control, $p < 0.01$) increase in the steady-state levels of MMP-9 mRNA in the presence of 10^{-8} M 17β-estradiol after 24 hours (Figure 27.4). No noticeable changes in the levels of MMP-9 mRNA were observed after 72 hours in the absence of 17β-estradiol stimulation; however, MMP-9 activity in mesangial cells increased markedly when treated with 17β-estradiol. After 24 hours, treatment with 10^{-8} M 17β-estradiol caused a $\sim$3.3-fold increase (328.4$\pm$73.4% of control, $p < 0.05$) in MMP-9 activity (Figure 27.4). After a 72 hours, there was a $\sim$2.4-fold (238.3$\pm$37.5% of control) increase in MMP-9 activity in the presence of 10^{-8} M 17β-estradiol (data not shown). These changes were abolished in the presence of the estrogen receptor antagonists, tamoxifen and ICI 182,780. Tamoxifen (10^{-6} M) and ICI 182,780 (10^{-6} M) blocked the 17β-estradiol-induced increase in MMP-9 activity in the mouse mesangial cells (60.1$\pm$15.4% and 59.9$\pm$10.4% of control, respectively) during a 24 hour incubation period. In addition, neither of these inhibitors significantly affected baseline MMP-9 activity (126.7$\pm$27.45% and 75.7$\pm$26.7%, respectively).

These studies demonstrated that 17β-estradiol upregulates MMP-9 expression in mesangial cells, which may have important implications for ECM turnover in diabetic nephropathy.

DISCUSSION

Role of MMPs in diabetic nephropathy

Several studies show that diabetic glomerulosclerosis is associated with a decrease in glomerular MMP levels. For instance, total MMP activity in glomeruli is decreased in diabetic rats (25). In rat and human mesangial cells, elevated glucose levels led to decreased MMP-2 levels (26,27). In the latter study, TIMP1 levels were moderately increased. Thus, the data from rat and human mesangial cells suggest that overall ECM degradation would be decreased in diabetics. This postulate is confirmed by recent data on glomeruli isolated from diabetic patients, where a decrease in MMP-2 mRNA was found (28). Coupled with the finding that post-menopausal women have a relative

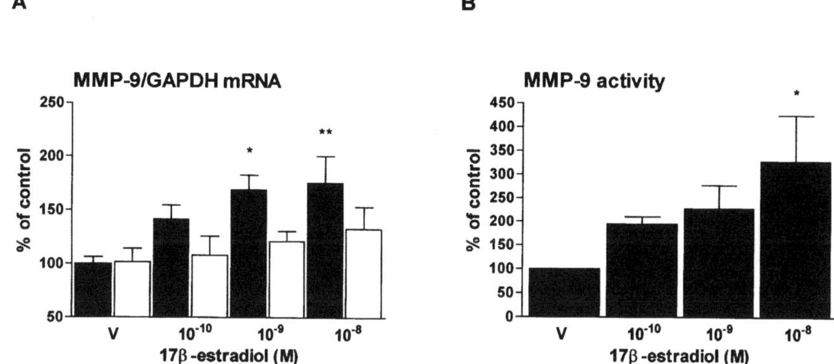

Figure 27.4. *Estradiol increases MMP-9 mRNA expression and activity.* Mesangial cells isolated from C57BL/6J mouse glomeruli were grown for 3 days in Phenol Red-free DMEM/F12 supplemented with 20% charcoal-stripped FBS. Medium was replaced with Phenol Red-free DMEM/F12 medium supplemented with 0.1% charcoal-stripped FBS and 17β-estradiol (10^{-10}–10^{-8} M) for 24 and 72 hours. (A) MMP-9 mRNA expression (normalized to GAPDH) in the presence of 17β-estradiol for 24 hours (closed bars) and 72 hours (open bars). (B) MMP-9 activity as assessed by zymography 24 hours after 17β-estradiol addition. Data are expressed as percentages of control (V, vehicle = 0.001% EtOH) at 24 hours. Shown are means±SE of three independent experiments. Statistical significance ($p < 0.01$ and $p < 0.05$) compared to baseline value (V) are indicated by [**] and [*], respectively

increase in diabetic nephropathy, these data suggest that there may be a link between estrogen status, MMP levels, and diabetic nephropathy.

MMP and TIMP function(s)

Remodeling of the extracellular matrix occurs in the normal maintenance of organ structure and function. Abnormalities in remodeling, as a result of a disease process, result in scarring. One important contributor to the turnover of ECM is a class of zinc-dependent proteases, the matrix metalloproteinases. Regulating the activity of the MMPs at the transcriptional, translational, secretion or extracellular activation levels is important in the maintenance of normal ECM. All MMPs possess conserved functional and structural protein domains, resulting in similar characteristics of activation, latency and enzyme activity (29). The amino-terminal (activation locus) and the catalytic site (Zn^{++} binding region) are the sites of greatest homology. The MMPs have been subdivided into five groups, based on substrate specificity (30). A new group of MMPs have been recently discovered, which are bound to cell membranes, the MT-MMPs (31–34). MT-MMP-1 is expressed predominantly in the kidneys, placenta, and GI tract (34). Its expression results in activation of pro-MMP-2 (pro-gelatinase A). It is blocked by molar excesses of TIMP-2, but not TIMP-1 (32). This could be an important observation for the mechanism(s) of glomerulosclerosis, since mesangial cells produce TIMP-2 (2).

Genetic basis of susceptibility to glomerulosclerosis

Multiple data suggest that the propensity to develop glomerulosclerosis is under genetic control. For instance, less than 40% of diabetics develop glomerulosclerosis resulting in end-stage renal disease (35,36). These observations led to the concept of sclerosis-prone and sclerosis-resistant backgrounds (37). In sclerosis-sensitive individuals, the response to injury is associated with progressive sclerosis, through a continuing excess synthesis of ECM and/or insufficient degradation. In sclerosis-resistant individuals, injury does not result in the progressive accumulation of ECM, suggesting that excess ECM synthesis is a transient event, appropriately balanced by MMP synthesis. The protection in sclerosis-resistant individuals is not absolute, as evidenced by the fact that very high levels of a sclerotic stimulus (i.e. 1000-fold excess growth hormone levels) results in the development of progressive glomerulosclerosis and renal failure in sclerosis-resistant mice transgenic for this hormone (38).

Role of estrogen in revealing genetic susceptibility to glomerulosclerosis

Estrogen status has also been shown to play a role in progressive glomerular lesions in rats. Severe glomerular lesions were observed in aging male rats but not in females (39). Similarly, subtotal nephrectomy in male and female Sprague–Dawley rats revealed that females had less proteinuria, less severe glomerulosclerosis and lower procollagen type IV levels than males, although systemic hypertension and glomerular hypertrophy were identical in both sexes (40). Female Munich–Wistar rats reportedly had fewer severe lesions than male rats (41). The frequency of renal impairment is less in female fawn-hooded rats than in males (42,43). These studies did not include analyses of the sex hormones. While metalloproteinase levels are not generally reported, higher glomerular metalloproteinase activity was found in mature adult female Munich–Wistar rats than in males with glomerulosclerosis (44). The authors concluded that testosterone was a causal agent in the sclerosis seen in males, and that the higher MMP levels in female rats contributed to the relative protection against the glomerulosclerosis found with aging in this rat strain. Not all investigators find that estrogen deficiency enhances renal disease. However, in the two known exceptions, the authors felt the results could be due to the marked elevation of plasma cholesterol, triglycerides and lipoproteins induced by estrogens in these analbuminemic rat models (45,46).

Regulation of sstrogen function(s) in mesangial cells

Estrogen action is mediated via estrogen receptor (ER) subtypes ERα and ERβ. We found that both ER subtypes were expressed and functional in human and mouse mesangial cells (MCs). In the presence of 17β-estradiol (10^{-10}–10^{-8} M), there was a progressive increase in the steady-state mRNA levels of both ERα and ERβ. ERα protein levels increased $\sim$three-fold after 24 hours and up to $\sim$8.5-fold after 72 hours. ERβ protein levels increased $\sim$1.6-fold in the presence of 17β-estradiol after 72 hours. Thus, the regulation of ER expression in mesangial cells was estrogen-dependent and estrogens may maintain or even increase the estrogen responsiveness of mesangial cells. The effect(s) of estrogens may account for their protective role in progressive glomerular disease. Glomerulosclerosis is largely due to excess of extracellular matrix and/or decrease of MMPs secreted by mesangial cells. We found that estrogen receptors increased MMP-9 mRNA and activity, thus accounting for part of the protective role of estrogens in diabetic nephropathy.

17β-estradiol enhances the release of matrix metalloproteinase-2 from human coronary artery and umbilical artery smooth muscle cells (47). In one study of rat mesangial cells, 17β-estradiol was shown to decrease total collagen synthesis by 30% (16). In a subsequent study these authors showed that 17β-estradiol blocked the agonist effects of TGFβ1 on transcription of the (α1 type IV collagen gene in a line of mouse mesangial cells (48).

Regulation of estrogen receptor expression and activity

We found both ERα and ERβ in human and mouse mesangial cells (6–9). We found that estrogen receptors are transcriptionally active in mesangial cells using an estrogen-responsive reporter construct (ERE) in transient transfection assays. The 1.5–2-fold increase of luciferase activity from a single ERE-driven reporter construct after 17β-estradiol stimulation (10^{-8} M) was in agreement with previously published data using supra physiologic doses of 17β-cstradiol (10^{-7} M) (4).

While estrogens are one of the most intensively studied modulators of estrogen receptor expression, little is known about the regulation of the estrogen receptor subtypes in vascular smooth muscle cells. Cell culture conditions have a profound impact on estrogen receptor levels. There was a change in the steady-state mRNA levels of the estrogen receptor subtypes after transfer of mesangial cells into charcoal-stripped FBS and phenol red-free medium. After an incubation period of 72 hours, ERα mRNA decreased, while ERβ mRNA increased.

Regulation of MMPs by estrogen

MMPs play an important role in ECM turnover and in tissue remodeling. MMP-9 belongs to a subgroup of matrix-degrading enzymes, which exhibit high activity against gelatin and type IV collagens (2,49). We found that 17β-estradiol induced MMP-9 mRNA expression and activity in a dose-dependent manner, and this was blocked by anti-estrogens (tamoxifen and ICI 182,780), suggesting that these effects were ER-mediated. In addition, we found that the response to estrogen stimulation was blunted in mesangial cells of certain sclerosis-prone mouse strains ($ROP^{+/+}$), and was essentially absent in others (NOD mesangial cells after the onset of diabetes mellitus). The molecular mechanisms by which estrogens regulate MMP-9 transcription in mesangial cells are unknown, and are the subject of current investigations in our laboratory. The rather complex nature of this promoter region may allow the cell to regulate MMP-9 expression under physiological and pathophysiological conditions. The importance of the present data is that estrogens activate MMP-9 expression in mesangial cells, which may contribute to the relative protection from diabetic nephropathy in premenopausal women.

SUMMARY

Mesangial cells express both estrogen receptor subtypes and estrogens positively regulate their transcription. The response to estrogens is blunted in sclerosis-prone mouse mesangial cells.

REFERENCES

1. Stamataki KE, Spina J, Rangou DB, Chlouverakis CS, Piaditis GP: Ovarian function in women with non-insulin dependent diabetes mellitus. *Clin Endocrinol* 45:615–621, 1996.
2. Lenz O, Striker LJ, Jacot TA, Elliot SJ, Killen PD, Striker GE: Glomerular endothelial cells synthesize collagens but little gelatinase A and B. *J Am Soc Nephrol* 9:2040–2047, 1998.
3. Lenz O, Elliot SJ, Stetler-Stevenson WG: Matrix metalloproteinases in renal development and disease. *J Am Soc Nephrol* 11:575–581, 2000.
4. Karas RH, Patterson BL, Mendelsohn ME: Human vascular smooth muscle cells contain functional estrogen receptor. *Circulation* 89:1943–1950, 1994.
5. US Renal Data System: *USRDS 1997 Annual Data Report*. Bethesda, MD: The National Institutes of Health, NIDDK, 1997.
6. Enmark E, Pelto-Huikko M, Grandien K *et al*: Human estrogen receptor beta-gene structure, chromosomal localization, and expression pattern. *J Clin Endocrinol Metab* 82:4258–4265, 1997.
7. Greene GL, Gilna P, Waterfield M, Baker A, Hort Y, Shine J: Sequence and expression of human estrogen receptor complementary DNA. *Science* 231:1150–1154, 1986.
8. Tremblay GB, Tremblay A, Copeland NG *et al*: Cloning, chromosomal localization, and functional analysis of the murine estrogen receptor beta. *Mol Endocrinolo* 11:353–365, 1997.
9. White R, Lees JA, Needham M, Ham J, Parker M: Structural organization and expression of the mouse estrogen receptor. *Mol Endocrinol* 1:735–744, 1987.
10. Hodges YK, Richer JK, Horwitz KB, Horwitz LD: Variant estrogen and progesterone receptor messages in human vascular smooth muscle. *Circulation* 99:2688–2693, 1999.

11. Karas RH, Patterson BL, Mendelsohn ME: Human vascular smooth muscle cells contain functional estrogen receptor. *Circulation* 89:1943–1950, 1994.

12. Karas RH, Baur WE, van Eickles M, Mendelsohn ME: Human vascular smooth muscle cells express an estrogen receptor isoform. *FEBS Lett* 377:103–108, 1995.

13. Lindner V, Kim SK, Karas RH, Kuiper GG, Gustafsson JA, Mendelsohn ME: Increased expression of estrogen receptor-beta mRNA in male blood vessels after vascular injury. *Circ Res* 83:224–229, 1998.

14. Mashiah A, Berman V, Thole HH *et al*: Estrogen and progesterone receptors in normal and varicose saphenous veins. *Cardiovasc Surg* 7:327–331, 1999.

15. Register TC, Adams MR: Coronary artery and cultured aortic smooth muscle cells express mRNA for both the classical estrogen receptor and the newly described estrogen receptor beta. *J Steroid Biochem Mol Biol* 64:187–191, 1998.

16. Kwan G, Neugarten J, Sherman M *et al*: Effects of sex hormones on mesangial cell proliferation and collagen synthesis. *Kidney Int* 50:1173–1179, 1996.

17. Striker GE, Striker L:Biology of disease: glomerular cell culture. *Lab Invest* 53:122–131, 1985.

18. Elliot SJ, Striker LJ, Hattori M *et al*: Mesangial cells from diabetic NOD mice constitutively secrete increased amounts of insulin-like growth factor-I. *Endocrinology* 133:1783–1788, 1993.

19. MacKay K, Striker LJ, Elliot S, Pinkert CA, Brinster RL, Striker GE: Glomerular epithelial, mesangial, and endothelial cell lines from transgenic mice. *Kidney Int* 33:677–684, 1988.

20. Fornoni A, Lenz O, Tack I *et al*: Matrix accumulation in mesangial cells exposed to cyclosporin A requires a permissive genetic background. *Transplantation* 2000 (in press).

21. Berthois Y, Katzenellenbogen JA, Katzenellenbogen BS: Phenol red in tissue culture media is a weak estrogen: implications concerning the study of estrogen-responsive cells in culture. *Proc Natl Acad Sci USA* 83:2496–2500, 1986.

22. Chomczynski P, Sacchi N: Single-step method of RNA isolation by acid guanidinium thiocyanate–phenol–chloroform extraction. *Anal Biochem* 162:156–159, 1987.

23. Jacot TA, Striker GE, Stetler-Stevenson MA, Striker LJ: Mesangial cells from transgenic mice with progressive glomerulosclerosis exhibit stable, phenotypic changes including undetectable MMP-9 and increased type IV collagen. *Lab Invest* 75:791–799, 1996.

24. Alarid ET, Bakopoulos N, Solodin N: Proteasome-mediated proteolysis of estrogen receptor: a novel component in autologous downregulation. *Mol Endocrinol* 13:1522–1534, 1999.

25. Reckelhoff JF, Tygart VL, Mitias MM, Walcott JL: STZ-induced diabetes results in decreased activity of glomerular cathepsin and metalloprotease in rats. *Diabetes* 42:1425–1432, 1993.

26. Anderson SS, Wu K, Nagase H, Stettler-Stevenson WG, Kim Y, Tsilibary EC: Effect of matrix glycation on expression of type IV collagen, MMP-2, MMP-9 and TIMP-1 by human mesangial cells. *Cell Adhes Commun* 4:89–101, 1996.

27. Leehey DJ, Song RH, Alavi N, Singh AK: Decreased degradative enzymes in mesangial cells cultured in high glucose media. *Diabetes* 44:929–935, 1995.

28. Del Prete D, Anglani F, Forino M *et al*: Downregulation of glomerular matrix metalloproteinase-2 gene in human NIDDM. *Diabetologia* 40:1449–1454, 1997.

29. Birkedal-Hansen H, Moore WG, Bodden MK *et al*: Matrix metalloproteinases: a review. *Crit Rev Oral Biol Med* 4:197–250, 1993.

30. Corcoran ML, Hewitt RE, Kleiner JrDE, Stetler-Stevenson WG: MMP-2: expression, activation and inhibition. *Enzyme Protein* 49:7–19, 1996.

31. Sato H, Takino T, Okada Y *et al*: A matrix metalloproteinase expressed on the surface of invasive tumour cells. *Nature* 370:61–65, 1994.

32. Takino T, Sato H, Shinagawa A, Seiki M: Identification of the second membrane-type matrix metalloproteinase (MT- MMP-2) gene from a human placenta cDNA library. MT-MMPs form a unique membrane-type subclass in the MMP family. *J Biol Chem* 270:23 013–23 020, 1995.

33. Takino T, Sato H, Yamamoto E, Seiki M: Cloning of a human gene potentially encoding a novel matrix metalloproteinase having a C-terminal transmembrane domain. *Gene* 155:293–298, 1995.

34. Will H, Hinzmann B: cDNA sequence and mRNA tissue distribution of a novel human matrix metalloproteinase with a potential transmembrane segment. *Eur J Biochem* 231:602–608, 1995.

35. Doria A, Warram JH, Krolewski AS: Genetic susceptibility to nephropathy in insulin-dependent diabetes: from epidemiology to molecular genetics. *Diabet Metab Rev* 11:287–314, 1995.

36. Striker GE, Peten EP, Carome MA *et al*: The kidney disease of diabetes mellitus (KDDM): a cell and molecular biology approach. *Diabet Metab Rev* 9:37–56, 1993.

37. Brown DM, Provoost AP, Daly MJ, Lander ES, Jacob HJ: Renal disease susceptibility and hypertension are under independent genetic control in the fawn-hooded rat. *Nat Genet* 12:44–51, 1996.

38. Yang CW, Striker GE, Chen WY, Kopchick JJ, Striker LJ: Differential expression of glomerular extracellular matrix and growth factor mRNA in rapid and slowly progressive glomerulosclerosis: studies in mice transgenic for native or mutated growth hormone. *Lab Invest* 76:467–476, 1997.

39. Elema JD, Arends A: Focal and segmental glomerular hyalinosis and sclerosis in the rat. *Lab Invest* 33:554–561, 1975.

40. Lombet JR, Adler SG, Anderson PS, Nast CC, Olsen DR, Glassock RJ: Sex vulnerability in the subtotal nephrectomy model of glomerulosclerosis in the rat. *J Lab Clin Med* 114:66–74, 1989.

41. Remuzzi A, Puntorieri S, Mazzoleni A, Remuzzi G: Sex related differences in glomerular ultrafiltration and proteinuria in Munich–Wistar rats. *Kidney Int* 34:481–486, 1988.

42. Gilboa N, Rudofsky U, Magro A: Urinary and renal kallikrein in hypertensive fawn-hooded (FH/Wjd) rats. *Lab Invest* 50:72–78, 1984.

43. Kreisberg JI, Karnovsky MJ: Focal glomerular sclerosis in the fawn-hooded rat. *Am J Pathol* 92:637–652, 1978.

44. Reckelhoff JF, Baylis C: Glomerular metalloprotease activity in the aging rat kidney: inverse correlation with injury. *J Am Soc Nephrol* 3:1835–1838, 1993.

45. Joles JA, van Goor H, Koomans HA: Estrogen induces glomerulosclerosis in analbuminemic rats. *Kidney Int* 53:862–868, 1998.

46. Sakemi T, Ohtsuka N, Shouno Y, Morito F: Effect of ovariectomy on glomerular injury in hypercholesterolemic female Imai rats. *Nephron* 72:72–78, 1996.

47. Wingrove CS, Garr E, Godsland IF, Stevenson JC: 17bβ-oestradiol enhances release of matrix metalloproteinase-2 from human vascular smooth muscle cells. *Biochim Biophys Acta* 1406:169–174, 1998.

48. Lei J, Silbiger S, Ziyadeh FN, Neugarten J: Serum-stimulated α 1 type IV collagen gene transcription is mediated by TGF-β and inhibited by estradiol. *Am J Physiol* 274:F252-F258, 1998.

49. Mott JD, Khalifah RG, Nagase H, Shield CF, Hudson JK, Hudson BG: Nonenzymatic glycation of type IV collagen and matrix metalloproteinase susceptibility. *Kidney Int* 52:1302–1312, 1997.

28

Pathophysiology of Diabetic Neuropathy: a Worrying Report

J. D. WARD and S. M. RAJBHANDARI

Department of Diabetic Medicine, Royal Hallamshire Hospital, Sheffield, UK

It is not the intention of this chapter to add to the numerous reviews of pathological pathways that may lead to damage to diabetic peripheral and autonomic nerve (1). Clinicians are well aware of the devastating effects of nerve damage in diabetes with regard to painful syndromes, neuropathic foot problems and impotence, along with the mercifully less common but very distressing syndromes of autonomic neuropathy. Sadly, the last three decades of research have not, as yet, led to an understanding of the mechanisms that allows any useful treatment to be offered to patients. Moreover, the pathways producing painful symptoms are likewise ill-understood and therapy for pain is not very effective. Much knowledge, but no understanding. The reason that real progress has been negligible is related to the enormous difficulties encountered in studying human nerve tissue—you cannot see it, biopsy opportunities are limited and surrogate tests tell us very little directly about the pathological process.

THEORIES BASED ON ANIMAL WORK

Many mainly metabolic theories of pathogenesis have been proposed from animal models. It is difficult to see the relevance of metabolic abnormalities found in young diabetic rats to the aged upright human being, and yet massive effort has been generated in the animal laboratories and taken by the pharmaceutical industry into clinical trials that have generally shown no

Diabetes in the New Millennium. Edited by U. Di Mario, F. Leonetti, G. Pugliese, P. Sbraccia and A. Signore.
© 2000 John Wiley & Sons, Ltd.

efficacy whatsoever, and maybe never will. The polyol pathway and aldose reductase theory has been on the move for nearly 30 years (2), followed by studies on growth factor in nerve (3) and protein kinase C (4), the process of oxidative stress and the possible benefits of antioxidant therapy (5), and the area of vasoactive factors relating to γ-linolenic acid (6). Moreover, it has been demonstrated that nerve protein is glycosylated (7), although the potent therapy that might reverse such glycosylation is not suitable in human subjects. It seems quite possible that all these factors are indeed relevant in human subjects, leading to nerve dysfunction and damage, and it would therefore be necessary to consider attacking the diseased nerve with therapies relating to all these abnormalities—perhaps the production of a composite compound 'neurosalve'. That further multiple pharmaceutical interests would be prepared to collaborate in such a project seems unlikely. However, the synergism between γ-linolenic acid and antioxidants, demonstrated by Cameron and Cotter (8) in respect to nerve blood flow and conduction velocities in rats, should lead to strong consideration of such a multipathogenetic approach to treatment.

THE HUMAN SITUATION

While it is not clear how rats suffer from diabetic nerve damage, humans clearly do. Much fine descriptive clinical work has characterized the many syndromes of diabetic peripheral and autonomic neuropathy (9). Such studies represent the very best in detailed clinical observation but such clinical classification gives no lead to pathogenesis, but rather raises very difficult problems. Why should different syndromes develop, and why in some patients and not others? No predictive factor or genetic input has yet been demonstrated as to why some subjects develop diabetic neuropathy. A personal observation is equally worrying. A male diabetic patient of 28, who presented with a totally paralysed bladder but who was not impotent, raises the question of how such highly selective nerve damage can occur. Numerous clinical and epidemiological studies have repeatedly shown that the age of the patient, the duration of the diabetes and the quality of the diabetic control are the main determinants of the development of neuropathy. Again, such observations give no lead to the mechanisms leading to the nerve damage. If we fully understood the pathways to neuropathy, we would then have to explain why one clinical syndrome develops rather than another.

A regular feature of diabetic neuropathy research has been the demonstration that electrical nerve conduction measurements improve as the blood glucose improves (10) and that the degree of electrophysiological deficit relates to the severity of the pathological change (11), but even these observations are unhelpful in understanding the pathogenesis. Further correlates of neuropathy with lipid status and blood pressure take us no further (12).

The possibility of more detailed analysis of human nerve in biopsy studies would seem very appealing in being able to elucidate pathogenetic mechanisms. However, in a clinical trial of aldose reductase therapy in diabetic neuropathy, where large numbers of sural nerve biopsies were performed before and after treatment, the assessment of fibre numbers and density showed considerable variation, which make it very difficult to see how clinical trials based on biopsy work can be of any value (2). The demonstration that regeneration of fibres is far more active in subjects with diabetic neuropathy with type 1 diabetes as opposed to type 2 diabetes indicates that clinical trials in the future should perhaps focus on either one of these types of diabetes, rather than mixing them together (13).

The literature bulges with papers on autonomic function tests and it seems very likely that abnormalities may relate to future mortality (14), yet we know little about the human autonomic nerve, apart from a suggestion that an autoimmune process may be at play. It is essential to understand whether autonomic fibre damage is a cause of early death.

THE MICROVASCULAR THEORY

Although the primary interest of the authors, it is not suggested that microvascular change in nerve is the one and only mechanism causing damage. The processes are complexly interrelated but there is ample visual evidence of small vessel disease in human diabetic peripheral nerve. There seems little dispute concerning the central role of microvascular abnormalities in the retinopathy and nephropathy, and many of the changes seen in nerve are identical to those in other tissues, and yet many authorities ignore the possibility of their role in nerve. Small vessels in human diabetic neuropathy show occlusion of the capillary lumen (15) and gross thickening of the basal lamina (16), indeed the thickest and most rigid-looking of all microvessels in human tissue. It is postulated that such extensive thickening of the basal lamina could be related to the upright posture and deficiency of vasoregulatory fibres which produce vasoconstriction on standing (17). Other changes on nerve show arterio-venous shunts of epineurial vessels (18) and gross ischaemia of nerve itself (19). Moreover, nerves from patients with painful neuropathy are ischaemic, while painless neuropathy is not associated with this ischaemia (20).

It is difficult to persuade oneself that by the time such changes are observed, they are not having a profound effect on nerve function, and whether they can ever be reversed seems unlikely. Once again, it is the pathways leading to such gross microvascular damage that need to be investigated, although this is an extremely difficult proposition.

CONCLUSION

The authors are open to the criticism that this review is negative and unhelpful. However, its realism can hardly be denied and to be realistic is to encourage more thought as to the different ways of approaching the problem. These may include nerve biopsy studies earlier in the course of the disease, with good prospective investigations; more detailed long-term clinical follow-up studies; non-invasive imaging of nerve to allow the sequence of metabolic change to be observed; and the possible intervention with multiple treatments relating to the known pathogenetic mechanisms in animals.

A point for the realistic physician — until more detailed understanding of pathogenesis leads to a logical therapy, then the central role of *blood glucose control* must be regarded as the only sure way of minimizing the development of nerve damage, placing neuropathy alongside all the other complications of diabetes as a major reason for provision of adequate clinical services to allow the achievement of the best possible blood glucose control in as many of our patients as possible.

REFERENCES

1. Boulton AJ, Malik RA: Diabetic neuropathy. *Med Clin N Am* 82(4):900–902, 1998.
2. Greene DA, Arezzo JC, Brown MB and the Zenarestat Study Group: Effect of aldose reductase inhibition on nerve conduction and morphometry in diabetic neuropathy. *Neurology* 53:580–591, 1999.
3. Anand P, Terenghi G, Warner G, Kopelman P, Williams-Chestnut RE, Sinicropi DV: The role of endogenous nerve growth factor in human diabetic neuropathy. *Nature Med* 2:703–707, 1996.
4. Nakamura J, Kato K, Hamada Y, Nakayama M, Chaya S, Nakashima E, Naruse K, Kasuya Y, Mizubayashi R, Miwa K, Yasuda Y, Kamiya H, Ienaga K, Sakakibara F, Koh N, Hotta N: A protein kinase C-beta-selective inhibitor ameliorates neural dysfunction in streptozotocin-induced diabetic rats. *Diabetes* 48(10):2090–2095, 1999.
5. Greene DA, Stevens MJ, Obrosova I, Feldman EL: Glucose-induced oxidative stress and programmed cell death in diabetic neuropathy. *Eur J Pharmacol* 375(1–3):217–223, 1999.
6. Jamal GA: The use of gamma linolenic acid in the prevention and treatment of diabetic neuropathy. *Diabet Med* 11(2):145–149, 1994.
7. Vlassara H, Brownlee M, Cerami A: Nonenzymatic glycosylation of peripheral nerve protein in diabetes mellitus. *Proc Natl Acad Sci USA* 78(8):5190–5192, 1981.

8. Cameron NE, Cotter MA: Comparison of the effects of ascorbyl gamma-linolenic acid and gamma-linolenic acid in the correction of neurovascular deficits in diabetic rats. *Diabetologia* 39(9):1047–1054, 1996.

9. Thomas PK: Classification, differential diagnosis, and staging of diabetic peripheral neuropathy. *Diabetes* 46 (Suppl 2):S54–57, 1997.

10. Ward JD, Barnes CG, Fisher DJ, Jessop JD, Baker RW: Improvement in nerve conduction following treatment in newly diagnosed diabetics. *Lancet* 1(7696):428–430, 1971.

11. Malik RA, Tesfaye S, Thompson SD, Veves A, Sharma AK, Boulton AJ, Ward JD: Endoneurial localisation of microvascular damage in human diabetic neuropathy. *Diabetologia* 36(5):454–459, 1993.

12. The EURODIAB Prospective Complication study (PCS) Group: Cardiovascular risk factors predict diabetic peripheral neuropathy in type 1 subjects in Europe. *Diabetologia* 42(Suppl 1):A50, 1999.

13. Bradley JL, Thomas PK, King RH, Muddle JR, Ward JD, Tesfaye S, Boulton AJ, Tsigos C, Young RJ: Myelinated nerve fibre regeneration in diabetic sensory polyneuropathy: correlation with type of diabetes. *Acta Neuropathol* 90(4):403–410, 1995.

14. Rathmann W, Ziegler D, Jahnke M, Haastert B, Gries FA: Mortality in diabetic patients with cardiovascular autonomic neuropathy. *Diabet Med* 10(9):820–824, 1993.

15. Timperley WR, Boulton AJ, Davies-Jones GA, Jarratt JA, Ward JD: Small vessel disease in progressive diabetic neuropathy associated with good metabolic control. *J Clin Pathol* 38(9):1030–1038, 1985.

16. Malik RA, Newrick PG, Sharma AK, Jennings A, Ah-See AK, Mayhew TM, Jakubowski J, Boulton AJ, Ward JD: Microangiopathy in human diabetic neuropathy: relationship between capillary abnormalities and the severity of neuropathy. *Diabetologia* 32(2):92–102, 1989.

17. Ward JD: Upright posture and the microvasculature in human diabetic neuropathy: a hypothesis. *Diabetes* 46 (Suppl 2):S94–97, 1997.

18. Tesfaye S, Malik R, Harris N, Jakubowski JJ, Mody C, Rennie IG, Ward JD: Arterio-venous shunting and proliferating new vessels in acute painful neuropathy of rapid glycaemic control (insulin neuritis). *Diabetologia* 39(3):329–335, 1996.

19. Newrick PG, Wilson AJ, Jakobowski J, Boulton AJM, Ward JD: Sural nerve oxygen tension in diabetes. *Br Med J* 293:1053–1054, 1986.

20. Eaton SEM, Ibrahim S, Harris ND, Selmi F, Patel KA, Tesfaye S, Ward JD: Difference in sural nerve haemodynamics in painful and painless diabetic neuropathy: clues to the cause of pain? *Diabet Med* 17 (Suppl 1):18, 2000.

29

Diagnosis and Treatment of Diabetic Neuropathy

VINCENZA SPALLONE and GUIDO MENZINGER
Department of Internal Medicine, University of Rome "Tor Vergata", Italy

Diabetic neuropathy can be defined as the presence of symptoms and signs of peripheral nerve dysfunction in diabetic patients after exclusion of other causes (1). Among different clinical syndromes characterizing diabetic neuropathy, polyneuropathy is the most common. Recently, due to a greater uniformity in diagnostic criteria, the amount of data available on the prevalence of this form has markedly increased. Based on clinical criteria, i.e. signs and symptoms, a prevalence of about 30% has been reported by several epidemiological studies in both type 1 and type 2 diabetes. Moreover, a large multicentre study in Italy has provided similar values of prevalence, 32% using clinical criteria, and 28% using clinical and electrodiagnostic criteria (2).

DIAGNOSIS OF PERIPHERAL DIABETIC NEUROPATHY

Twelve years ago, the San Antonio Conference on Diabetic Neuropathy organized by the American Diabetes Association (1) provided recommendations to fully classify diabetic polyneuropathy, indicating the need to perform at least one measure from each of the following five categories: (a) clinical symptoms; (b) clinical examination; (c) electrodiagnostic studies; (d) quantitative sensory testing; (e) autonomic function testing. This approach requires experienced personnel and specialized equipment. It is appropriate for research purposes but less practical for routine clinical settings, where simplicity, rapidity and a wide availability of techniques are necessary. Thus, Feldman *et*

Diabetes in the New Millennium. Edited by U. Di Mario, F. Leonetti, G. Pugliese, P. Sbraccia and A. Signore.
© 2000 John Wiley & Sons, Ltd.

al. (3) developed a two-step quantitative clinical and electrophysiological assessment. In the first step, called the Michigan Neuropathy Screening Instrument, patients initially undergo a questionnaire and screening examination, and in the case of positive findings, a further quantitative neurological examination coupled with nerve conduction studies, together called the Michigan Diabetic Neuropathy Score. A similar two-step approach was used in a multicentre Italian study on 8757 diabetic patients (2). Finally, international guidelines on the outpatient management of diabetic peripheral neuropathy were developed in London in 1995 from an international consensus meeting and approved by the Neuropathy Study Group of the EASD in 1997 (4). They propose a simplified diagnostic protocol to be used by practising clinicians in primary or hospital care, based on patient history and neurological symptoms, inspection of feet, and neurological examination (pin-prick test, light touch, vibration test, ankle reflex, pressure perception).

Clinical measures

In order to allow a complete, systematic, rapid, and quantitative assessment of symptoms, questionnaires with scoring systems have been developed such as the Neurological Symptom Score of Dyck *et al.* (5), a validated standardized scale, particularly useful in clinical trials. Shorter questionnaires are also available which focus on more common neuropathic symptoms and are aimed at screening purposes. Validated pain scales are useful for quantifying pain severity over time, but positive symptoms do not necessarily correspond to the degree of nerve fibre damage.

Neurological examination evaluates sensory and motor deficit. Scoring systems are available, such as the Neurological Disability Score of Dyck *et al.* (5), that improve standardization and reproducibility. Short versions of neurological examinations have been developed for outpatient diagnostic evaluation and include basic assessment of vibration with a 128 Hz tuning fork on the big toe, of light touch with a cotton wisp, of pain with disposable dressmaker's pins, of pressure perception with a 10 g monofilament, of ankle reflex, and of muscle strength (walk on heels and foot extension). Inspection of the feet is essential for identifying feet at risk for ulceration. It is easy and quick, and represents a mandatory component of routine clinical evaluation of diabetic patients.

Quantitative sensory testing

Instrumental procedures have been introduced that allow a quantitative assessment of somatosensory function (QST). They are based on the evaluation of evoked sensation in response to measurable physical stimuli that activate cutaneous sensory receptors. They are psychophysical somatosensory tests that evaluate the function of the whole afferent nervous pathway from the receptor to the brain. Thus, they are psychodependent and influenced by both the attention and motivation of the patient. Although there are problems of standardization, reproducibility, specificity and cost, these tests represent a valid adjunct to the clinical examination, as they are very sensitive and non-invasive (6). Elevated thresholds are the correlate of clinical sensory loss, and are associated with neuropathological abnormalities, with neuropathic symptoms, with deficits and with reduced conduction velocity (5). They are related to clinical end-points of diabetic neuropathy and have been shown to be independent predictors of foot ulcerations.

Vibration perception testing is the most widely used method. It has good reproducibility, it is easy to perform and uses low-cost equipment of small size (biothesiometer). A vibration perception threshold (VPT) higher than 25 V identifies patients at increased risk for foot ulceration.

Assessment of the thermal perception threshold (TPT) is the selective measure of C fibres. Its impairment is common and early, probably due to the high susceptibility of small fibres to damage. Several devices have been developed to test the TPT. However, they are quite expensive, time-consuming and have low reproducibility.

Pressure perception cutaneous threshold (PPCT) can be measured very easily using Semmes–Weinstein monofilaments. Absence of sensation in the foot to the filament of 10 g has proved to be a prognostic marker of the risk of foot ulceration.

The Computer Assisted Sensory Examination (CASE) systems are automated microprocessor-controlled systems that deliver appropriate and quantified stimuli, using algorithms of testing and finding thresholds. The CASE IV system evaluates vibratory, cooling and warming thresholds and heat-pain, thus exploring large- and small-fibre sensory function. Sensory abnormalities as measured by CASE provide a reliable, reproducible and sensitive index of diabetic neuropathy. The availability of normative values in more than 300 healthy subjects allows comparison of patient values to those of a control group. Variability of thresholds with site, age, sex, body mass index and body surface area has been documented in healthy subjects (5). Thus, CASE IV is a very effective device, although somewhat expensive and too time-consuming for routine clinical settings. Its results have been used as end-points in clinical trials, especially those with NGF.

Electrodiagnosis

Electrodiagnostic assessments provide a direct evaluation of neural activity and correlate with clinical neurological deficits, with underlying pathophysiological changes and with QST to a variable degree.

Needle electromyography is the most sensitive indicator of motor axonal degeneration. It documents denervation in muscles secondary to myelinic or axonal neural damage, axonal loss and functional alterations. Due to its relative invasiveness, it is usually reserved for diagnostic evaluation in the individual patient.

Nerve conduction studies with surface electrodes obtain measure of motor and sensory conduction velocity, distance latency, evoked-response amplitude and F wave latency. While conduction velocity depends on fibre diameter and myelin integrity, amplitude correlates to the number of active axons, i.e. to fibre density, thus corresponding better to the early pathophysiological changes. A major limit of electrodiagnosis is represented by its ability of studying exclusively large-diameter myelinated fibres ($A\alpha$ and $A\beta$), whereas thinly myelinated ($A\delta$) or unmyelinated fibres (C) are those involved at an earlier stage. Moreover, since the rate of decrease in conduction velocity is rather slow in the natural history of diabetic neuropathy (0.5–0.7 m/s per year), this parameter could not be a very sensitive marker of the onset of diabetic neuropathy (7). However, its greater sensitivity compared to clinical measures has been documented, together with a reproducibility excellent for groups and good for individuals (7). On the other hand, no electrodiagnostic abnormalities are specific for diabetic neuropathy, indicating a need to identify, in any case, other possible causes of nerve dysfunction. Recommendations for standardization have been provided (6) and considerable progress has been achieved in standardization and interpretation of the results (7). Electrodiagnosis has proven to be an effective endpoint in several trials in diabetic neuropathy.

Diagnosis of diabetic neuropathy in patients with unusual problems might need a full electrodiagnosis with electromyography and conduction studies in upper and lower limbs, while for epidemiological purposes or for clinical trials it can be sufficient to perform conduction velocity studies only on one side.

The assessment of response area instead of amplitude, the measurement of distribution of velocities or of current thresholds needed to elicit a response, and multistimulus collision techniques, are some methodological innovations proposed to increase sensitivity of electrodiagnosis, but which have not actually been implemented (7).

In conclusion, in a diagnostic approach to diabetic neuropathy, it is important to distinguish between different purposes, i.e. epidemiological studies, pharmacological trials or clinical diagnosis in individual patients, to identify increased risk of ulceration or to properly classify diabetic neuropathy. The multimodal approach suggested by the San Antonio Conference is the best way to fully classify neuropathy and to better evaluate pharmacological effects in clinical trials. The use of composite scores, such as NIS(LL) + 7, developed by Dyck *et al.* (5), a score that includes Neuropathy Impairment Score (NIS) for lower limbs and seven electrophysiological, quantitative sensory and autonomic tests, is a preferable method of combining information from multiple measures in a single score, to use for longitudinal studies. Simpler scoring systems have been developed by Feldman *et al.* (3) and by Arezzo *et al.* (7). Simplified approaches aimed at the identification of patients at risk for ulceration include symptoms evaluation, foot inspection and a brief neurological examination, according to the guidelines for outpatient management of diabetic neuropathy (4). The inclusion of QST with biothesiometer or monofilament may become routine clinical practice.

New technical developments in peripheral neuropathy testing

Skin-punch biopsy and immunostaining with specific antibodies to human protein gene product 9.5, substance P and calcitonin gene-related peptide is a new technique of morphological evaluation of peripheral nerve damage, with the advantage of minimal trauma to the patient compared to whole-nerve biopsy. It provides reliable staining of small axons innervating the skin and allows quantification of fibre density with good interobserver agreement and demonstrated correlation with clinical degree of diabetic neuropathy (7). Criticism has been expressed about the actual meaning of this technique, i.e. how well it detects all nerve fibres and what degree of change over time corresponds to a clinical change (5).

Motor function in diabetic neuropathy has recently been reviewed by Andersen (8). Muscle strength is commonly evaluated by testing the ability to stand on heels and toes and to arise from a kneeling position, or by dynamometry. Dynamometry shows a moderately impaired strength and working performance of the lower extremity in long-term type 1 diabetic patients, but an unexplained increased muscular endurance. Movement performance, gait and postural stability are also impaired in neuropathic diabetic patients (9). Magnetic resonance imaging of the lower limbs has allowed documentation of reduced muscle volume of the ankle extensors and flexors, with a clear distal–proximal gradient of muscular atrophy (8). Finally, quantitative electromyography with the specialized techniques of single fibre electromyography and macro-EMG has shown a close and inverse relationship between muscle strength and signs of reinnervation, suggesting that reinnervation is insufficient in diabetic neuropathy (8).

DIAGNOSIS OF AUTONOMIC NEUROPATHY

Cardiovascular reflex tests

The development of simple non-invasive cardiovascular reflex tests has allowed extensive evaluation of diabetic autonomic neuropathy, now recognized as an earlier and more frequent diabetic complication than previously thought, with a prevalence of 16–22% in both type 1 and type 2 diabetes (10,11). Although in recent years much has been done for the standardization of these tests, many questions still remain unresolved. Regarding the choice of tests, the Ewing battery of five tests was recommended by the San Antonio conference on diabetic neuropathy (1), while in the Proceedings of a more recent consensus, only three tests were proposed (6). Nevertheless, the tests most widely used, validated and best known in their physiological bases, are heart rate (HR); variation on deep breathing, lying-to-standing and Valsalva manoeuvre; and the blood pressure (BP) response to standing. Also for these tests there are some problems with the techniques, measurements and indices used for assessment, in particular for deep breathing and lying-to-standing tests (11–13). The development of computer-assisted systems will probably allow easier and more standardized procedures in the performance of tests and in the calculation of results.

Many authors have emphasized the need for age-related normal limits to define test results, since using the non-age-related normal values proposed by Ewing (12), false-negatives are possible in younger and false-positives in older patients. Probably, provided that more than one test and the classification proposed by Ewing are used, in the age range of diabetic patients commonly undergoing autonomic function assessment, Ewing's limits of normality retain validity for clinical purposes.

Confounding factors in cardiovascular tests

Cardiovascular tests measure the end-organ response to the activation of a neural reflex arc. An abnormal response may result from an alteration in any step of the reflex arc. Thus, adequacy of the stimulus, the patient's collaboration, instruction and familiarization with the test are necessary to achieve a standardized stimulus. Other factors, such as cardiovascular disease or volume status, may influence the tests by affecting end-organ function. Moreover, many drugs, such as antihypertensive drugs, diuretics and antidepressants, may interfere with tests, either inhibiting or exciting the cardiovascular responses, with non-homogeneous effects even within the same class (13).

Recommendations for standardization of testing have recently been provided (6), including the avoidance of many possible confounding factors for 8–12 hours before the test, such as physical exercise, stress, alcohol, hypoglycaemia, food, coffee, smoking, metabolic derangement, insulin and drugs. In particular, caffeine, alcohol, smoking and insulin can acutely modify the tests based on BP (13).

In conclusion, the recommendations of the American Diabetes Association consensus conference (6) to use for diagnostic purposes at least three among standard cardiovascular tests, i.e. deep breathing, Valsalva manoeuvre and postural hypotension, are still valid. In the presence of cardiovascular disease, especially in young patients, or when drugs cannot be withdrawn, some caution is needed in interpreting the results.

Sympathetic function tests

A limit of the standard cardiovascular tests is a rather poor sensitivity of blood pressure (BP) tests, whose impairment generally follows that of HR variation tests. Moreover, the sustained handgrip test has poor reproducibility. The mental arithmetic stress test has been described as being more sensitive than the sustained handgrip and postural hypotension tests. The cold pressor test probably shows too low reproducibility to be accepted as a standard test. The squatting test has recently been introduced as a non-invasive test of both parasympathetic and sympathetic function. Squatting-induced bradycardia would be mediated by the vagus nerve, whereas cardio-acceleration from squatting to standing would express a sympathetic activation triggered by a sustained fall in BP on standing. Early simultaneous involvement of both components of autonomic nervous system are described in diabetic patients (11–13).

Baroreflex sensitivity testing

A rapid rise in arterial BP, induced by an α-adrenoceptor stimulant such as phenylephrine, elicits a reflex bradycardia; the rise in systolic BP and the lengthening of the RR interval are linearly related, and the slope of this relationship may be taken as an index of baroreflex sensitivity (BRS) (14). Another method to study BRS is by analysing the spontaneous fluctuations of BP in steady-state conditions through the 'sequences' method or the 'α angle'. The 'sequences' method is based on continuous recording of BP and HR and on identifying sequences of at least three successive beats, where progressive increase in systolic BP is associated with progressive decrease in HR or vice versa. Such sequences are considered to be baroreflex-mediated and the regression coefficient of the sequences is an index of BRS. The 'α angle' analyses the gain of the baroreflex loop on the assumption that, given the presence of a significant relationship between BP and HR documented by the coherence function, fluctuations produced on HR by BP are baroreflex-mediated. Thus, when applying spectral analysis to BP and HR signals, the 'α angle' is the ratio between RR interval and BP spectral powers at each frequency (15).

Baroreflex-mediated bradycardia is impaired in diabetic patients. Animal studies have attributed this impairment to a selective defect in parasympathetic control of HR during increases in BP, and more precisely to a defect in the activation of central parasympathetic pathways. The index α in diabetic patients when supine and after tilting has indicated a progressive loss of baroreflex loop gain. A reduction in baroreflex gain assessed using the 'sequences' method and the 'α angle' has been increasingly reported, with the characteristic of a greater sensitivity in comparison with standard cardiovascular tests (15). The significance of these early abnormalities, i.e. if structural or functional in nature, is not completely clear as to the utility of these tests for clinical use. However, increasing evidence points to the prognostic value of BRS for cardiovascular mortality in the general population in chronic heart failure and in myocardial infarction, thus supporting a prognostic significance of impaired BRS also in diabetic patients (13–15).

Prolongation of the QT interval

Prolongation of the QT interval has been reported in diabetic autonomic neuropathy and associated with poorer survival prognosis in diabetic patients (11–13). This ECG abnormality is considered to be a marker of electrical instability, possibly leading to life-threatening ventricular arrhythmias. Although several reports have linked QT prolongation to diabetic autonomic neuropathy, QT lengthening now seems to be related also to other factors, such as female gender and genetic factors (16). Moreover, a correlation between QTc (rate corrected QT) and standard cardiovascular tests has been reported to be weak and not constant, so that the use of QT interval as a reliable single index of autonomic dysfunction should be made with caution. However, although the aetiopathogenesis of QT prolongation in diabetes appears to be quite complex, there is a growing evidence regarding its significance as an independent predictor of cardiac deaths in various cardiac diseases, in alcoholic liver disease, in dysautonomias, in diabetic nephropathy and so on. In type 1 diabetic patients with overt nephropathy, a prolonged QTc was associated with an increased mortality risk, independently of the presence of autonomic neuropathy. In type 2 diabetes the role of QTc as a prognostic marker of mortality is less obvious, whereas QT dispersion might be more important. QT dispersion (the difference between the longest and shortest QT interval from any lead of a 12-lead ECG) reflects a sort of spatial heterogeneity of repolarization and is an independent marker of arrhythmogenic potential. Increased QT dispersion has been found to be a major determinant of total mortality risk in type 2 diabetic patients, but it seems to be more linked to structural factors and focal ischemia than to autonomic neuropathy *per se*.

Imaging of myocardial sympathetic innervation

Non-invasive methods for the *in vivo* evaluation of the myocardial sympathetic activity have been recently developed. They measure the postganglionic presynaptic noradrenergic uptake of noradrenaline analogues, such as ^{123}I meta-iodobenzylguanidine (^{123}I-MIBG), with single photon emission computed tomography (SPECT) gamma scintigraphy, or ^{11}C-hydroxyephedrine (^{11}C-HED) with positron emission tomographic (PET). Reduced myocardial ^{123}I-MIBG accumulation and ^{11}C-HED retention independent on coronary flow defect have been shown in diabetic patients as in various cardiac diseases and also in dysautonomias. A relationship between these uptake abnormalities and indexes of cardiac autonomic function, such as cardiovascular tests, QT interval and HR variability, has been described in diabetic patients, but at a weaker degree than expected and inconstantly, at least in part indicating a greater sensitivity than indirect autonomic function testing. Whether the reduced ^{123}I-MIBG uptake always reflects true structural changes or reversible functional abnormalities in cardiac sympathetic innervation is not elucidated, in particular when considering the reports of myocardial sympathetic dysinnervation in newly-diagnosed type 1 diabetic patients, and of a potential reversibility of ^{123}I-MIBG uptake and ^{11}C-HED retention defects by near-normoglycaemia (11,13). Another interesting point regards distribution of sympathetic dysinnervation, which is commonly heterogeneous and involves predominantly posterior or inferoposterior regions, or apical, inferior and lateral walls, according with a distal–proximal gradient. Furthermore, proximal hyperinnervation associated with distal denervation has been recently shown by Stevens *et al.* (17) and considered a source of electrical instability, possibly triggering arrhythmogenic activity.

Heart rate variability

Analysis of HR variability has been used as a measure of cardiac autonomic control. It can be performed by statistical operations on RR intervals (time domain analysis) or by spectral analysis of a series of successive RR intervals (frequency domain analysis). Both analyses can be performed on short RR sequences or on 24 hour ECG recordings (12).

A number of time domain indices can be obtained from RR intervals. Standard deviation (SD), coefficient of variation (CV) for a given RR interval sequence, or for a sequence of successive RR interval differences, and also the mean square (MSSD) or the root mean square of successive RR interval differences (RMSSD). The RMSSD and counts method, first introduced by Ewing (12), would be more specific for vagal activity. The counts method measures the number of larger differences ($> 50\,\mathrm{ms}$) in successive RR intervals. It is considered to be easy, relatively insensitive to artefacts, rather reproducible, and more sensitive than standard cardiovascular tests (12). The widespread use of 24 hour ECG recordings in cardiology has led to a number of studies in which 24 hour HR variability indices were shown to be a prognostic marker after myocardial infarction for all-cause mortality, for sudden deaths, and for arrhythmic events (18). Low 24 hour HR variability has been interpreted as the expression of a shift in sympathovagal balance in favour of sympathetic activity with arrhythmogenic effect. A decrease in 24 hour HR variability measured by time domain indices has been observed in diabetic patients, being more pronounced in those with cardiovascular test impairment (12).

Spectral analysis of HR variability allows the evaluation of both components of the autonomic nervous system in steady-state conditions and has a greater ability in differentiating vagal and sympathetic modulation of HR than time-domain methods. Abnormalities in spectral parameters with reduction in both low- (LF) and high-frequency (HF) components of the power spectrum seem to occur before clear alterations in the standard cardiovascular tests, and document, in addition to a parasympathetic involvement, an early impairment of sympathetic heart control. Also, spectral analysis of BP and peripheral flow signals would indicate in diabetic patients an impaired sympathetic outflow to vessels. Thus, neural control of both HR and BP could be altered early in the course of diabetes (11,13).

Circadian rhythms of cardiovascular parameters

Twenty-four hour ECG recordings have shown a progressive flattening of the normal 24 hour heart rate pattern in diabetic patients with increasing degree of autonomic damage, resulting in a complete loss of the nocturnal fall (12). Also, the night-time increase in HR variability is attenuated in diabetic patients (19).

As in patients with primary autonomic failure, tetraplegia, uremic neuropathy and cardiac transplantation, a blunted or reversed circadian pattern of BP has been described in diabetic patients. Although it has been also reported in macro- and microalbuminuric type 1 diabetic patients, this abnormality seems to be most likely linked to autonomic neuropathy. A reduced BP nocturnal fall has also been associated with higher left ventricular mass index in normotensive diabetic patients with autonomic neuropathy (13). Moreover, in diabetic patients a reversed circadian pattern of BP has been found to be associated with an increased risk of fatal and non-fatal vascular events, especially in type 2 diabetic patients.

Spectral analysis of HR variability applied to 24 hour ECG recordings, has shown a circadian rhythm of sympathovagal balance in the general population. There is a day-time prevalence of the LF component, a marker of sympathetic activity, and a prominent increase of the HF component, a marker of vagal activity, during the night, with a consequent decrease from day to night in the LF:HF ratio, an index of sympathovagal balance. In diabetic patients with autonomic neuropathy there is a blunting in the nocturnal increase of the HF component (19), indicating the persistence of a sympathetic dominance during the night. A relationship between this circadian sympathovagal imbalance and the loss of the nocturnal BP fall has been shown (13). It might represent an additive cardiovascular risk factor and modify the circadian distribution of cardiovascular events, accounting for the reported high incidence of myocardial infarction during the night in diabetic patients.

Twenty-four hour evaluation of HR variability has greater sensitivity and a better intraindividual reproducibility than short-term evaluation (18). It provides data on the circadian rhythm of sympathovagal activity, and thus on autonomic control mechanisms linked to the sleep cycle, which can be affected earlier and differently from those involved in cardiovascular reflex tests. Furthermore, the information obtained could have prognostic implications and offer therapeutic opportunities aimed at restoring the most favourable balance throughout the 24 hour period. On the other hand, there are still many problems of standardization with these methods. In addition, sensitivity, specificity and prognostic value of

HR variability assessment have to be determined in large longitudinal studies in the general and in the diabetic population (18).

TREATMENT OF DIABETIC NEUROPATHY

That hyperglycaemia is a requisite condition for the development and progression of diabetic neuropathy has been clearly demonstrated in many animal studies and in man in the DCCT study (20). The same study clearly shows the benefit of strict glycaemic control on the progression of neuropathy. Thus, meticulous control of blood glucose is certainly the mainstay in the prevention and treatment of diabetic neuropathy.

However, it must be recognized that even strict glycaemic control, as achieved in the DCCT, does not obtain regression but at best a stabilization of existent neuropathy. In the most advanced degree of metabolic control obtainable with pancreas transplantation, there has been a doubtful degree of regression in composite scores of neuropathy in a follow-up study of 10 years, with more stabilization in autonomic parameters. In any case, significant differences between transplanted and non-transplanted patients began to appear after 42 months with a clear separation after 10 years (21). These findings suggest that any proposed treatment for diabetic neuropathy will probably need 5 years of clinical trials before a difference between treated and untreated patients is significantly established. Such a long period of observation requires that the proposed treatment be absolutely free from serious side effects.

In general, aetiologic treatment of diabetic neuropathy has been discouragingly unsuccessful in man, even when apparently highly effective in animals.

The main lines of pathogenesis around which treatments have been set up include metabolic changes, ischaemic alterations and growth factor deficiency. These pathogenetic mechanisms interact with each other and the most probable theory is that neuropathy recognizes a multifactorial origin.

The main metabolic pathways identified in experimental studies as being associated with the development of diabetic neuropathy are: (a) increased activity of the polyol pathway through aldose reductase activation; (b) auto-oxidation of glucose, leading to reactive oxygen species (ROS); (c) formation of advanced glycosylation end products by non-enzymatic glycosylation of proteins; (d) inappropriate activation of protein kinase C.

In the presence of hyperglycaemia, sorbitol is formed through the action of aldose reductase, and then converted to fructose by sorbitol dehydrogenase. The first reaction involves the oxidation of NADPH to $NADP^+$, whereas the second reaction involves the reduction of NAD^+ to NADH. The decreased availability of NADPH associated with the flux through the polyol pathway has some important consequences. The first concerns the detoxification of reactive oxygen species (ROS), such as the superoxide anion and the hydroxyl radical. A key enzyme in detoxification is superoxide dismutase, which induces the catalysis of superoxide into hydrogen peroxide, which in turn is reduced in the mitochondria by reduced glutathione (GSH), which is converted to oxidized glutathione (GSSG). Regeneration of GSH by glutathione reductase requires NADPH. Lack of NADPH results in mitochondrial damage by ROS. Mitochondrial dysfunction then causes reduced production of ATP, that is required for *de novo* synthesis of GSH, thus further impairing defence against ROS. A similar mechanism also may limit the activity of the NADPH-dependent nitric oxid synthase (NOS), leading to decreased production of the potent vasodilator nitric oxide, vasoconstriction, nerve ischemia, increased ROS production and mitochondrial damage (22).

In the presence of elevated levels of glucose, proteins undergo non-enzymatic glycosylation leading to the formation of the advanced glycosylation end-products (AGEs). The production of AGEs is enhanced by ROS and in their turn AGEs enhance the generation of ROS through a process known as auto-oxidative glycosylation.

The role of protein kinase C (PKC) in diabetic neuropathy is probably more complex than in other complications, as PKC is reported to be reduced rather than increased in diabetic rat sciatic nerve, while increased aldose reductase pathway activity promotes diacylglycerol synthesis by diverting dihydroxya-cetone phosphate towards formation of α-glycerophosphate, which is known to increase PKC activity. Activation of PKC would then promote vasoconstriction and nerve ischaemia (22).

Several vascular abnormalities expression of nerve ischaemia have been documented in diabetic neuropathy, both morphological changes, such as thickening or occlusion of endoneurial and epineurial blood vessels, and functional impairment, as decreased neural blood flow and pO_2, and increased vascular resistance (23). Many vasodilating agents have been shown to be effective in experimental neuropathy (24), and some encouraging data have recently appeared on the use of the ACE inhibitor trandolapril in patients with diabetic neuropathy (25).

Deficiencies in growth factors have been reported in diabetes. A reduction of insulin-like growth factor (IGF) gene expression has been observed in rodents, and a reduction of circulating IGFs has been reported in type 1 diabetic patients with neuropathy. A decrease in nerve growth factor (NGF) concentration and axonal transport in rat sciatic nerve and in the skin of diabetic patients has been reported. Other growth factors are being studied (26,27).

Deficiency of γ-linolenic acid (GLA) has been observed in rodent diabetic nerve, which leads, through an imbalance between lipo-oxygenase and cyclo-oxygenase, to a defective production of vasodilating prostaglandins and then to vasoconstriction, nerve ischemia and abnormalities in conduction velocity (26).

Attempts at treatment of diabetic neuropathy have for a long time concentrated on what seemed a key passage in the metabolic changes leading from hyperglycaemia to nerve damage, that is on the inhibition of the enzyme regulating access to the polyol pathway, aldose reductase. Notwithstanding notable successes with ARIs in experimental neuropathy, however, clinical experimentation has been largely unsuccessful. This may have been associated with problems of duration of the studies, neural penetration of drugs and toxicity, whereas some long-term trials with new ARIs with a promising profile are still going on.

Another logical step in the aetiologic treatment of diabetic neuropathy is to interfere with the ROS mechanism of damage through the use of antioxidants. In animal studies, various antioxidants, such as α-tocopherol, α-lipoic acid and probucol, have been shown to improve neural blood flow and conduction velocity (22,24,26). In humans a large clinical trial of α-lipoic acid is in progress. There have also been many reports of positive effects of α-lipoic acid in the German literature (α-lipoic acid having been on the market there for some time) (28).

The administration of GLA in diabetic patients has been moderately successful in improving nerve conduction velocity without symptomatic improvement (26). The production of AGEs can be inhibited by aminoguanidine with increase in conduction velocity in experimental diabetes. However, clinical trials started in man did not reach significant effects or were interrupted before completion (26).

The perception that neuropathy is the outcome of complex interactions between various pathways leading to nerve dysfunction is prompting experiments with combinations of drugs acting with different mechanisms. For instance, a marked synergy of action has been recently observed in animal studies by the combination of GLA and antioxidants such as α-lipoic acid. Similar synergies have also been observed between ARIs and GLA (26).

TREATMENT OF PAINFUL DIABETIC NEUROPATHIES

Neuropathic pain is present in many of the clinical syndromes of diabetic neuropathy with possible different behaviour in terms of localization, duration and natural history. Thus, before starting a pharmacological treatment of painful diabetic neuropathies, a correct diagnosis should be made in order to obtain prognostic information (29).

Symptomatic treatment of painful polyneuropathies is still problematic due to incomplete effectiveness of the drugs available and to the difficulty in evaluating therapeutic response. Because of the great variability and unpredictibilty of individual responsiveness to drugs, the results of significant pain relief and amelioration of quality of life with tolerable side-effects can be obtained only by ensuring an adequate trial for each drug prescribed. Each trial should be conducted for a sufficient length of time and at adequate dosage, beginning with the lowest dosage and then increasing it every 5–7 days until significant pain relief or intolerable side-effects occur.

Given the documented clinical relationship between rapid worsening or amelioration of glycaemic control and onset of acute painful neuropathies, the first step in management of these neuropathies is to attempt a stable optimal glycaemic balance and to avoid glycaemic oscillations. Non-steroidal anti-rheumatic agents can be only used for short-term or for slightly painful neuropathies. Tricyclic antidepressants are the first-line drugs, acting by blocking reuptake of noradrenaline and serotonin, thus enhancing the nociceptive-modulation system in the brainstem. The efficacy of amitriptyline, imipramine and desipramine has been proved in several placebo-controlled trials with a percentage of responders at about 60%. Desipramine is better tolerated, with less anticholinergic and sedative effects than the best studied, amitriptyline. A meta-analysis of antidepressants in neuropathic pain syndromes has confirmed their efficacy in painful diabetic neuropathy, indicating a number needed to treat of 3.2 and an odds ratio when comparing active to placebo treatment of 3.6. On the other hand, there were no benefits using fluoxetine, paroxetine or mianserin, compared to placebo (30). Among anticonvulsants, carbamazepine was used with a certain efficacy but with common side-effects, especially in the past. A new anticonvulsant, gabapentin, has been recently proposed for painful diabetic neuropathy. This drug acts through complex and unknown mechanisms involving its structural similarity with GABA, in both the central and peripheral nervous systems. In an 8 week placebo-controlled study in 165 diabetic patients with chronic painful polyneuropathy at a dosage of 3600 mg/day, it was proved to obtain a significant pain relief with limited side-effects (31).

Local anaesthetic agents, such as intravenous lidocaine and oral mexiletine, have been used in some placebo-controlled studies, with particular efficacy in subsets of patients with symptoms of burning, heat or stabbing or with night-time pain and sleep disturbances. They act by blocking sodium channels and spontaneous firing in regenerating fibres. Mexiletine is contraindicated in second- or third-degree atrioventricular blockade, and should be used with caution in presence of cardiac diseases, but in general at a maximal dose of 10 mg/kg body weight/day it is well tolerated without cardiovascular side-effects (30).

Tramadol, a centrally acting analgesic with low-affinity to μ-opioid receptors and weak inhibition of noradrenaline and serotonin reuptake, has been used in a double-blind randomized trial in 131 diabetic patients, showing, at a dosage of 210 mg/day, greater efficacy than placebo, with minor adverse events (32).

Among trials in diabetic neuropathy with drugs acting on pathogenetic mechanisms, two studies with antioxidant α-lipoic acid deserve to be mentioned because pain was included among the end-points. In the ALADIN study, 260 type 2 diabetic patients with symptomatic neuropathy were given α-lipoic acid intravenously over 3 weeks at a dosage of 600 mg/day

Table 29.1.   Management of painful diabetic neuropathies

Correct diagnosis
Glycaemic control
Pharmacological treatments
   Tricyclic antidepressant
      Amitriptyline: 10–150 mg/day at bedtime
   Anticonvulsant agents
      Gabapentin: 900–3600 mg/day
   Opioids
      Tramadol: 50–400 mg/day in four doses
   Anaesthetic–antiarrhythmic agents
      Mexiletine: 150–10 mg/kg body weight in three doses after meals
Physical adjuvant measures
   TENS
   Physiotherapy

---

with a significant effect on pain and without major side-effects. However, in a successive study (ALADIN III), a 3-week intravenous treatment with α-lipoic acid followed by a 6-month oral treatment (600 mg/day) failed to obtain any effect on neuropathic symptoms (28).

Isolated reports in small groups of patients suggest a possible utility of transcutaneous electrical nerve stimulation (TENS) and spinal cord electrical stimulation. The former is safe and has also been used in combination with amitryptiline; the latter should be reserved for severe cases unresponsive to conventional therapies.

In conclusion, after correct diagnosis, a possible treatment algorithm of painful diabetic neuropathy includes an attempt to reach a stable optimal glycaemic control, and then a trial with tricyclic antidepressants, which have to be replaced, in the case of intolerance or inefficacy, with gabapentin, tramadol or mexiletin. A possible adjuvant role of TENS should not be undervalued, and physical therapies are useful in the patient's functional recovery (Table 29.1).

SYMPTOMATIC TREATMENT OF AUTONOMIC NEUROPATHY

Although rigorous glycaemic control in type 1 diabetic patients can prevent the development and delay the progression of autonomic neuropathy (20), no or only slight improvement of cardiovascular tests can be obtained with combined kidney and pancreas transplantation after several years (21). Thus, treatment of clinical autonomic neuropathy becomes almost exclusively symptomatic.

Orthostatic hypotension should be treated only when symptomatic, with the aim of minimizing cerebral hypoperfusion in the upright posture. Non-pharmacological measures have to be applied first, such as: (a) avoiding drugs that potentially exacerbate symptoms, alcohol, large carbohydrate rich meals, heat exposure; (b) supplementary salt intake to ensure water retention; (c) full-length elastic stockings; (d) physical manoeuvres, increasing venous return, such as leg-crossing, bending forward, or squatting. Head-up tilt during the night can be useful to correct excessive nocturnal diuresis and natriuresis, and the consequent morning hypotension. In the uncommon forms non-responsive to these measures, pharmacological treatment is indicated.

Fludrocortisone is the most widely used drug, at a dose of 0.1–0.4 mg/day. Supine hypertension and fluid retention are common side-effects, sometimes leading to drug withdrawal. Recently, erythropoietin (25–50 U/kg × 3/week) is increasingly being used in dysautonomic patients with orthostatic hypotension, for the finding of anoemia with relative erythropoietin deficit, which is responsive to erythropoietin treatment, with associated improvement in symptoms of postural hypotension and well-being (33). It is not known whether this beneficial effect of erythropoietin is consequent to anoemia correction or to other direct cardiovascular actions. Caffeine (250 mg before meal) and octreotide, a somatostatin analogue (0.2–0.4 µg/kg s.c. before breakfast) have been used for orthostatic and post-prandial hypotension. Other drugs used in treatment of postural hypotension are midodrine, a peripheral α1-agonist, although with limited effects, and desmopressine, a vasopressin analogue, now available also in tablets to take at bedtime to correct nocturnal polyuria (33,34).

A more relevant problem could be the treatment in neuropathic patients of clinostatic nocturnal hypertension associated with orthostatic hypotension. There is a generical practice of using a short-acting vasodilator (ACE inhibitors, calcium antagonists, hydralazine) just before bedtime, possibly associated with a vasoconstrictor agent during the day. However, this condition remains very difficult to treat, often evolving in later stages into spontaneous attenuation concomitantly with the progression of the usually associated diabetic nephropathy and of fluid retention.

Gastroparesis

Delayed emptying of solid and/or nutrient liquid meals is reported in 30–50% of long-standing type 1 and type 2 diabetic patients. This abnormality may be associated with upper gastrointestinal symptoms, although there is a poor correlation between symptoms and delay in gastric emptying, with impaired glycaemic control, and with delayed oral drug absorption.

Scintigraphy is the method of choice for the measurement of gastric emptying, with the disadvantages of exposure to radiation and of requiring expensive equipment with limited availability. Ultrasound scanning is a time-consuming procedure that needs a skilled operator. Magnetic resonance imaging allows simultaneous assessment of both meal and secretion volumes and of the stomach morphology without exposure to radiation, but its application is limited by the cost. Breath tests are increasingly being used as easy non-invasive diagnostic methods in gastroenterology also for gastric emptying, in particular the ^{13}C-acetate breath test and the ^{13}C-octanoic acid breath test. They may be useful for screening purposes, although the ^{13}C-octanoic acid breath test compared to scintigraphy was found to be sufficiently sensitive, specific and reliable in diabetic patients.

The diagnostic assessment of gastroparesis is complicated by the inhibitory effects of hyperglycaemia on motor gastric activity and emptying in both normal subjects and type 1 diabetic patients. Moreover, insulin-induced hypoglycemia increases the rate of gastric emptying in both normal subjects and type 1 diabetic patients. In addition, there is conflicting evidence of a possible direct inhibitory effect of insulin on gastric motility. Finally, in type 2 diabetic patients in early stages of the disease and in the absence of autonomic neuropathy, a faster gastric emptying for liquid and solid meals has been described, whereas long-standing type 2 diabetic patients and/or those with autonomic neuropathy share the behaviour of type 1 diabetic patients, showing a delayed gastric emptying (35,36).

Treatment of gastroparesis is indicated only in symptomatic forms, after exclusion of other reversible causes. Current treatment includes the use of four gastrointestinal prokinetics, listed in Table 29.2. Due to its sustained effect during chronic administration, cisapride was the drug of first choice until a clear association between use of cisapride and serious cardiac events (QT interval prolongation and ventricular arrhythmias) was evidenced. This fact has led several national health organizations to recommend caution in prescribing the drug and not to authorize its use in infants and children. In particular, the risk of developing serious adverse events is increased by preexisting pro-arrthymogenic conditions, such as QT lengthening, or by concomitant medication with other drugs that affect the QT interval or inhibit cisapride metabolism, or by the use of grapefruit juice. Thus, combined use of cisapride and erythromycin must be avoided. Moreover, diabetic patients with gastroparesis are probably for several reasons, at increased risk of serious cardiac side-effects from cisapride.

Diabetic diarrhoea is a troublesome neuropathic symptom, mostly affecting long-standing type 1 diabetic patients. Its diagnosis can be made only after exclusion of other possible causes. First of all, diarrhoea must be distinguished from fecal incontinence on the basis of daily stool weight (above 200 g). Then, pharmacological causes, general diseases and infectious causes must be excluded. In the presence of steatorrhoea (stool fat above 6 g/day), possible causes of malabsorption should be evaluated, in particular coeliac sprue, pancreatic insufficiency and bile salts deconjugation due to bacterial overgrowth. An increase in exhaled $^{14}CO_2$ in the ^{14}C-D-xylose breath test or in the bile acid breath test, or increased breath H_2 in the glucose H_2 breath test

Table 29.2. Pharmacological treatment of symptomatic diabetic gastroparesis

Drug	Mechanism	Dosage	Side effects
Metoclopramide	Dopamine antagonist (peripheral and central), central anti-emetic, enhanced acetylcholine release	10–20 mg × 4/day*	Restlessness, somnolence, weakness, extrapyramidal symptoms, hyperprolactinaemia
Domperidone	Dopamine antagonist (peripheral)	10–20 mg × 4/day*	Hyperprolactinaemia
Cisapride**	Enhanced acetylcholine release	10 mg × 4/day*	Abdominal cramping, diarrhoea, headache *Serious cardiac arrhythmias (see text)*
Erythromycin	Motilin agonist	3 mg/kg i.v.*** 250 mg × 3/day	Gastrointestinal symptoms, hepatitis, hypersensitivity

*15–30 min before meals and at bedtime.
**Long-term efficacy: *never use in combination with erythromycin* (see text).
***Only in severe cases.

suggest the diagnosis of bacterial overgrowth. Finally, if steatorrhoea is absent, and upper gastrointestinal endoscopy, radiograph with a small bowel follow-through and colonscopy are negative, diabetic diarrhoea is a possible diagnosis.

Treatment of diabetic diarrhoea usually starts with broad spectrum antibiotics, such as tetracycline, paramomycin or metronidazole, which if successful can be prolonged by intermittent, rotating treatment (10 days each month) to avoid resistance to antibiotics. Opiate antidiarrhoeal agents such as codeine, dyphenoxilate or loperamide are potentially useful, although they affect the number of bowel movements more than stool weight. Cholestiramine (4–12 g/day) has some utility in the presence of bile salt malabsorption or resistance to antibiotics. Somatostatin analogues such as octreotide have an inhibitory effect on intestinal water secretion and gastrointestinal hormone secretion. Octeotride has been used (50–75 μg × 2/day s.c.) in several studies with benefits and occasional side-effects (abdominal pain and malabsorption). One case of severe hypertension has been recently observed with the long-acting somatostatin analogue, sandostatin. The use of clonidine, an α_2-adrenergic agonist, was also described as effective in some cases, with possible side-effects avoided with topical treatment (34).

REFERENCES

1. American Diabetes Association and American Academy of Neurology: Consensus statement: report and recommendations of the San Antonio Conference on Diabetic Neuropathy. *Diabet Care* 11:592–597, 1988.
2. Fedele D, Comi G, Coscelli C, Cucinotta D, Feldman EL, Ghirlanda G, Greene DA, Negrin P, Santeusanio F: A multicenter study on the prevalence of diabetic neuropathy in Italy. Italian Diabetic Neuropathy Committee. *Diabet Care* 20:836–843, 1997.
3. Feldman EL, Stevens MJ, Thomas PK, Brown MB, Canal N, Greene DA: A practical two-step quantitative clinical and electrophysiological assessment for the diagnosis and staging of diabetic neuropathy. *Diabet Care* 17:1281–1289, 1994.
4. Boulton AJM, Gries FA, Jervell JA: Guidelines for the diagnosis and outpatient management of diabetic peripheral neuropathy. *Diabet Med* 15:508–514, 1998.
5. Grant IA, O'Brien P, Dyck PJ: Neuropathy tests and normative results. In *Diabetic Neuropathy*, 2nd edn. Dyck PJ, Thomas PK, Eds. Philadelphia, PA: WB Saunders, 1999, pp. 123–141.
6. Kahn R: Proceedings of a consensus development conference on standardized measures in diabetic neuropathy. *Diabet Care* 15:1081–1103, 1992.
7. Arezzo JC: New developments in the diagnosis of diabetic neuropathy. *Am J Med* 107:9S–16S, 1999.
8. Andersen H. Motor function in diabetic neuropathy. *Acta Neurol Scand* 100:211–220, 1999.
9. Uccioli L, Giacomini PG, Monticone G, Magrini A, Durola L, Bruno E, Parisi L, Di Girolamo S, Menzinger G: Body sway in diabetic neuropathy. *Diabet Care* 18:339–344, 1995.
10. Neil HAW: Epidemiology of diabetic autonomic neuropathy. In *Autonomic Failure*, 3rd edn. Bannister R, Mathias CJ, Eds. Oxford, UK: Oxford Medical Publications, 1992, pp. 683–697.
11. Ziegler D: Diabetic cardiovascular autonomic neuropathy: prognosis, diagnosis, and treatment. *Diabet Metab Rev* 10:339–383, 1994.
12. Ewing DJ: Analysis of heart rate variability and other non-invasive tests with special reference to diabetes mellitus. In *Autonomic Failure*, 3rd edn. Bannister R, Mathias CJ, Eds. Oxford, UK: Oxford Medical Publications, 1992, pp. 312–333.
13. Spallone V, Menzinger G: Diagnosis of cardiovascular autonomic neuropathy in diabetes. *Diabetes* 46 (Suppl 2):S67–S76, 1997.
14. Wieling W, Karemaker JM: Measurement of heart rate and blood pressure to evaluate disturbances in neurocardiovascular control. In *Autonomic Failure*, 4th edn. Mathias CJ, Bannister R, Eds. Oxford, UK: Oxford University Press, 1999, pp. 196–210.
15. Parati G, Di Rienzo M, Omboni S, Mancia G: Computer analysis of blood pressure and heart rate variability in subjects with normal and abnormal autonomic cardiovascular control. In *Autonomic Failure*, 4th edn. Mathias CJ, Bannister R, Eds. Oxford, UK: Oxford University Press, 1999, pp. 211–223.
16. Veglio M, Borra M, Stevens LK, Fuller JH, Perin PC, EURODIAB IDDM Complications Study Group: The relation between QTc interval prolongation and diabetic complications. The EURODIAB IDDM Complications Study Group. *Diabetologia* 42:68–75, 1999.
17. Stevens MJ, Raffel DM, Allman KC, Dayanikli F, Ficaro E, Sandford T, Wieland DM, Pfeifer MA, Schwaiger M: Cardiac sympathetic dysinnervation in diabetes. Implications for enhanced cardiovascular risk. *Circulation* 98:961–968, 1998.

18. Task Force of the European Society of Cardiology and the North American Society of Pacing and Electrophysiology: Heart rate variability. Standards of measurement, physiological interpretation, and clinical use. *Circulation* 93:1043–1065, 1996.

19. Bernardi L, Ricordi L, Lazzari P, Soldà PL, Calciati A, Ferrari MR, Vandea I, Finardi G, Fratino P: Impaired circadian modulation of sympatho-vagal activity in diabetes: a possible explanation for altered temporal onset of cardiovascular disease. *Circulation* 96:1443–1452, 1992.

20. The Diabetes Control and Complications Trial Research Group: The effect of intensive diabetes therapy on the development and progression of neuropathy. *Ann Intern Med* 122:561–568, 1995.

21. Navarro X, Sutherland DER, Kennedy WR: Long term effects of pancreatic transplantation on diabetic neuropathy. *Ann Neurol* 42:727–736, 1997.

22. Feldman EL, Russel JW, Sullivan KA, Golovoy D: New insights into the pathogenesis of diabetic neuropathy. *Curr Opin Neurol* 12:553–563, 1999.

23. Vinik AI: Diabetic neuropathy: pathogenesis and therapy. *Am J Med* 107:17S–26S, 1999.

24. Cameron NE, Cotter MA: Metabolic and vascular factors in the pathogenesis of diabetic neuropathy. *Diabetes* 46(Suppl 2):S31–S37, 1997.

25. Malik RA, Williamson S, Abbott C, Carrington AL, Iqbal J, Schady W, Boulton AJM: Effect of angiotensin-converting enzyme (ACE) inhibitor trandolapril on human diabetic neuropathy: randomised duble-blind controlled trial. *Lancet* 352:1978–1981, 1998.

26. Ward JD: Improving prognosis in type 2 diabetes. *Diabet Care* 22 (Suppl 2):B84–B88, 1999.

27. Apfel SC: Neurotrophic factors in the therapy of diabetic neuropathy. *Am J Med* 107:34S–42S, 1999.

28. Ziegler D, Hanefeld M, Ruhnau K-J, Hasche H, Lobisch M, Schütte, Kerum G, Malessa R, The ALADIN III Study Group: Treatment of symptomatic diabetic polyneuropathy with the antioxidant α-lipoic acid. *Diabet Care* 22:1296–1301.

29. Thomas PK: Painful diabetic neuropathy: mechanisms and treatment. *Diabet Nutr Metab* 7:359–368, 1994.

30. Benbow SJ, Cossins L, MacFarlane IA: Painful diabetic neuropathy. *Diabet Med* 16:632–644, 1999.

31. Backonja M, Beydoun A, Edwards KR, Schwartz SL, Fonseca V, Hes M, LaMoreaux L, Garofalo E: Gabapentin for the symptomatic treatment of painful neuropathy in patients with diabetes mellitus: a randomized controlled trial. *J Am Med Assoc* 280:1831–1836, 1998.

32. Harati Y, Gooch C, Swenson M, Edelman S, Greene D, Raskin P, Donofrio P, Cornblath D, Sachdeo R, Siu CO, Kamin M: Double-blind randomized trial of tramadol for the treatment of the pain of diabetic neuropathy. *Neurology* 50:1842–1846, 1998.

33. Watkins PJ, Edmonds ME: Diabetic autonomic failure. In *Autonomic Failure*, 4th edn. Mathias CJ, Bannister R, Eds. Oxford, UK: Oxford University Press, 1999, pp. 378–386.

34. Menzinger G, Frontoni S: Symptomatic treatment of autonomic neuropathy in diabetic subjects. *Diabet Nutr Metab* 7:349–358, 1994.

35. Spallone V, Menzinger G: Autonomic neuropathy: clinical and instrumental findings. *Clin Neurosci* 4:346–358, 1997.

36. Horowitz M, Wishart JM, Jones KL, Hebbard GS: Gastric emptying in diabetes: an overview. *Diabet Med* 13:S16–S22, 1996.

30

Diabetic Complications in Pregnancy

FRANCESCO FALLUCCA, ESMERALDA BORRELLO,
NICOLINA DI BIASE, ANGELA NAPOLI, ANGELA SABBATINI
and ERNESTA SCIULLO
Policlinico Umberto 1, Clinica Medica II, Rome, Italy

Diabetic pregnancy tends to focus upon the fetus. Perinatal management emphasizing strict metabolic control has markedly improved perinatal outcome. Using the White classification in pregnancy (1), classes F, R, T and H (with serious diabetic complications), previously discouraged by obstetricians, now often results in a successful outcome.

Although medical advances may have markedly reduced short-term maternal complications, the long-term sequelae of diabetic vascular disease still prevent many mothers from surviving long enough to provide needed nurturance to their children. Despite the the recognition that pregnancy superimposes a condition with marked hormonal and circulatory changes in a woman with a disease characterized by metabolic derangement and complicated by anatomic dysfunction of the micro- and macrocirculation, surprisingly little information has been gathered in a systematic fashion. The majority of observations concern the effect of pregnancy upon diabetic retinopathy or nephropathy. There is information available about the effects of pregnancy upon these complications, as well as the effects of these complications upon the pregnancy. In addition there is scant information about the effect of pregnancy upon women with macrovascular diseases. In a large series published from the Joslin's Clinic (2), the majority of the women with vascular disease had also eye and kidney disease, associated with a poorer perinatal survival of their infants. The reason for the slightly lower perinatal survival in women with micro- and macrovascular disease is not well known, but presumably would be related to alterations in uteroplacental flow, leading to growth retardation or hypoxia. It should also be noted that hypertension has an adverse effect on pregnancy outcome. This is true in all women with diabetes, whether they do or do not have diabetes. Hypertension in women with diabetes may be an independent risk factor or may accompany renal disease. The one maternal complication about which remarkably little is known is diabetic neuropathy. The pathophysiology is currently felt to have to do with metabolic derangements in the nerve and in disturbances in the handling of sorbitol and myoinositol. Since pregnancy is associated with changes in solute content and with syndromes of compression neuropathy, the silence of the literature on the interaction of diabetes and pregnancy is even more striking.

In this chapter we focus our attention on the microvascular diabetic complications (retinopathy, nephropathy and neuropathy) and hypertension in diabetic pregnant women.

DIABETIC RETINOPATHY

It is now clearly established that retinopathy is not a contraindication to pregnancy, although the effect of pregnancy on retinopathy is less clear. As recently as 1971, White advised termination of pregnancy in patients with progressive proliferative retinopathy. The results of the Diabetic Retinopathy Research Group's report in 1976 clearly indicated that proliferative diabetic retinopathy is treatable by photocoagulation (3), and shortly after that the first report on effective photocoagulation of diabetic retinopathy during pregnancy appeared (4). Until the 1980s, very few studies were performed that could have clearly indicated the relationship between pregnancy and retinopathy. The first careful study, which compared pregnant diabetic patients with a control group who were not pregnant, came from Dublin (5). Among the pregnant patients, one with background retinopathy deteriorated to proliferative level, and most others with background retinopathy showed advance of their lesions. There was a remarkable improvement in the post-partum period, so that this careful study clearly indicated worsening of retinopathy during pregnancy, with regression of lesions post partum. Using fluorescein angiograms (which most people would consider contraindicated during pregnancy), Soubrane and co-workers (6) noted that microaneurysm numbers increased during pregnancy and reduced after delivery. In the Wisconsin epidemiological study, a progression of retinopathy related to pregnancy was found (7). Thus, both the descriptive reports and the controlled studies indicate that retinopathy tends to deteriorate during pregnancy, with many improving in the post-partum period.

The pathogenetic mechanisms well recognized in diabetic retinopathy are three: hormonal, metabolic and hemodynamic. Pregnancy is associated with a number of hormonal changes, and some are exaggerated in diabetic patients.

The beneficial effect of strict diabetic control on the fetus has been well known for a long time. Could the rapid normalization of blood glucose in previously poorly controlled diabetic patients be detrimental to retinopathy? In the controlled studies of the Steno Hospital (8), the Kroc study (9) and the Oslo study (10), it was noted that during the first few months following the introduction of good or even excellent blood glucose control, retinopathy deteriorated in some, though not all, patients. The lesions tended to regress, or at least not to advance, after the first few months. The deterioration of retinopathy with improved control in pregnancy does not militate against introduction of such control, but emphasizes the importance of good control even before pregnancy, and suggests that in patients in whom control was poor prior to pregnancy retinal surveillance should be more frequent. The hemodynamic changes of pregnancy may have a role in the deterioration of retinopathy in diabetic women, as observed by Chen and coworkers (11). The increased blood flow which, in diabetics, could be due to high blood glucose, elevated blood pressure or impaired autoregulation associated with pericyte loss, is itself detrimental to diabetic retinopathy (12). In pregnancy all the known pathogenetic mechanisms for deterioration of diabetic retinopathy are involved and worsened, therefore it is not astonishing that in many patients the retinopathy deteriorates more rapidly.

Our experience

Our study (13) on diabetic retinopathy in pregnancy was on the correlation between electroretinographic, ophthalmologic and clinical parameters in 20 diabetic women (11 IDDM, six NIDDM and three GDM). Adaptoelectro-retinography (AERG) was used as the main monitoring parameter, and in particular the relationship between the cone-mediated (b1) and rod-mediated (b2) components of the 'b' wave (b2/b1 ratio) was studied. A significant correlation was demonstrated both between the type of diabetes and AERG responses and between metabolic control (HbA_{1c} value) and AERG alterations. A higher maternofetal complication rate in those patients with more severe and frequent AERG alterations during pregnancy was also found (Table 30.1).

Management

The management of retinopathy should start in the preconception period, improving diabetic control (so that deterioration of retinopathy associated with rapid improvement of control does not occur), and treating any lesions (if

Table 30.1. AERG and maternal–fetal complications

AERG	Fetal status			
	Normal	Jaundice	Malformation	Abortion
Normal	8/8	0/8	0/8	0/8
1 Altered	3/5	1/5	1/5	0/5
$\geqslant$2 Altered	0/9	5/9	1/9	3/9

$\chi^2 = 376.19$; $p = 0.0001$.

present) by photocoagulation. Pregnant patients should have an eye examination at their first visit (better if antenatal). If there is any retinopathy, the eye examination should be repeated frequently. If there is no deterioration, 2-monthly examinations will suffice. Patients with proliferative retinopathy should have early photocoagulation (also during pregnancy).

Diabetic nephropathy

Of all maternal diabetic complications, diabetic renal disease has the most serious consequences for the fetus. While perinatal mortality in diabetic pregnancies has continued to decline over recent decades, it still tends to be high for mothers with diabetic nephropathy.

Overt clinical diabetic nephropathy is characterized by proteinuria (total protein excretion $>0.5\,\text{g}/24$ hours) or urinary albumin excretion $>200\,\mu\text{g/min}$ or $>300\,\text{mg}/24$ hours), hypertension, declining glomerular filtration rate and eventual end-stage renal failure with uremia (14). Incipient diabetic nephropathy is diagnosed when urinary albumin excretion (known as microalbuminuria) is found to be 20–$200\,\mu\text{g/min}$ or 30–$300\,\text{mg}/24$ hours (14). A large percentage (about 85%) of diabetic patients with microalbuminuria progress to diabetic nephropathy (15,16). Factors that may influence the susceptibility to diabetic nephropathy include genetic predisposition (17) or familial clustering of other influences, such as poor glycemic control, hyperlipidemia or hypertension (17).

The effect of pregnancy on the glomerular filtration rate (GFR) and effective renal plasma flow (ERPF) was disputed for many years. Serial studies performed in the 1950s convincingly demonstrated that both GFR and ERPF increase during pregnancy (18). More recently, investigators have studied the course of renal hemodynamics in pregnancy (19). These studies indicate that GFR markedly increases early in pregnancy and the increment is maintained, at least until the last month of gestation. ERPF also increases markedly during gestation and is as high as 50–80% above prepregnancy levels during the initial two trimesters (19). Near term, however ERPF seems to decrease approximately 25% (19), but it remains considerably above non-gravid values. The reason that renal hemodynamics increase during gestation is obscure, but there are a number of cardiovascular, volume and endocrine changes in normal pregnancy that could conceivably influence renal function. On the other hand, plasma albumin decreases early in pregnancy, and the concomitant decrease in oncotic pressure, which may enhance glomerular filtration, is sustained to term (20). Endocrine changes during gestation include increases in the production and circulating levels of aldosterone, deoxycorticosterone, progesterone, prolactin, cortisol and parathyroid hormone, as well as placental lactogen and chorionic gonadotropin. Finally, it has been observed that renal hemodynamics increase in pseudo-pregnant rats, suggesting that factors that trigger the gestational increase in GFR are independent of the products of conception (21). The increase in GFR has important clinical consequences. Increments in clearances of creatinine and urea lead to reductions in their plasma levels. Sims and Krantz (22) observed that serum creatinine concentration averaged 0.67±14 (mg/dl) in non-pregnant women and 0.46±0.13 (mg/dl) during pregnancy. The implication of all these observations is that values considered normal in non-pregnant women may reflect decreased renal function during gestation. Concentrations of serum creatinine and urea nitrogen exceeding 0.8 (mg/dl) and 13 (mg/dl), respectively, should alert the physician to evaluate renal function further.

Diabetic nephropathy is a progressive disorder in absence of pregnancy. There is no evidence that pregnancy hastens the progression. The diagnosis of diabetic nephropathy during pregnancy is usually made on the basis of the same parameters reported outside pregnancy. The presence of nephropathy in pregnant women with diabetes compounds the risk to the mother and fetus.

As recently as 1977, Pedersen (23) stated that not only should these pregnancies be discouraged but that therapeutic termination should be offered to patients with nephropathy, in particular those with renal failure and pre-existing hypertension. He further mentioned that the prognosis for the infant was poor, with an extraordinarily high perinatal mortality rate, an increased incidence of congenital malformations and a substandard 'quality' of the surviving infant. However, more recently, studies by Kitzmiller (24), Jovanovic (25), Nesler (26) and Reece (27) have demonstrated that perinatal outcome has significantly improved in women with diabetic nephropathy. In these studies, creatinine clearance was not worsened by the course of pregnancy in the majority of the women with renal disease. Proteinuria increased dramatically in the third trimester and the degree of proteinuria was associated with poor perinatal outcome, especially when linked to hypertension and low creatinine clearance.

On the other hand, a proportion of non-proteinuric insulin-dependent diabetic patients (without overt nephropathy) varying from 6% to 20% depending on the study and population selected (28), excreted albumin at rates well above normal but below the detection limit of usual routine tests. These

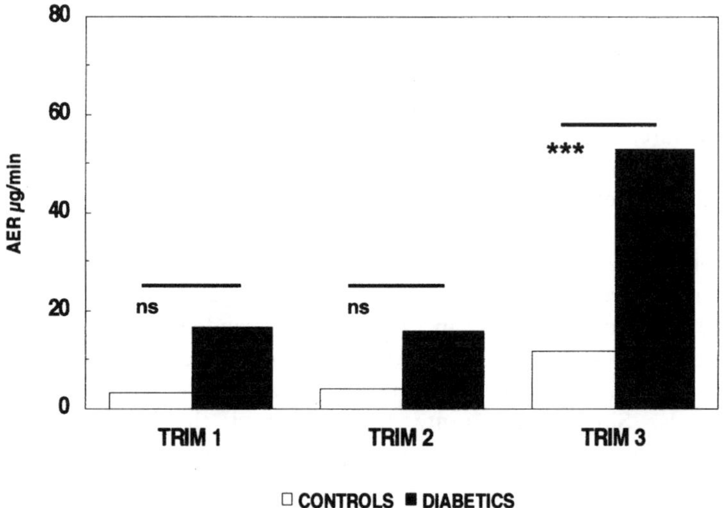

Figure 30.1. *AER during pregnancy in diabetic and non-diabetic women.* TRIM, trimester of pregnancy

subclinical elevations of albumin excretion are of 30–300 mg/24 hours and are defined as microalbuminuria. Up to now, very few studies have been performed concerning microalbuminuria in diabetic pregnancy (29,30), showing a similar rate in diabetic pregnancy as in non-pregnant diabetics.

Our experience

Our own studies (29,31) on the microalbuminuria in diabetic pregnancy was done in 124 diabetic (38 GDM, 28 type 2 and 58 type 1) and 52 non-diabetic women during pregnancy. Microalbuminuria increased during pregnancy in diabetic as well as in non-diabetic women, although in the latter it never reached values above 20 mg/dl (Figure 30.1). In the diabetic women microalbuminuria was correlated with the degree of diabetes (WHO or White classification), diabetes duration (Figure 30.2), metabolic control and blood pressure values.

The evaluation of the better prognostic value of microalbuminuria in pregnancy indicated a value of 50 µg/min (irrespective of the trimester of pregnancy), greater than that observed in non-pregnant diabetic women. Microalbuminuric values over 50 vs. under 50 µg/min were associated with greater maternal complications and feto-neonatal complications (greater occurrence of perinatal mortality and congenital malformations) (Table 30.2, Figure 30.3).

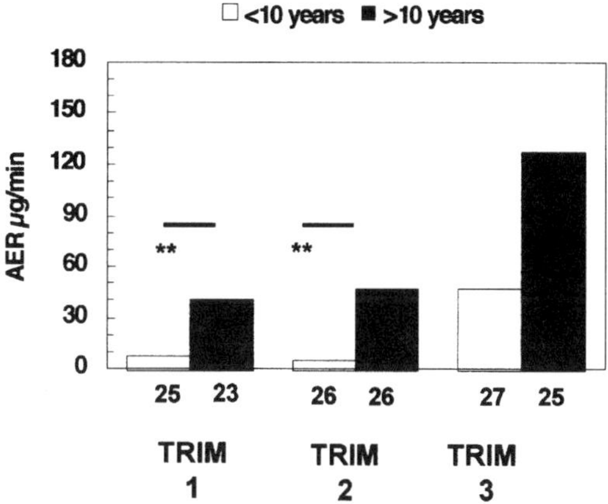

Figure 30.2. *AER during diabetic pregnancy and diabetes and duration.* TRIM, trimester of pregnancy

Table 30.2. Correlations of microalbuminuria concentrations over 50 μg/min vs. under 50 μg/min with metabolic control (FPG, HbA$_{1c}$, insulin need), kidney function (plasma creatinine) and blood pressure (systo-diastolic)

AER μg/min	Trimester	< 50 μg/min (102)	> 50 μg/min (22)	$p <$
FPG (mg/dl)	I	128.4±5.3	168.2±17	0.0025
	II	114.9±3.8	140.1±9.4	0.005
	III	110.6±31	123.6±8	0.05
HBA$_{1c}$ (%)	I	6.1±0.2	6.8±0.6	ns
	II	6.1±0.2	7.1±0.6	0.025
	III	5.6±0.2	7.6±0.6	0.0005
Plasma creatinine	I	0.75±0.03	0.77±0.04	ns
	II	0.75±0.02	0.82±0.05	ns
	III	0.77±0.02	0.87±0.04	0.025
Systolic BP (mmHg)	I	115.4±1.4	122±4	0.05
	II	117±1.4	114.3±3.6	ns
	III	118.6±1.3	124.5±3	0.05
Diastolic BP (mmHg)	I	72.9±0.9	77.9±2.7	0.025
	II	7.28±0.9	75.2±1.6	ns
	III	76.1±1.2	78.5±1.8	ns
Insulin need (Ul/day)	III	45±3	68±8	0.0025

These complications were even more significant when microalbuminuria was present from the first trimester of pregnancy. This observation suggests that fetal complications are more correlated with pre-existing microangiopathy than microalbuminuria itself. These considerations, associated with the knowledge that pregnancies in non-diabetic women with kidney disease are characterized by a less favorable fetal prognosis (32), with increased risk of

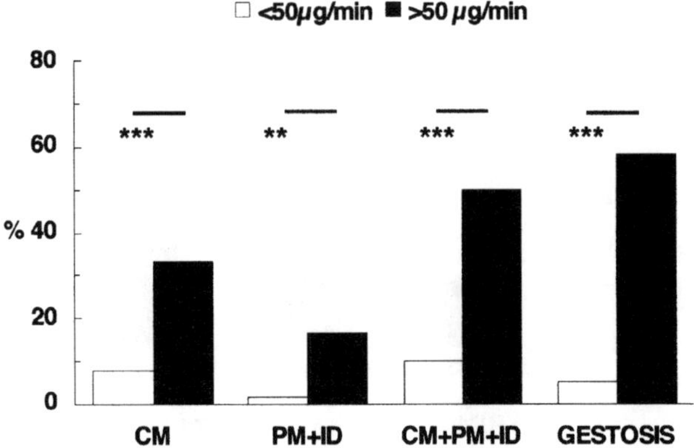

Figure 30.3. Fetal and maternal complications in diabetic pregnancy according to the first trimester AER values: <50 (96 cases) and 50 (12 cases). CM = congenital malformation; PM = perinatal morbidity; ID = intrauterine death

prematurity, fetal growth retardation and intrauterine death, especially when proteinuria is present at conception or early in pregnancy (32), also suggests that an early kidney impairment may have an unfavorable effect on fetal development. On the other hand, it is well known that intrauterine growth is impaired and the risk of perinatal mortality increases when EPH gestosis supervenes in both non-diabetic and diabetic women (33,34). These considerations strongly suggest that in diabetic pregnancy an impairment of both placental perfusion and fetoplacental circulation, on the one hand, and a poor maternal metabolic control, on the other, can independently cooperate in damaging the conceptus.

Management

All trials are consistent in showing that good metabolic control can often prevent the progression from incipient to overt nephropathy. On the other hand, the maternal and perinatal benefits of intensified diabetes treatment before and during pregnancy are well known. In addition to metabolic control, antihypertensive treatment is required. ACE inhibitors are contra-indicated in pregnancy. The α1-receptor blockers and calcium antagonists may be preferred in pregnancy, but the data on their potential teratogenicity are inadequate, so alternative agents should be used in the first trimester. Therefore, α-methyldopa as the first-line agent, with the addition of clonidine and/or β-blockers if additional therapy is needed at the beginning of pregnancy, are preferred. Finally, dietary protein should be restricted to 0.6–0.8 mg/kg/day in women with overt nephropathy in the non-pregnant state. During pregnancy the minimum amount acceptable for fetal development seems to be a protein intake of 60–80 g/day in women with clinical diabetic nephropathy.

Diabetic neuropathy

The importance of diabetic neuropathy derives from its frequency and potential involvement of any organ system in the body. Although neuropathy may occur in the course of diabetes, it is not so frequently studied in pregnancy. For this reason, little has been written on the relatioship between pregnancy and diabetic neuropathy. Since every innervated organ system may be affected by diabetic neuropathy, a future discovery of a profound effect of diabetic neuropathy on pregnancy would not be a surprise.

Hypertension in pregnancy

Hypertension and proteinuria have long been recognized to be important complications of pregnancy, but agreement on their classification and definition is still lacking.

Hypertension is a physical sign, not a disease entity, and may be due to a number of different underlying causes. In obstetric practice the arterial BP is nearly always measured by sphygmomanometry. The systolic BP is more variable than the diastolic BP and, although valuable in management, it does not add to the diagnostic or prognostic significance of hypertensive disorders of pregnancy. The definition of hypertension is therefore based solely on the diastolic BP, as it has the advantage of being both simple and unequivocal. To minimize variations caused by exercise and posture, it is recommended that the BP should be measured with the patient lying on a bed or couch on the right side at 30 degrees of lateral tilt, normally being taken in the right arm.

The BP normally falls in pregnancy and reaches its lowest level in the second trimester, when diastolic BP is, on average, 15 mmHg lower than before pregnancy. The fall occurs in both normotensive women and in women with chronic hypertension. The BP also normally rises in the third trimester and reaches pre-pregnancy levels by term. A rise in BP that has been used in previous definition of hypertension in pregnancy, of up to 30–40 mmHg, may thus fall within the normal statistical range (35).

Any definition of hypertension that is based on a particular level of BP is inevitably arbitrary, but the use of a diastolic BP (phase IV) of $\geqslant 90$ mmHg on two or more occasions during pregnancy as a diagnostic criterion has the advantages of: (a) simplicity, precision and convenience; (b) correspondence with defined statistical limits; (c) a defined relationship to perinatal mortality. It has been suggested that different levels of diastolic blood pressure should be used for the diagnosis of hypertension in the different stages of pregnancy and in different communities. The use of different criteria at different stages of pregnancy, in different populations and at different centers, would similarly lead to confusion and vitiate any comparison of results.

The term 'gestational hypertension', meaning pertaining to pregnancy, labor or the puerperium, is applied to all hypertensive and/or proteinuric conditions that develop during pregnancy or labor in a previously normotensive, non-proteinuric woman. It is preferred to 'pregnancy-induced hypertension', which may be taken to imply that pregnancy is the sole cause of the condition, whereas in some instances the hypertension is primarily caused by an underlying latent tendency to essential hypertension which becomes overt during pregnancy. It is also preferred to the term 'pregnancy-associated hypertension', which tends to imply that the development of hypertension or proteinuria is purely coincidental, whereas in other cases the hypertension may be caused entirely by pregnancy. The term 'gestational' in this classification is not intended to have any etiologic or pathologic implication, but is intended simply to mean that hypertension and/or proteinuria developed during pregnancy and disappeared after delivery. Gestational hypertension may be caused by a number of different causes or underlying conditions, including latent essential hypertension, 'pregnancy-induced hypertension', or 'supra-normal' or 'physiologic' hypertension.

Gestational proteinuric hypertension may be regarded as synonymous with 'pre-eclampsia', because the development of proteinuria and hypertension in pregnancy is closely correlated with the finding of specific 'pre-eclamptic' changes in the renal glomeruli (36). Gestational proteinuric hypertension also includes acute nephritis and an exacerbation of chronic nephritis, but these conditions are so rare that the occurrence of gestational proteinuric hypertension may be presumed to be 'pre-eclampsia' until proved otherwise. Gestational hypertension, proteinuria and proteinuric hypertension are further subdivided according to whether the hypertension and/or proteinuria develop antenatally, for the first time in labor, or for the first time after delivery. The subdivision of gestational hypertension, proteinuria and proteinuric hyperten-sion by the time of the first occurrence antenatally, in labor, or in the puerperium also overcomes the difficulties in previous classifications, where terms such as 'transient' or 'transitory' hypertension were used.

Chronic hypertension is diagnosed as the finding of hypertension at the first booking visit before the twentieth week of pregnancy in the absence of trophoblastic disease, at any stage of pregnancy in women with known chronic hypertension, or at >6 weeks after delivery. Chronic hypertension may be due to essential hypertension or to other causes.

Hypertension and diabetes mellitus are interrelated diseases. Hypertension is approximately twice as common in people with diabetes as in those without (37). An elevated blood pressure is often noted before or during pregnancy in women with type 1 diabetes who have diabetic nephropathy or chronic pyelonephritis. Many type 2 patients are both obese and hypertensive. Pregnancy-induced and/or accentuated hypertension (pre-eclampsia, toxemia) is more common in diabetic women.

The classic studies of Priscilla White (38) founded the dictum that the insulin-dependent diabetic mother is at increased risk for developing hypertension during pregnancy. Pedersen's work (39) confirmed this belief and further suggested that insulin-dependent diabetic patients who develop pregnancy-induced hypertension (PIH) have a significantly higher perinatal mortality and morbidity rate. Furthemore, Kitzmiller *et al* (40) have demonstrated that the proteinuric diabetic patient may have a large increase in her 24 hour urinary protein loss with advancing gestation, without ever developing hypertension. A definite relationship between PIH and glycemic control before the development of this complication has been found (41), as well as an association with advanced White class. Cousins (42) reviewed the English literature from 1965–1985 and reported an average rate of 11.7%, highly correlated with advanced White classes. Advanced diabetic class and poor glycemic control in pregnancy may be important factors correlated with PIH in the diabetic patient. It seems that the pregnancy-induced vascular adaptation of the uteroplacental bed involves two stages: rapid proliferation of cytotrophoblastic cells which reach the inner myometrial layer before the end of the first trimester (43), and subsequently the conversion of maternal spiral arteries to large sinusoidal vessels, which open into intervillous space (43). The extent of these physiologic changes is restricted in pregnancies complicated by hypertensive disorders (43).

The successful diagnosis of hypertension in pregnancy, and the decision arising from it regarding investigation, treatment, prognosis and epidemiological conclusions depend on accurate measurements. Current definitions of hypertension in pregnancy give an illusion of precision where none exists. Hypertension is categorized by either an absolute threshold or by a BP increase from baseline in the first half of pregnancy. It has been known for decades that the BP pattern in normal and hypertensive patients is subject to marked circadian fluctuations. The changes in systemic BP that occur according to the time of the day in healthy pregnant women, as well as in women with hypertensive complications, have only been recognized in the last two decades. The studies on BP variability in pregnant women that have been carried out so far have used different methods of BP monitoring measurement under different conditions. In normal pregnancies, or in pregnant women with pre-existing hypertension or mild pre-eclampsia, the circadian rhythm of BP is maintained, with a nocturnal decrease in BP (44). Since hypertensive disease of pregnancy remains a major cause of maternal and perinatal morbidity, any technique that can potentially give insight into hypertensive disease of pregnancy is therefore to be welcomed. There are relatively few studies on BP change in normal pregnancy.

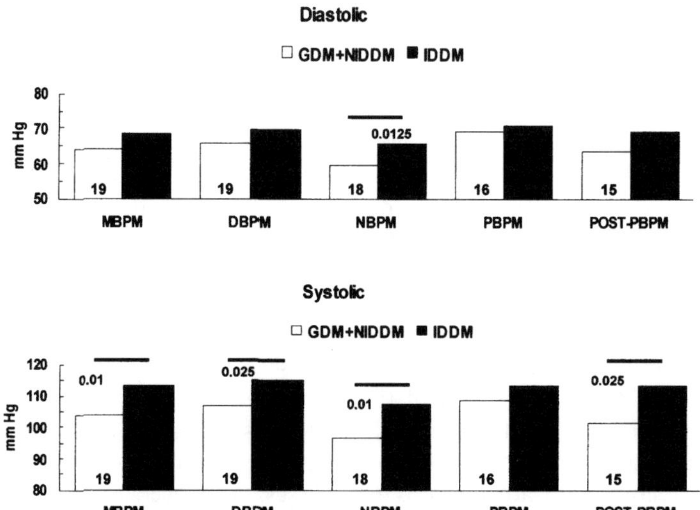

Figure 30.4. *Time-period of BP monitoring in the third trimester of pregnancy in diabetic women.* MBPM, mean BP monitoring; DBPM, diurnal BP monitoring; NBPM, nocturnal BP monitoring; PBPM, prandial BP monitoring; POST-PBPM, post-prandial BP monitoring

The inadequacy of single readings of BP suggests that ambulatory blood pressure monitoring (ABPM) appears to be a very satisfactory way of overcoming the large sampling and measurement errors associated with the commonly used methods of casual BP determinations.

In our preliminary study (45–47) we investigated ABPM in 70 diabetic (14 GDM, 13 NIDDM: nine WC B and four WC C; 43 IDDM: 12 WC B, eight WC C, 23 WC DF) and 21 non-diabetic women. The 24 hour periods were investigated as: (a) 24 hour BP profile (MBPM); (b) systo-diastolic 24 hour mean BPM (DBPM); (c) daytime mean BPM; (d) night-time mean BPM (NBPM); (e) pre-prandial BPM (PBPM); and (f) post-prandial BPM (post-PBPM). The results were studied taking into account the metabolic evaluation and the clinical findings.

Among the diabetic women, the systo-diastolic 24 hour ABPM values were correlated with the degree of diabetes (IDDM > NIDDM > GDM), being the differences more evident in late gestation, where, in addition, the circadian nocturnal decrease of BP was impaired in IDDM and preserved in both NIDDM and GDM women. Evaluation of the different time-periods investigated confirmed more elevated BP values in IDDM than in NIDDM + GDM patients (Figure 30.4). Among IDDM women, BP values were correlated with diabetes duration (> 10 vs. < 10 years) (Figure 30.5). Moreover, BP values were found to be correlated with the patient's weight gain

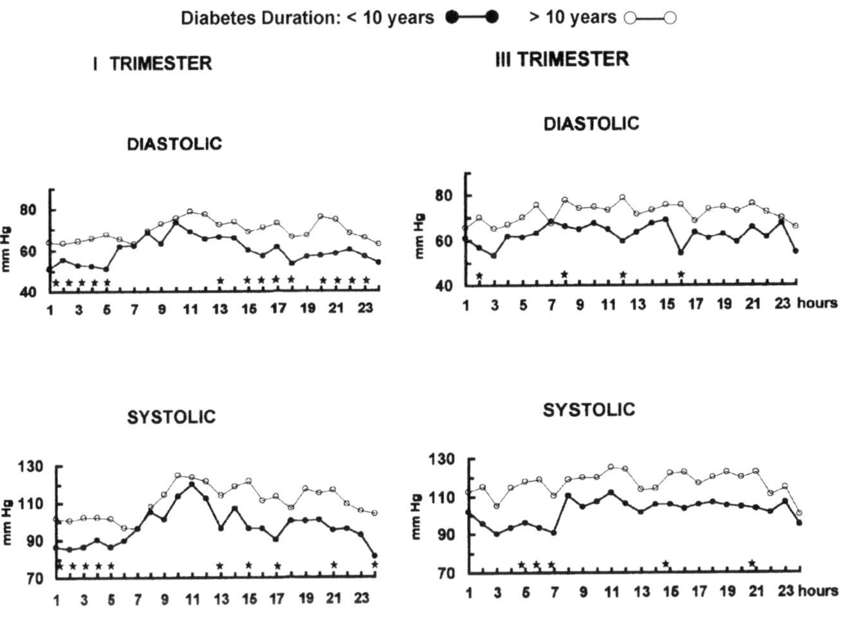

Figure 30.5. *24 hour BPM during pregnancy in IDDM patients*

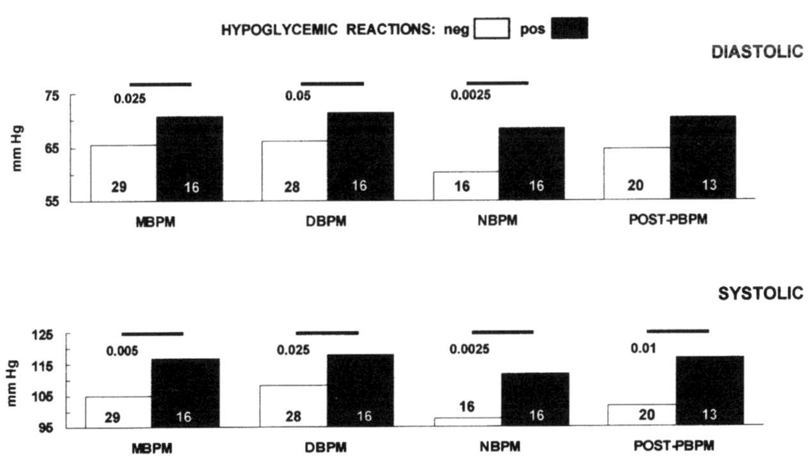

Figure 30.6. *Repeated hypoglycemic reactions during diabetic pregnancy and BP monitoring.* For abbreviations, see Figure 30.5

($>12\,kg$), the BMI (>23), daily insulin requirement, a poorer metabolic control and repeated hypoglycemic reactions during pregnancy (Figure 30.6). In addition, an impairment of ABPM was associated with increased plasma creatinine levels, a greater prevalence of microalbuminuria and retinopathy, a higher occurrence of EPH gestosis, a shorter time of gestation, with lower birth weight and an increased occurrence of fetal morbidity.

These results, in agreement with a few other investigations in diabetic pregnancy, indicate that the usual measurements taken during the day may miss the most relevant changes. In our opinion it may be necessary to modify existing pregnancy classifications of hypertension for ambulatory monitoring. Absolute values may be replaced by behavioral patterns, both over a 24 hour ABPM and 24 hour time periods, with longitudinal follow-up during pregnancy. Since diabetes is associated with an increased risk of pregnancy and fetal complications, ambulatory 24 hour BP monitoring from a research tool to implementation in clinical practice is strongly auspicious in diabetic pregnancy.

EPH-gestosis (pre-eclampsia)

Because of inconsistencies in the definition of pre-eclampsia, differences in the criteria used for its diagnosis, and differences in the composition of patients reported in regard to the diabetes degree, it becomes difficult to assess the exact incidence of pre-eclampsia in diabetic pregnancies, although an average incidence of approximately 12–15% may be estimated (48). Some predisposing factors may trigger the disease, including multiple pregnancies, hydatidiform mole, hydramnios and diabetes mellitus.

The diagnosis of pre-eclampsia in diabetic pregnancies is made using the same criteria used in non-diabetic pregnancies. In those patients with underlying nephropathy or hypertension, superimposed pre-eclampsia is often difficult to diagnose, since the hypertension and the proteinuria usually worsen in the second half of pregnancy. Microangiopathy is a typical vascular lesion of diabetes mellitus, therefore it is not surprising that the prevalence and severity of toxemia are greater in diabetic pregnancy. An incidence of 14.8% has been found by us (34) in a consecutive series of 135 diabetic pregnancies. On the other hand, perinatal losses and fetal morbidity in diabetic and non-diabetic patients increase when toxemia occurs during pregnancy.

Characteristics of severe pre-eclampsia are: hypertension ($BP>170/110$, or 60/30 rise); proteinuria ($>5g/24$ hours); oliguria ($<500\,ml/24$ hours); edema (massive, generalized, pulmonary edema); severe thrombocytopenia or hemolysis; disseminated intravascular coagulation; epigastric or right upper quadrant pain with hepatocellular damage. The ideal management is prevention. Increased periods of bed rest with or without dietary sodium restriction and low dose of aspirin may help in reducing the incidence of pre-eclampsia.

CONCLUSION

Planning one's family with appropriate spacing of childbearing, such that control of pre-existing diabetes is optimum, is vital to reduce morbidity and complications in such pregnancies. High glucose concentrations *in vitro* cause abnormal embryos by altering prostaglandin metabolism and by the generation of free oxygen radicals (49). Glycated hemoglobin assays were introduced in the late 1970s. Miller *et al* (50) showed *in vivo* that women whose hemoglobin was less than 8.5% before 14 weeks' gestation had a 3.4% risk of malformation, whereas those whose HbA_{1c} was over 8.5% had a 22.4% risk. In Denmark 75% of pregnancies were planned in diabetic women between 1982 and 1986, the frequency of congenital malformations being much lower in planned than in unplanned pregnancies (51). The abnormality rate was close to that of the non-diabetic population. Similarly, those attending pre-pregnancy clinics have a lower rate of congenital abnormality in their offspring than that of non-attenders (52). Poor first trimester glycemic control is significantly associated with congenital abnormalities, maternal vasculopathy being another risk factor. Kitzmiller's study (52) indicated that women seen before conception for a median of 17 weeks had a congenital abnormality rate of 1.2% in their infants, as compared with 10.9% in mothers who presented late in pregnancy. A mean blood glucose level of 3.3–7.8 mmol/l was obtained in half of the women before pregnancy occurred. The purpose of pre-pregnancy counseling is to educate not only regarding the adverse outcomes that can be reduced by meticulous diabetic control, such as encouraging the latter, but also to advise regarding medical suitability for pregnancy and suggest contraceptive methods appropriate to the individual woman and her partner.

REFERENCES

1. Hare JW, White P: Gestational diabetes and the White Classification. *Diabet Care* 3:394, 1980.
2. Hare JW, White P: Pregnancy in diabetes complicated by vascular disease. *Diabetes* 26: 953–955, 1977.
3. The Diabetic Retinopathy Study Research Group. Preliminary report on effects of photocoagulation. *Am J Ophthalmol* 81:383–390, 1976.
4. Cassar J, Kohner EM, Hamilton AM: Diabetic retinopathy and pregnancy. *Diabetologia* 15:105–111, 1978.
5. Maloney JBM, Drury MI: Diabetic retinopathy during pregnancy. *Am J Ophthalmol* 93:745–756, 1982.
6. Soubrane G, Canivet J, Coscas G: Influence of pregnancy on the evolution of background retinopathy. *Int Ophthalmol* 8:249–255, 1985.
7. Klein BEK, Moss SE, Klein R: Effect of pregnancy on progression of diabetic retinopathy. *Diabet Care* 13:34–40, 1990.

8. Lauritzen T, Larse KF, Larsen HW *et al*: Effect of one year near normal blood glucose on retinopathy in insulin-dependent diabetics. *Lancet* I:200–203, 1983.
9. The Kroc Collaborative Study Group. Blood glucose control and the evolution of diabetic retinopathy and albuminuria. *N Engl J Med* 311:365–372, 1984.
10. Brinchmann-Hansen O, Dahl-Jorgensen K, Hanssen KF: Effects of intensified insulin treatment on various lesions of diabetic retinopathy. *Am J Ophathlmol* 100:644–653, 1985.
11. Chen HC, Newsom RSB, Patel V *et al*: Retinal blood flow changes during pregnancy in women with diabetes. *Invest Ophthalmol Vis Sci* 1994, 35:3199–3208, 1994.
12. Patel V, Rassam SMB, Newsome RSB *et al*: Retinal blood flow in diabetic retinopathy. *Br Med J* 230:221–225, 1992.
13. Vingolo AM, Rispoli E, Zicari D, Pannarale L, Iannaccone A, Fallucca F: Electro-physiologic monitoring of diabetic retinopathy in pregnancy. *Retina* 13:99–106, 1993.
14. Mogensen CE, Shmitz O. The diabetic kidney: from hyperfiltration and microalbuminuria to end-stage renal failure. *Med Clin North Am* 72:1465–1492, 1988.
15. Viberti GC, Hill RD, Jarrett RJ *et al*: Microalbuminuria as a predictor of clinical nephropathy in insulin-dependent diabetes mellitus. *Lancet* I:1430–1432, 1982.
16. Mogensen CE, Christensen CK: Predicting diabetic nephropathy in insulin-dependent patients. *N Engl J Med* 311:89–93, 1984.
17. Seaquist ER, Goetz RC, Rich S, Barbosa J: Familial clustering of diabeteic kidney disease: evidence for genetic susceptibility to diabetic nephropathy. *N Engl J Med* 320:1161–1165, 1989.
18. Lindheimer MD, Katz AI: Renal physiology in pregnancy. In *The kidney: Physiology and Pathophysiology*. Seldin DW, Giebisch G, Eds. New York:Raven, 1985, pp. 2017–2041.
19. Davison JM, Dunlop M: Renal hemodynamics and tubular function in normal human pregnancy. *Kidney Int* 18:152–161, 1980.
20. Lindhemeier MD, Katz AJ: *Renal Functions and Disease in Pregnancy*. Philadelphia, PA: Lea & Febiger, 1977.
21. Baylis C: Glomerular ultrafiltration in the pseudopregnant rat. *Am J Physiol* 234: F300–305, 1982.
22. Sims EAH, Krantz KE: Serial studies of renal function during pregnancy and the puerperium in normal women. *J Clin Invest* 37:1764–1774, 1958.
23. Pedersen J: *The Pregnant Diabetic and Her Newborn*. 2nd edn. Copenhagen: Munksgaards, 1977.
24. Kitzmiller JL, Brown ER, Philippe M, Stark AR, Acker D, Kaldany A, Singh S, Hare JW: Diabetic nephropathy and perinatal outcome. *Am J Obstet Gynecol* 141:741–751, 1981.
25. Jovanovic R, Jovanovic L: Obstetric management when normoglycemia is maitained in diabetic pregnant women with vascular compromise. *Am J Obstet Gynecol* 149:617–623, 1984.
26. Nesler CL, Sinclair SH, Schwartz SS, Gabbe SG: Diabetic nephropathy in pregnancy. *Clin Obstet Gynecol* 28:528–535, 1985.
27. Reece AE, Coustan DR, Hayslett JP *et al*: Diabetic nephropathy: pregnancy performance and fetomaternal outcome. *Am J Obstet Gynecol* 159:56–66, 1988.
28. Gatling A, Knight C, Mullee MA, Hill R: Microalbuminuria in diabetes: a population study of the prevalence and an assessment of three screening tests. *Diabet Med* 5:343–347, 1987.

29. Napoli A, Bueti A, De Vecchis P *et al*: Microalbuminuria during diabetic pregnancy: correlation with fetal morbidity. *Diabet Nutr Metab* 3(suppl 2):101–104, 1990.

30. Winocour PH, Taylor RJ: Early alterations of renal function in insulin-dependent diabetic pregnancies and their importance in predicting pre-eclamptic toxemia. *Diabet Res* 10:154–164, 1989.

31. Fallucca F, Napoli A, Bueti P *et al*: Microalbuminuria in diabetic pregnant women: its prognostic value for mother and fetus. *Diabetes* 40(suppl. 1): abstract 14th ADA's Annual Meeting, 1991.

32. Katz AI, Davison JM, Hayslett JP, Singson E Lindhemeier MD: Pregnancy in women with kidney disease. *Kidney Int* 18:192–206, 1980.

33. Janish H, Dadak CH: Perinatal mortality in EPH-gestasis. In *Perinatal Care and Gestosis*. Suzuki M, Furuhashi N, Eds. International Congress Series 686, Amsterdam, Excerpta Medica, pp. 3–10, 1985.

34. Pach A, Fallucca F, Gerlini G, Scarciotta O, Maggi E, Gargiulo P, Di Mario U, Troili F: Metabolic and immunological aspects in diabetic pregnancy with and without toxemia. In *Recent Advances in Pathophysiological Conditions in Pregnanacy* Schenker JG, Ripman ET, Weinstein D, Eds. Amsterdam: Elsevier, pp. 45–48, 1984.

35. Davey DA, MacGillivray I: The Classification and definition of the hypertensive disorders of pregnancy. *Am J Obstet Gynecol* 158:892–898, 1988.

36. King GE: Taking the blood pressure. *J Am Med Assoc* 209:1902–1904, 1969.

37. Epstein M Sowers JR: Diabetes mellitus and hypertension. *Hypertension* 19:403–418, 1992.

38. White P: Pregnancy complicating diabetes. *Am J Med* 7:609–616, 1949.

39. Pederen J, Pedersem LM: Prognosis of the outcome of pregnancies in diabetics. *Acta Endocrinol* 50:70–78, 1965.

40. Kitzmiller JL, Brown ER, Philippe M *et al*: Diabetic nephropathy and perinatal outcome. *J Pediatr* 105:149–150, 1984.

41. Siddiqi T, Rosenn B, Mimouni F, Khoury J, Miodovnik M: Hypertension during pregnancy in insulin-dependent diabetic women. *Obstet Gynecol* 77:514–519, 1991.

42. Cousins L: Pregnancy complications among diabetic women: review 1965–85. *Obstet Gynecol Surv* 12:140–149, 1987.

43. Robertson WB, Brosens I, Dixon G: Uteroplacental vascular pathology. *Eur J Obstet Gynecol Reprod Biol* 5:47–65, 1975.

44. Oney T, Meyer-Sabellek: Variability of arterial blood pressure in normal and hypertensive pregnancy. *J Hypertension* 8:suppl 6, S77-S81, 1990.

45. Fallucca F, Sabbatini A, Montanari G, Di Biase N, Sciullo E, Mazziotti F, Napoli A: Blood pressure monitoring in diabetic pregnancies. 2nd International Symposium on Diabetes and Pregnancy in the 90s, Jerusalem, 19–23 March, 1995, pp 94.

46. Napoli A, Di Biase N, Mazziotti F, Marceca M, Sabbatini A, Fallucca F: Blood pressure monitoring in diabetic pregnancy. *Annali Ist Sup Sanità* 33:337–342, 1997.

47. Napoli A, Sabbatini A La Torre R, Di Biase N, Fallucca F: Blood pressure monitoring in diabetic women. Their pregnancy outcome. *Diabetolcgia* 40:(Suppl 1), A 230, 1997.

48. Martin TR, Allen AC, Stinson D: Overt diabetes in pregnancy. *Am J Obstet Gynecol* 133:275, 1979.

49. Eriksson UJ, Borg LA: Protection by free oxygen radicals scavenging enzymes against glucose-induced embryonic malformations *in vitro*. *Diabetologia* 34:325–331, 1991.

50. Miller E, Hare JW, Cloherty JP *et al*: Elevated maternal HbA1c in early pregnancy and major congenital anomalies in infants of diabetic mothers. *N Engl J Med* 304:1331–1334, 1981.
51. Damm P, Molsted-Pedersen L: Significant decrease in congenital malformations in newborn infants of an unselected population of diabetic women. *Am J Obstet Gynecol* 161:1163–1167, 1989.
52. Kitzmiller JL, Gavin LA, Gin GD *et al*: Preconception care of diabetes: glycemic control prevents congenital anomalies. *J Am Med Assoc* 265:731–736, 1991.

31

Impact of Pancreas/Islet Transplantation on the Course of Diabetic Complications

R. LANDGRAF, W. MÜLLER-FELBER, W. PIEHLMEIER
and C. DIETERLE

Diabetes Center, Department of Internal Medicine Innenstadt, University of Munich,
Munich, Germany

Over the years, few therapeutic interventions offered to diabetic patients have been subjected to so much discussion as pancreatic transplantation, which has been greeted partly with great enthusiasm but also with critical scepticism, despite the fact that there is increasing evidence that it has become a highly efficacious procedure in restoring long-term normalization of glucose metabolism, and has a number of other benefits for diabetic patients with severe diabetic complications. In this mini-review we would like to summarize recent evidence favoring pancreatic grafting in highly selected type 1 diabetic individuals, as a single organ transplant or as simultaneous or consecutive kidney/pancreas transplantation. In addition, simultaneous pancreas/kidney transplantation might even be a therapeutic option in young type 2 diabetic patients with end-stage renal disease (1).

SURVIVAL OF PATIENTS AND TRANSPLANTED ORGANS

Long-term experience in organ retrieval, improved surgical procedures (bladder drainage and, more recently, enteric drainage of the exocrine fluids), improvements in preoperative patient selection and disease manage-

Diabetes in the New Millennium. Edited by U. Di Mario, F. Leonetti, G. Pugliese, P. Sbraccia and A. Signore.
© 2000 John Wiley & Sons, Ltd.

ment, better perioperative patient care, as well as new immunosuppressants (monoclonal antibodies for induction treatment and the introduction of tacrolimus and mycophenolate mofetil) have led to patient and organ survival rates which are very much comparable to those of other solid organ transplantations. In the International Pancreas Transplant Registry, 11 422 pancreas recipients have been registered since May 1999. The 1-year patient survival has been reported to be 94% and the 1-year pancreas survival is, for simultaneous pancreas/kidney (SPK; 86% of all pancreas transplantations) 83% (for the kidney 90%), for pancreas after kidney (PAK) 71% and for pancreas alone (PTA) 64%. Long-term survival rates have also been improved dramatically. However, pancreas transplantation can lead to a number of serious perioperative complications (e.g. graft thrombosis, acute graft rejections, wound infections, fistulas, urological complications, infections due to immunosuppression and chronic graft failure), which can be minimized by centralizing pancreas transplantation activities to those centers with a high number of transplantations, where the staff are prepared to deal with all potential complications that may occur with pancreas grafting.

Despite a higher perioperative morbidity after SPK in comparison to kidney transplantation alone (KTA), there is now evidence that the long-term survival of SPK patients is significantly better than for kidney-transplanted diabetic patients (Table 31.1). The study of Navarro *et al* (2) compared patients after SPK, patients after SPK but with early loss of the pancreas (<3 months after transplantation), and patients without pancreas grafting but with a similar neuropathy score. After 5 years patient survival was similar in the two transplanted groups, but less in the non-grafted group. At 11 years, however, the difference between the three groups of patients was highly significant, and a patient with a functioning pancreas and kidney had much better survival than those patients who lost their pancreas graft early post-transplant. Three other institutions also reported a much better outcome in pancreas transplant recipients when compared with diabetic patients who received only a kidney (Table 31.1) (3–5).

In a small prospective study with 11 SPK and 10 KTA patients with an observation time of 69±37 and 70±33 months, respectively, progression of macrovascular disease in both groups of patients was seen (6). It is important to stress that much longer follow-up periods (see Table 31.1) are necessary to demonstrate the beneficial effects of pancreatic grafting on macroangiopathic complications (4).

Therefore, when considering kidney transplantation in diabetic patients with end-stage renal disease, it should be primarily planned as an SPK, provided that there are no major contraindications, such as severe macroangiopathic complications. Careful and critical patient appraisal prior to transplantation is absolutely necessary for optimal patient selection and reduction of perioperative morbidity and mortality (7).

Table 31.1. Patient survival in diabetic pancreas/kidney (SPK) vs. kidney alone (KTA) recipients or no transplantation (NoTX)

Observation time mean, years	SPK (%)	KTA (%)	NoTX (%)	Reference
10	79	20		Tyden *et al* (4)
11	91	70	20	Navarro *et al* (2)
13	78	35		Smets *et al* (3)
13	90	35		Becker *et al* (5)

REDUCTION OF THE VASCULAR RISK

Long-term survival of the grafted organs, together with normalization of glucose metabolism and reduction of other vascular risks, e.g. by improving hyperlipidemia and hypertension, are main prerequisites for prevention, retardation or reversal of secondary complications. Is there a long-term normalization of glucose metabolism? The longest metabolic follow-up studies cover only the first 5 years (8). Recently, observation times of up to 18 years in pancreas recipients with euglycemia and adequate insulin secretory reserves have been reported (9; our unpublished data). Although daily blood glucose and glycated hemoglobin may be entirely normal, glucose metabolism may not be completely normalized and only 60–80% of pancreas transplant recipients have normal oral glucose tolerance. This fact is mainly due to: the number of islets (segmental pancreas graft, islet destruction perioperative and β cell loss due to chronic graft dysfunction of various causes); systemic insulin delivery with loss of first-pass insulin clearance in the liver, leading to peripheral hyperinsulinemia; the complex chronic immunosuppression, which may lead to insulin resistance and/or β cell dysfunction and the denervation of the pancreas graft. All factors together result in most patients in normal daily blood glucose profiles, but there might be a greater insulin secretory demand due to reduced glucose uptake, while in most cases hepatic glucose production and splanchnic glucose metabolism are in the normal range [for review, see (10)] (Table 31.2).

There are beneficial effects of pancreas transplantation on lipids and lipoproteins (10,11), but there are still disturbances in lipid metabolism, such as increased non-HDL-cholesterol and total cholesterol, although higher levels of large-sized HDL (HDL$_2$)-cholesterol and LDL particles and normal lipoprotein lipase activity, as well as fasting and post-prandial triglycerides, have been reported. This metabolic constellation is considered to be less atherogenic.

Recently, fibrinogen has been identified as an independent vascular risk factor. Mellinghoff *et al* (12) found that fibrinogen and plasma viscosity are

Table 31.2. Metabolic consequences of successful SPK transplantation

Parameter	Outcome
Oral glucose tolerance	Normal in 60–80% Often hyperinsulinemia
Intravenous glucose tolerance	Normal in 80–90% Biphasic insulin release
Intravenous glucagon	Insulin release improved or normal
Intravenous arginine	Near-normal insulin release and glucose-potentiated insulin secretion
Oscillations in insulin release	Normal high- and low-frequency insulin pulses present
Proinsulin	Higher levels of proinsulin and proinsulin-like peptides
Negative feedback of insulin release	Yes
Pancreatic glucagon release	Often basal hyperglucagonemia; glucose-induced suppression sometimes blunted; sometimes higher responses after stimulation (e.g. arginine)
Lipid metabolism	Improvement to less atherogenic potential
Effects of immunosuppression on intermediary metabolism	Complex

still much higher in successfully transplanted pancreas recipients than in healthy controls.

Hypertension is a major risk factors for atherosclerosis and for promoting diabetic vascular complications. Most patients waiting for a pancreas/kidney transplant are hypertensive. After successful grafting, the number of patients with hypertension is reduced or the patients are more effectively treatable (12,13).

In summary, pancreas transplantation leads to a significant reduction of the vascular risk profile, which in fact, as already mentioned, is reflected by the lower incidence of cardiovascular mortality after SPK when compared to diabetic KTA recipients (2–5).

Hypoglycemia can be a life-threatening complication in the management of diabetes and strict metabolic control increases the incidence of hypoglycemic episodes in type 1 diabetic patients. Especially in those patients with hypoglycemia unawareness and a defective counter-regulation, strict metabolic control is dangerous and limited. Therefore, PTA or SPK is generally accepted as an indication for pancreatic grafting. Several studies have shown that hypoglycemia still occurs in as many as 50% of successful pancreas-grafted patients, but they are mostly mild (10) and can be avoided by many patients with adequate dietary counseling.

SPECIAL RISKS OF PANCREAS TRANSPLANTATION

Besides the numerous benefits of organ grafting, chronic immunosuppression may lead to risks which need a specialized close follow-up of the patient in order to adequately detect and treat such complications as opportunistic infections.

In addition, there is an increased risk of neoplasia, which has been recently reviewed for renal transplant recipients (14,15). Since graft recipients survive much longer, there is a clear necessity for closer investigation and life-long surveillance of these patients.

Due to secondary hyperparathyroidism and undetected hypogonadism, bone mass is often already reduced prior to transplantation. Specific for these patients is the development of a post-transplant osteoporosis, which is mainly dependent on the time and dosage of the immunosuppressive therapy and which is most pronounced during the first 6–12 months after transplantation. Without therapy, the fracture rate ranges up to 65%. Therefore, pre- and post-transplant screening and prophylactic and early therapeutic treatment is necessary (16). An especially high rate of posttransplant fractures was seen in type 1 diabetic patients when compared to non-diabetic kidney recipients (40% vs. 11%) (17).

Recently, a new immunosuppressive-associated complication has been identified in organ recipients using cyclosporin or tacrolimus—leukoencephalopathy. Manifestation of this syndrome—mainly with seizures, mental alterations and visual abnormalities—is rather early post-transplant (82% occurred within 90 days) (18). Again, early detection can reverse the signs and symptoms on cessation or drastic reduction of these immunosuppressive drugs.

THE IMPACT OF PANCREATIC GRAFTING ON DIABETIC SECONDARY COMPLICATIONS

Diabetes-specific vascular and neurological complications lead to excess morbidity and mortality as well as to a dramatically reduced quality of life. Therefore, one major goal of pancreas transplantation is to reduce, retard, prevent or reverse secondary complications, to improve quality of life and to restore psychosocial integrity. Recently there has been a comprehensive review dealing with this topic (19).

DIABETIC EYE DISEASE

Chronic hyperglycemia is the most important risk factor for the development and progression of retinopathy. Therefore, normalization of glucose metabolism by pancreatic grafting should lead to marked amelioration of retinopathy. The data available, however, suggest that advanced retinopathy might not benefit from pancreas transplantation. One has to keep in mind that almost all studies here have had rather short observation times (< 5 years), the number of patients under study has been quite small and at least 80% of the graft recipients have received pan-retinal laser treatment or were even blind prior to transplantation. In fact, laser coagulation has been demonstrated to lead to stable retinal function and therefore any additional therapeutic intervention is difficult to interpret (19). One recent study from Australia (20) examined successful pancreas/kidney recipients ($n = 46$) and patients with failed pancreas transplants but with a functioning kidney graft ($n = 8$) for up to 10 years post-transplant. Pancreatic grafting together with appropriate laser therapy stabilized active to inactive proliferative retinopathy.

Cataract is the major cause of visual disturbance after transplantation. Cataract becomes more common 2 years after SPK transplantation and lens abnormalities were virtually universal at 6–10 years. The main risk factors for the development of the predominantly seen nuclear and posterior subcapsular cataracts were older age, chronic hemodialysis and high-dose pulses of glucocorticoids, and probably also the use of cyclosporin (21).

PERIPHERAL MICROCIRCULATION

Peripheral microcirculatory disturbances contribute to nutritional and infectious complications, especially in the lower extremities. Numerous studies using non-invasive methods to measure nutritional and total blood flow (transcutaneous oxygen tension, Doppler fluxmetry) or skin temperature demonstrated the beneficial effects of blood glucose normalization on the microcirculation. Also microvascular leakage in nailfold capillaries, using sodium fluorescein-labeled albumin for its quantification, could be rapidly reversed after successful pancreas transplantation [for review, see (19)]. Recently our group has studied the long-term effect of glucose normalization on skin microcirculation using laser Doppler fluxmetry. Forty-two type 1 diabetic patients after SPK, 28 diabetic kidney recipients and 13 diabetic patients waiting for organ replacement were compared with 33 matched healthy controls (data unpublished). Resting blood flow, post-occlusive hyperemia, the microangiopathic index and reactive vasoconstriction during a cold pressure test in the SPK patients were similar to the healthy controls and were worse in the diabetic patients on chronic dialysis. However, even after a mean post-transplant period of 50 months in the SPK group, the microcirculatory parameters were not normalized completely, which is in line with a number of previous studies (19).

A computer-assisted intravital microscopy study on conjunctival micro-circulation revealed that 18 months after SPK, but not after KTA, there were significant improvements of diabetic microangiopathy, such as decrease of the diameter of the venules, increase of arteriole length/area, vascular perfusion and blood flow velocity (22).

Since many of the described positive changes in microcirculation occur relatively early after transplantation and do not improve further after a longer observation time, it can be speculated that blood glucose normalization leads to functional rather than to morphological ameliorations.

NEUROPATHY

The only strategy shown to be consistently beneficial in the treatment of diabetic neuropathy is meticulous control of blood glucose. Indeed, numerous studies have reported improved neurological parameters of neuropathy, considering group comparisons as well as intraindividual longitudinal data in pancreas transplant recipients [for review, see (19,2)]. An extensive analysis of diabetic neuropathy has been performed, comparing SPK ($n = 44$) and KTA ($n = 9$) patients as long as >6 years (longest observation time 8 years) ($n = 19$) post-transplant (23). Nerve conduction velocity improved in a biphasic manner, with a rapid initial recovery and a subsequent stabilization. The recovery of the nerve action potential amplitude, however, was monophasic and continued to ameliorate with time. Predictors for improvement in nerve function were time after transplantation, baseline nerve function, HLA mismatch, use of nifedipine, and the ratio of fasting insulin to glucose and body weight. Unfortunately no details about metabolic control were given in this analysis. In a small number of patients, long-term analysis of neuropathy was reported (4). The electroneurographic index, as well as the measurement of cardiac autonomic neuropathy (RR variation), were not different at 2 years post-transplant between SPK ($n = 14$) and KTA ($n = 15$) patients. After 4 years a significant difference was found between the two groups, which widened after 8 years, being significantly better in the SPK group. In a study which has recently finished, 12 SPK recipients were compared to seven KTA patients and were followed neurologically for more than 10 years (Müller-Felber *et al*; unpublished data). Neurophysiological parameters and clinical neurological deficits were stabilized in both groups. After 10 years there was a trend in favor of the SPK group concerning neurological status, expressed by the Dyck score (SPK, $+1$ vs. KTA, -2), motor nerve compound action potentials (SPK, $+1.2$ mV vs. KTA, -1.1 mV) and motor nerve conduction velocities, but there was no significant difference between the groups, which is in contrast to the data of Tyden *et al* (4). One important reason might be that the metabolic control of our PTA patients was much better than that of Tyden *et al* (HbA$_{1c}$,

6.5±0.5% vs. around 10%), stressing again the importance of optimal metabolic control also in diabetic kidney transplant recipients.

In summary, peripheral sensorimotor neuropathy as well as autonomic neuropathy stabilize, and in many patients ameliorate, after successful pancreas and pancreas/kidney transplantation. The interpretation of the various studies is difficult, however, especially in patients with SPK, since elimination of uremia and diabetic metabolism is achieved at the same time, both contributing to a non-quantifiable degree to the improvement of neuropathy, which is most impressive in the first 3–4 years post-transplant. The studies are also difficult to compare because the protocol varies considerably, and many investigations compare the neurological function at different times to prior transplantation with data post-transplant. Others use neurological data 1–3 months post-transplant as the baseline for their prospective analyses. In addition, there are mostly no detailed data on metabolic control, especially in diabetic kidney recipients. High HbA_{1c} levels in diabetic kidney recipients will make the impact of pancreas grafting on the improvements in nerve function even more significant.

NEPHROPATHY

Nephropathy is one of the most devastating complications in type 1 diabetic patients, often leading to end-stage renal disease with the necessity of kidney replacement therapy. Kidney transplantation is the best option in these patients and the survival of the kidneys has improved considerably (24). With very good organ survival rates, the chance of the development of diabetic renal lesions in the grafted kidney becomes a possibility for graft deterioration. Unfortunately, there are only a few studies with a limited number of patients addressing this question in histomorphometric analyses [for review, see (19)]. In summary, long-term normalization of glucose metabolism by pancreas transplantation can prevent or slow the progression of typical signs and lesions of diabetic nephropathy in kidney allografts. Since the function and morphology of native and transplanted kidneys can be severely changed by cyclosporin, which exerts specific nephrotoxicity, the results of these studies have to be interpreted with caution. In patients with incipient nephropathy who have not received a kidney transplant, pancreas transplantation does not improve established lesions of diabetic nephropathy within 5 years after transplantation. When the kidney function and renal biopsies were studied before and 5 and 10 years after pancreatic grafting, normalization of glucose metabolism by pancreas transplantation was able to reverse lesions of nephropathy: microalbuminuria decreased, creatinine clearance remained constant between years 5 and 10, the thickness of the glomerular and tubular basement membranes, which were similar at year 5, decreased significantly 10 years post-transplant, and the mesangial matrix was reduced at 10 years (25). Although the number of patients was low ($n = 8$), this study is a milestone in diabetology, since it demonstrates that in patients with rather advanced diabetic lesions (micro- and macroalbuminuric individuals), glucose normalization can reverse functional as well as structural abnormalities in a main target organ of diabetes. But it takes between 5 and 10 years to demonstrate this beneficial effect.

QUALITY OF LIFE

One of the major goals in the treatment of chronic diseases is to improve life-expectancy *and* quality of life. Since major restrictions in life-style and rapid life-threatening progression of vascular complications are still the major problems in the management of diabetes, pancreas transplantation offers both meticulous metabolic control and reduction of the vascular risk. Despite the limitations of recent reports [for review, see (19,26)], there is sufficient evidence to suggest that pancreas transplantation improves quality of life in type 1 diabetic patients with end-stage renal disease. Greater satisfaction with life and vitality, more feelings of control and independence, better physical, social and mental health and functioning, as well as better overall quality of life are the main areas of improvement. It has to be stressed that similar improvements have also been reported in diabetic kidney recipients, and it is hard to prove that pancreas transplantation adds very much to the overall increase in quality of life in these severely ill patients. Recent data from a prospective study using the self-administered SF-36 questionnaire showed that the improvement in quality of life occurs between the time of chronic dialysis and within 2 years of successful transplantation. In the long-term follow-up (>9 years) of SPK or TKA recipients, no further improvement could be demonstrated (own unpublished data so far).

All studies on quality of life so far available have important shortcomings: most are cross-sectional and not longitudinal, the observation time is mostly too short and the number of patients under study too small, the patients in the different groups are rather heterogenous, comparing the degree of secondary complications prior to and after transplantation, as well as gender and social status which have not been analyzed separately. Since the statistical power of these studies — using also different instruments for measuring quality of life — is not high enough, additional large-scale prospective studies are urgently needed in the field of pancreas transplantation.

Pancreas/kidney transplantation is able to restore fertility in uremic female type 1 diabetic patients. Nineteen successfully completed pregancies have been reported to the International Pancreas Transplant Registry up to 1996 (27). Although there is a wish for many young couples to have children after successful transplantation, pregnancies are still high-risk and detailed counseling prior to and after transplantation about all potential complications for the mother and the child are highly recommended.

ISLET TRANSPLANTATION

Islet transplantation is a highly attractive option for replacing insulin-producing and glucose-sensing tissue in type 1 diabetic individuals. The potential advantages in comparison to whole pancreas transplantation are obvious. According to the International Islet Transplant Registry (from 31 December 1999), the success rate is limited to only a very few patients and the survival rate of the implanted material is short. In allograft islet recipients, the 1 year patient survival is 96%, the partial success rate (i.e. lower exogenous insulin requirement, measurable C-peptide levels (>0.5 ng/ml), more stable glucose metabolism) is 31–39% and the full success (i.e. insulin independence) is 8% (11 of 172 patients). The longest insulin independence is 70 months. Very recently, Lakey *et al* (28) reported a series of eight type 1 diabetic patients in which solitary islet transplantation was performed using a steroid-free immunosuppression. In all patients insulin independence could be achieved in a median follow-up of 6 months using a modified immunosuppressive protocol, a larger number of islets ($>12\,000$ islets/kg body weight) and freshly prepared islets from two to four donors. Whether this new protocol is a real breakthrough in islet transplantation remains to be seen.

There are no data available to show that successful islet transplantation has any beneficial influence on secondary complications. However, recent data suggest that C-peptide replacement by partially or fully functioning implanted islets may prevent or retard diabetic complications (29).

REFERENCES

1. Sasaki TM, Gray RS, Ratner RE, Currier C, Aquino A, Barhyte DY, Light JA: Successful long-term kidney–pancreas transplants in diabetic patients with high C-peptide levels. *Transplantation* 65:1510–151, 1999.
2. Navarro X, Kennedy WR, Aeppli D, Sutherland DER: Neuropathy and mortality in diabetes: influence of pancreas transplantation. *Muscle & Nerve* 19:1009–1016, 1996.
3. Smets YFC, Westendorp RGJ, Van der Pijl JW, De Charro FT, Ringers J, De Fijter JW, Lemkes HHPJ: Effect of simultaneous pancreas–kidney transplantation on mortality of patients with type 1 diabetes mellitus and end-stage renal failure. *Lancet* 353: 1915–1919, 1999.
4. Tyden G, Bolinder J, Solders G, Brattström C, Tibell A, Groth CG: Improved survival in patients with insulin-dependent diabetes mellitus and end-stage diabetic

nephropathy 10 years after combined pancreas and kidney transplantation. *Transplantation* 67: 645–648, 1999.

5. Becker BN, Brazy PC, Becker YT, Odorico JS, Pintar TJ, Collins BH, Pirsch JD, Leverson GE, Heisey DM, Sollinger HW: Simultaneous pancreas–kidney transplantation reduces excess mortality in type 1 diabetic patients with end-stage renal disease. *Kidney Int* 57:2129–2135, 2000.

6. Biesenbach G, Margreiter R, Königsrainer A, Bösmüller C, Janko O, Brücke P, Gross C, Zazgornik J: Comparison of progression of macrovascular diseases after kidney or pancreas and kidney transplantation in diabetic patients with end-stage renal disease. *Diabetologia* 43: 231–234, 2000.

7. Landgraf R: Pancreas–kidney transplantation with end-stage renal disease? *Int Diabetes Monitor* 1999; 11:4–6.

8. Robertson RP, Sutherland DER, Kendall DM, Teuscher AU, Gruessner RW, Gruessner A: Metabolic characterization of long-term successful pancreas transplants in type 1 diabetes. *J Invest Med* 44:1–7, 1996.

9. Robertson RP, Sutherland DER, Lanz KJ: Normoglycemia and preserved insulin secretory reserve in diabetic patients 10–18 years after pancreas transplantation. *Diabetes* 48:1737–1740, 1999.

10. Christiansen E: Metabolic consequences of successful simultaneous pancreas–kidney transplantation in humans. *Diabet Rev* 7:187–216, 1999.

11. Föger B, Königsrainer A, Ritsch A, Lechleitner M, Steurer W, Margreiter R, Patsch JR: Pancreas transplantation modulates reverse cholesterol transport. *Transpl Int* 12:360–364, 1999.

12. Mellinghoff AC, Reininger AJ, Wurzinger LJ, Landgraf R, Hepp K: Impact of pancreas and kidney transplantation on determinants of blood and plasma viscosity. *Clin Hemorrheol Microcirc* 18: 175–184, 1998.

13. La Rocca E, Gobbi C, Ciurlino D, Di Carlo V, Pozza G, Secchi A: Improvement of glucose/insulin metabolism reduces hypertension in insulin-dependent diabetes mellitus recipients of kidney–pancreas transplantation. *Transplantation* 65:390–393, 1998.

14. London NJ, Farmery SM, Will EJ, Davison AM, Lodge JPA: Risk of neoplasia in renal transplant patients. *Lancet* 346: 403–406, 1995.

15. Danpanich E, Kasiske BL: Risk factors for cancer in renal transplant recipients. *Transplantation* 68: 1859–1864, 1999.

16. Stempfle HU, Werner C, Wehr U, Meiser B, Angermann CE, Rambeck WA, Gärtner R: Prevention of osteoporosis after cardiac transplantation. A prospective, randomized, double-blind trial with calcitriol. *Transplantation* 68: 523–530, 1999.

17. Nisbeth U, Lindh E, Ljunghall S, Backman U, Fellström B: Increased fracture rate in diabetes mellitus and females after renal transplantation. *Transplantation* 67: 1218–1222, 1999.

18. Singh N, Bonham A, Fukui M: Immunosuppressive-associated leukoencephalopathy in organ transplant recipients. *Transplantation* 69: 467–472, 2000.

19. Landgraf R: Impact of pancreas transplantation on secondary complications and on quality of life. *Diabetologia* 39:1415–1424, 1996.

20. Chow VC, Pai RP, Chapman JR, O'Connell PJ, Allen RD, Mitchell P, Nankivell BJ: Diabetic retinopathy after combined kidney–pancreas transplantation. *Clin Transplant* 13: 356–362, 1999.

21. Pai RP, Mitchell P, Chow VC, Chapman JR, O'Connell PJ, Allen RD, Nankivell BJ: Posttransplant cataract: lessons from kidney–pancreas transplantation. *Transplantation* 69: 1108–1114, 2000.

22. Cheung ATW, Perez RV, Chen PCY: Improvements in diabetic micrangiopathy after successful simultaneous pancreas–kidney transplantation: a computer-assisted intravital microscopy study on the conjunctival microcirculation. *Transplantation* 68: 927–932, 1999.
23. Allen RDM, Al-Harbi IS, Morris JGL, Clouston PD, O'Connell PJ, Chapman JR, Nankivell BJ: Diabetic neuropathy after pancreas transplantation: determinants of recovery. *Transplantation* 63: 830–838, 1997.
24. Ojo AO, Hanson JA, Wolfe RA, Leichtman AB, Agodoa LY, Port FK: Long-term survival in renal transplant recipients with graft function. *Kidney Int* 57: 307–313, 2000.
25. Fioretto P, Steffes MW, Sutherland DER, Goetz FC, Mauer M: Reversal of lesions of diabetic nephropathy after pancreas transplantation. *N Engl J Med* 339:69–75, 1998.
26. Gross CR, Limwattananon C, Matthees BJ: Quality of life after pancreas transplantation. *Clin Transplant* 12: 351–361, 1998.
27. Barrou BM, Gruessner AC, Sutherland DER, Gruessner RWG: Pregnancy after pancreas transplantation in the cyclosporine era. *Transplantation* 65: 524–527, 1998.
28. Shapiro AM, Lakey JR, Ryan EA, Korbutt GS, Toth E, Warnock GL, Kneteman NM, Rajotte RV: Islet transplantation in seven patients with type 1 diabetes mellitus using a glucocorticoid-free immunosuppressive regimen. *N Eng J Med* 343:230–238, 2000.
29. Wahren J, Ekberg K, Johansson J, Henriksson M, Pramanik A, Johansson BL, Rigler R, Jornvall H: Role of C-peptide in human physiology. *Am J Physiol Endocrinol Metab* 278: E759–768, 2000.

Index

Note: Page references in *italics* refer to Figures; those in **bold** refer to Tables

Index compiled by Annette Musker